2LP 7M

2545
7 —

Three Simple Steps to Healthy Pets

The Holistic Animal Care LifeStyle™

by
Lisa S. Newman, N.D., Ph.D.

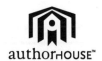

authorHOUSE™

1663 LIBERTY DRIVE, SUITE 200
BLOOMINGTON, INDIANA 47403
(800) 839-8640
WWW.AUTHORHOUSE.COM

First published by AuthorHouse 09/19/05

ISBN: 1-4208-8246-5 (e)
ISBN: 1-4208-6383-5 (sc)

Library of Congress Control Number: 2005905442

Printed in the United States of America
Bloomington, Indiana

This book is printed on acid-free paper.

Cover photo by Vern Pilling.

Dr. Newman's Holistic Animal Care LifeStyle™

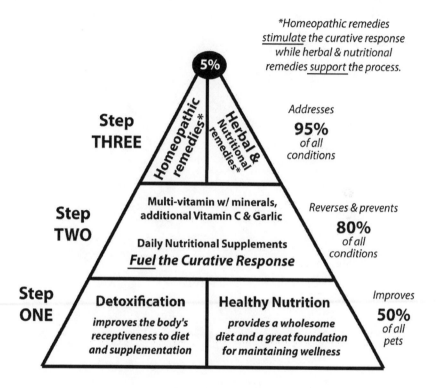

Homeopathic remedies stimulate the curative response while herbal & nutritional remedies support the process.

Step THREE

Homeopathic remedies*

Herbal & Nutritional remedies*

5%

Addresses
95%
of all conditions

Step TWO

Multi-vitamin w/ minerals, additional Vitamin C & Garlic

Daily Nutritional Supplements
Fuel the Curative Response

Reverses & prevents
80%
of all conditions

Step ONE

Detoxification
improves the body's receptiveness to diet and supplementation

Healthy Nutrition
provides a wholesome diet and a great foundation for maintaining wellness

Improves
50%
of all pets

This systematic approach was created to eliminate the guesswork associated with natural pet care. As you take each step, you reach a greater depth of wellness and symptom reversal. The use of Dr. Newman's naturopathic protocols with specific nutritional, herbal and homeopathic products is proven to promote rapid, reliable and long-term results. If an animal fails to improve on the next Step, taken with a proven product, then it is likely the body failed to respond rather than the product failed to work. This allows you to uncover the true weakness, based on the symptoms you witness, and adjust the protocol as needed, rather than simply supplementing blindly.

5% of chronically ill pets will still need medication. The LifeStyle™ approach will help prevent toxic build-up and provide support to maintain health while lessening the need for higher doses and possibly, the drug itself. It is not uncommon, for instance with diabetic pets, that insulin need is cut in half from previous use, and within months possibly eliminated.

DISCLAIMER:

The principles of The Holistic Animal Care LifeStyle™, Azmira® products and other products as described should not be used in lieu of, but as support to, proper veterinary care. This book is not intended to diagnose illness, prescribe medical treatment, make any claims nor imply any guarantees other than to educate. We feel that sharing information on the proven non-medical, safe, natural alternatives available to your pet will help you provide optimum care for them. Dr. Newman simply helps you to help your pets help themselves.

Please inform your Veterinary Doctor of any serious health concerns, observations or questions that you might have, and do rely on a clinical diagnosis, blood work, x-rays, medication, fluids, etc., when needed. Above all, please do honor yourself and your animals. Trust in what you are observing or sensing, while examining all sides of the issue. There are many sources of information available, but it is up to you to decide what is best for you and your pet.

DEDICATION:

I am grateful for all the people and animals that have made my life special.

Marcy Merin for her unwavering love and support; Linda Pilling and Rob Carr for helping to make Azmira Holistic Animal Care® a reality; Doris Dorfman for her patient editing; Lisa Marie Davis for her task mastering; Kevin Leehey, M.D. for making all things possible; my friends and family who have supported my dreams; Zaezar, my first Rottie, for showing me the need; the other animals I have loved, personally and professionally, who have proven that living The Holistic Animal Care LifeStyle™ works and Gloria Dodd, D.V.M., Founding President of the American Holistic Veterinary Medical Association, for her pioneering work and encouragement.

What Some of Dr. Newman's Satisfied Animal Caregivers Had to Say:

"I have had the opportunity to work with Dr. Newman on several problem cases that were not responding to standard medical treatment. Many of these cases responded favorably with the addition of Dr. Newman's holistic care. **This success has stimulated my interest in holistic medicine.**"
LuAnn Groves, DVM
San Marcos, TX

"With never less than 1500 animals to care for... It is such a blessing to be able to consult with you on some of our more difficult cases that are not responding to a traditional approach. **Your remedies are truly miraculous.**"
Estelle Munro
Best Friends Animal Sanctuary
Kanab, UT

"She has dedicated her life to helping you care for your animal companions – we can all benefit from her years of experience.
We are living in a time of great change, especially in the realm of health care. As a practicing veterinarian for more than two decades, I have witnessed both myself and my clients begin to seek less invasive, more natural methods for healing our dogs and cats. **Dr. Newman will show you the way so that you can be empowered as a healer.**"
Deborah C. Mallu, DVM, CVA
Flagstaff, AZ

"Within a month, my cat went from being on death's door to returning to her normal healthy playfulness. **The transformation I have witnessed is truly a miracle.** I could not have done it without the support and knowledge provided by (Dr. Newman) and without the products you carry."

Penelope Gedeon
Tucson, AZ

"During my shepherd's recovery from a car accident, his kidneys began to fail. Our veterinarian suspected it was triggered by weeks of high dose corticosteroids and Phenobarbital administered to control brain inflammation, which was resulting in seizures. Although the seizures had not subsided much, occurring sometimes 20 times per day, we had several other negative side-effects such as weight gain and lack of coordination.

Initially I called (Dr. Newman) to help with the kidneys, and appreciated the (kidney-specific) supplement which **helped him void normally again within a day. The most amazing thing though was, within three days of starting on (Step Two plus Step Three's anti-inflammatory and brain function supplements) there was a noticeable reduction in his seizure activity,** so we discontinued all the other medication and within another few days he was eating on his own, moving about the house again and practically seizure free! **Thanks for saving his life."**

John and Pat Roscott
Long Island, NY

"I have a miniature dachshund named Lucy, she was **unable to move from the waist down** (three herniated discs). I took her to a specialist who wanted to do immediate surgery to the tune of $2000.00, no guarantees.

He put her on prednisone and she stayed on it for eight weeks with no results.

(After using Azmira® products one week with Dr. Newman's paralysis protocol) …at nine weeks **with no prior movement or results, she started walking, and now, she's running!** Thank you so much!"

Brenda De Souzh
Tucson, AZ

"Our cat, Pretty Boy, was diagnosed with skin cancer in October 2000. The **vet that found the cancer said it was a fairly aggressive type** and there was really nothing we could do for him. He told us to take our cat home, make him comfortable and we probably had 6 months to possibly a year left with our cat.

(Started Dr. Newman's cancer protocol) Since that time, we have changed his routine a little bit (Step Three) by adding or subtracting different types of (Azmira®'s nutritional, herbal and homeopathic remedies), but I have never taken him off the Azmira® pet food – **that was three years ago. Pretty Boy today, appears to be a healthy and happy cat.** He has not lost any of his 18 pounds and his personality has not been altered."

Kimberley Young
Tucson, AZ

"Eighteen months ago I contacted (Dr. Newman) because my Bichon, Buttons, **had suffered from bladder stones**. The stones had been passed through a very painful and lengthy process administered by a veterinarian. **Although the stones no longer existed, Buttons was still in tremendous pain and was passing blood in her urine.** The vet's "cure" was to keep her on (prescription diet), which she had been on for years, and take an x-ray every six months to see if new stones had developed. He was baffled by the pain she was experiencing and stated that the blood in her urine was due to cystitis, something she would have to take drugs for the rest of her life.

With your help in developing a nutritional diet, supplements and remedies for Buttons she is now completely recovered. Her energy is incredible and she is more alert and happier than she has ever been.

Dusty, our poodle, had **suffered from allergies for years**. In June of 1992 I called upon (Dr. Newman) again to correct this situation. **With your help Dusty is now free of allergies, his energy level is high, and he feels great!**

The cost of your service, including supplements, remedies and vitamins runs a little less over a year's period than we were spending buying (prescription diets) from the vet and the (prescription diets) didn't help their problems. **Your advice and nutritional expertise are well worth it.** Had we continued with the veterinary services for the above problems with both dogs the cost would have been tremendous AND the vet was unable to make any difference in the general health of our "babies." I strongly recommend your services and products to anyone wishing a healthier, happier life for their "friends."

Charly Ritcheson
Scottsdale, AZ

"After three years of antibiotic and steroid use to suppress terrible skin outbreaks that resulted in staph infections, thousands of dollars spent on testing, veterinary care, supplements and diet changes, and very little to show for it, we finally found (The Holistic Animal Care LifeStyle™ and Azmira®).

Not only has your staff been the most supportive and informed we ever dealt with, your products have worked quickly! **The results we saw within the first month were impressive, but now, six months later, we have a new dog and the cycle of problems has been broken.** I never thought this would be so easy, but your help made it so."

Carnie Green
Charlotte, NC

"My Boxer puppy was diagnosed with H.O.D. I was skeptical at first that these (Azmira®) products would work…**He is running around like a puppy again – not bad considering the vet thought he would have to put him to sleep.**"

Gayann Jones
Tucson, AZ

"My ferret Swoopy was diagnosed with an adrenal problem 6 months ago and was losing the fur on his tail and belly. I began using (Dr. Newman's adrenal protocol and Azmira® products) … now Swoopy's **fur is growing back and thicker and darker than before – he has also gained weight and is doing much better than before.**"

Lisa Needham
Tucson, AZ

"I called Lisa Newman, a holistic animal care practitioner, when my regular **vet told me nothing could be done to help my cat** and that the best course of action was to just watch him closely and when the time came when he could no longer function to let him die in peace. My cat is an older neutered male whose **kidneys… One was enlarged and not functioning at all: the other one was just starting to fail.**

The end result of her care and (Dr. Newman's protocols) is a contented cat well on his way to recovery and a long, quality rich life. Just several months in his (protocol), his coat looks soft and healthy rather than lifeless and dull. His energy level seems limitless, and he runs and plays as he hasn't done for a long time.

I shall forever be grateful to Lisa for restoring my cat to health and giving him the opportunity to enjoy his "golden" years."

Helen Weber
Tucson, Az

"I think in today's world the good things of **carefully prepared products such as your own** must be well explained so that the people should know the ingredients, preparation..."
Stefanie Powers, actress
London, UK

"Thank you for being so attentive to my questions. By the way, **(Azmira® was) the first one to respond so readily and happily to my questions (three other major natural pet food companies) have not.** This means you have a sincerely dedicated serious line to answering customer or future customer questions.

I am happy to know you have a very qualified (Dr. Newman) to advise and oversee your line of pet foods and products. Thanks."
Cathy Baderick (e-mail)

"My other female German Shepherd **has allergies to so many things** that I would need a ream of paper to list them all. **Thanks to (Dr. Newman's Holistic Animal Care LifeStyle™ and Azmira® products); she has never had to take any kind of drugs to keep her allergies in check.** I am proud of the fact that she is four years old now and has never had to go on steroids. Her coat is so soft and beautiful, **that the vets find it hard to believe she has any problems at all.** All my sheps have coats that are so soft, I am always asked what I do to get them that way."
Lynn Eastman
Tucson, AZ

"After **seven months of spraying, our vet informed us that no medical problem existed and our cat suffered from a learned behavioral problem that could not be helped.** After adjusting his diet and supplementing him as (Dr. Newman) recommended, we also used your homeopathic spraying formula. It took a while at first, but **now it has been almost two months and he hasn't sprayed for three weeks!** Besides, his attitude is so much better than it ever was, he doesn't seem so intense anymore."
James McFarland
San Francisco, CA

"Sammy **was diagnosed with tick fever, his titer was at the highest level possible.** We spent the next eighteen months giving Sammy one antibiotic after another prescribed by the veterinarian, with no results. He was still sick, with the highest titer count possible.

The regimen you put Sammy on was effective and after seven weeks, his tick fever report came back negative. He was cured!!"
Tom and Kathern Johnson
Tucson, AZ

"I was treating four cats for **chronic viral infections**, three of the four had been on cephalexin (medication)… if I would stop the cephalexin they would be so sick I would have to put them on a stronger antibiotic. I put them on (Dr. Newman's viral protocol and Azmira® products) and **it has been three months since they have been off all antibiotics.** Presently all housed in this no-kill shelter receive (The Holistic Animal Care LifeStyle™ Step Two's recommended Azmira® daily supplements).

The most remarkable results are by a seven year old German Shepard named Nitro. After going through emergency surgery in June 1996, he had **his spleen and a portion of his stomach removed.** He was diagnosed a month later with a deteriorating spinal disorder. By December 1996, **we contemplated euthanization, because he could barely walk.** I put him on (Dr. Newman's anti-inflammatory and tissue repair protocol and Azmira® products). All sores are healed and his hair has grown back. He can run, play and gets into trouble just like he used to.

Thanks to your wonderful products, these animals are now living a much healthier and happier life."
Melanie Friedman
Burlington, WI

"Angie is not your typical German Shepherd. I have raised GSD dogs for thirty years and have **never seen one as hyper** as this girl. When she gets real excited there is no getting through to her. It's as if she tunes the whole world out except, for the object of her excitement.

I have worked with vets, both holistic and traditional. We have been to behaviorist and have tried everything I could think of… with no results. While reading a book on amino acids, I came across the description of l-Tryptophan and read what it has done for humans, with personality disorders. I ordered your L-TryptoPet … **Well I must tell you that your products have worked wonders for my dogs again."**
Lynn Eastman
Tucson, AZ

"...my two years old, female Persian, Muffin went in for routine spay... following surgery my cat got progressively sicker.

...**had lost half her body weight, and had no red blood platelets**... After kidney dialysis, blood transfusions and surgery it was found Muffin had her ureters tied off so her kidneys could not make urine.

...**she also refused to eat** her normal "gourmet" cat food. The veterinary hospital gave us (a prescription) "special" low protein diet. Muffin absolutely refused to eat this, so I gave her turkey. She still had no real appetite and only gained an ounce back at a time. I went to a local pet store and the owner told us all about Azmira®. **As soon as Muffin and Robear had the Azmira® they loved it. Muffin started eating several times per day.**

Muffin has **always had running eyes,** Persians typically have brown dripping that runs over their face and stains it. I thought this was normal because all Persians have it. **Since starting the Azmira®, Muffin's eyes have stopped dripping,** her face is always clean now. She has **gained weight,** her fur is growing back and she is playing like a kitten; **she has more energy now than she did before her medical accident.**

Robear is 13 years old, he has been **very lethargic and cranky,** he had started hitting Muffin when she got near him. Since starting the Azmira® food Robear has been running around and playing again, jumping over the balcony, before the Azmira® he couldn't jump on the kitchen table. He is also friendly towards Muffin again, and they share food from the same plate. **Both cats have nicer fur, more energy and a better disposition all due to having Azmira®....REAL FOOD."**

Kristin Vernon (e-mail)

"...Austin is a 3 years old West Highland White Terrier whom we RESCUED from horrid conditions.

...who LOVES your food. **He has even lost 3 pounds** – YIPPEE.

... and is a HAPPY – HEALTHY little boy who **has his SPUNK back!!!"**

Artiz (from e-mail)

"I learned of the Azmira® cat food through a friend. **Her cat had gone through an amazing change.** Her fur was beautiful. **My two cats now eat Azmira® canned, and dry food. They love it! And I noticed a difference in their fur in just over a week!** I told another family member about the food, and they now feed it to their dog. They are **extremely happy with the results.** I will gladly recommend your product to anyone."

Crystal Ohlhausen
New Westminster, BC, Canada

"Just a quick note to let you know about the marvelous news I got from the vet about Saavik. I took her to the vet this past week and as a safety measure I had a blood profile done on her. **Well the vet called me up yesterday and in a somewhat astounded voice told me that Saavik has the blood work he would expect to see in a dog 5 years old!!! Saavik will be 14 years old (next month).**

Last year Saavik had the normal readings a dog her age should have, however she also had only just started getting (Dr. Newman's recommended Azmira® products). What is great is that Saavik has been exclusively on the Azmira® dry and canned food two months prior to the blood work. Yes, I have stopped making her dog food for her, as an experiment to see how long she could go without it. So far, so wonderful!!!

To have Saavik finally doing so well makes all the effort we have put in her worth it all. **The rest of my motley crew is doing fine, they are so healthy, it's boring! With having your food to eat, I've no doubt that they will outlive me!"**

Juanita Alvarez
Tucson, AZ

"One of our cats is 14 years old and was diagnosed with diabetes about 4.5 years ago, **the diagnosis was a little late** and his diabetes was discovered when his hind legs would not support his weight. **He eventually lost one eye and the other started to look cloudy,** then I found Azmira® on the web, we put all the cats on Azmira®, **after a few months we noticed that Merry's eye – that was cloudy before – was now clear, bright and very healthy looking, his coat was silky and he was more alert and sociable.**

The **veterinarian is surprised that he is doing so well after several years of being diabetic,** he takes insulin daily but we feel the real reason for his comeback and general good health is the diet."

David Brillo
Kissimee, FL

"…all the tests came back negative. The vet blamed the aggression on the fevers (Twinky) had his first three years of life, **fighting what may have been FIP… he still has an elevated titer.**

After two weeks (of following Dr. Newman's recommendations and Azmira® products) I can't believe the change! Minnie is digesting food and Twinkie is very mellow and happy. **The change in their health is**

very remarkable. The cats used to growl and fight with each other, now they are content.

Beth Bailey
Tucson, AZ

"The vet wanted to do surgery (cruciate repair on a Lhasa Apso) to the tune of about $2000.00 ...he said a 50/50 chance of using her leg again. Thanks to (Dr. Newman Holistic Animal Care LifeStyle™ and Azmira® products) and lots of prayers, her leg was healed in less **than 1½ months!**"

Margie Riester
Tucson, AZ

"Last March, my 16½ year old cat became extremely ill. The vet said she was **having problems with her liver, kidneys and heart**... to keep her on (prescription) diet the rest of her life. After two weeks of this diet, I grew desperate. **She was slowly dying.**

...I was very impressed with your abilities. My prayers had been answered.

My best friend is still going strong. I can't thank Lisa Newman enough for her wonderful products. My cat has a better life and I'm not paying high vet bills. Thank You!"

Sheri Horton
Tucson, AZ

"I have been working with Lisa Newman in treatment of my cat, Kali, for the past two years. **Kali was originally treated by a vet and was diagnosed as having 20% use of her kidneys and no treatment possibilities or potential for recovery of any kind. He gave her a very limited lifespan as well.**

I then worked with Lisa and through (her Holistic Animal Care LifeStyle™ protocols and Azmira® products) Kali has gone through a very significant recovery. She has no kidney problems... She has become a mellower cat since Lisa has been working with her physical and emotional well being.

Because of the results I have seen in Kali, I have become totally confident that any problems or conditions that any of the animals in my life may incur I would and will turn to Lisa for advice and treatment."

Joanie Trussel
Tucson, AZ

TABLE OF CONTENTS

Introduction

When I considered writing my ninth book on natural pet care, I first asked myself—what more could I share with you to make it worth your time to read it and worth the financial investment? I soon realized that over the years I have been perfecting a specific and unique approach to natural pet care based on *a systematic progression* of curative reactions. It is an approach which simplifies the process of applying remedies by using modalities in stages to encourage healing, as nature intended.

I will introduce you to three simple steps and explain their potential to quickly create wellness in your pet, which encourages a long life, and self-healing when needed. I will help you learn to read your own animal's symptoms and unravel the mysteries of a curative response versus healing crisis; I separate the two, so you can learn how to address the symptom successfully. Knowing the most logical approach to healing: what to expect and which remedy is needed to stimulate a series of symptom changes based on your pet's individual symptom progression promotes a quicker, long term recovery. Following my protocols will also help you avoid chasing chronic symptoms with one remedy or drug after another and will eliminate suffering major relapses. This approach can lessen the cost of general chronic health care as you will know when it is necessary to rely on veterinary medical care to avoid unnecessary bills. It will also eliminate unnecessary use of medications, vaccinations, monthly pest control drugs and chemical topical treatments. You will also learn that when these are used, they are known to cause a variety of symptoms and poor health conditions, including cancer.

In addition, you will learn when the body needs energy to deal with a toxic drug or substance, there is not enough energy left to direct toward maintaining wellness and healing. The immune system and other organs become compromised. The body loses nutrients fighting off drug or chemical toxicity instead of being able to use these nutrients to fuel rejuvenation. Only through full cellular regeneration can there be symptom reversal, and without the proper fuel, rejuvenation cannot be completed—the body fails to reach a state of strengthening and ultimately, wellness maintenance.

Symptom *suppression* can also be achieved with natural remedies and the result is the same. When suppression is achieved through drugs, or even natural remedies, symptoms often return within weeks once the protocol has ended. Holistic-minded clients may soon feel betrayed and give up on all alternative care, allowing their pets to suffer needlessly while believing this is the best they can achieve. My specific approach, called The Holistic Animal Care LifeStyle™, has been clinically documented since 1986 to help support the body in preventing and reversing poor health conditions. It has been proven by several generations of pets to be safe and effective while quickly addressing specific underlying weaknesses, or symptoms. My hope now is to share with you this simple three step plan and the products I guarantee can help you to be in full control of your pet's wellness and comfort.

Certainly, if you have read other authors' books on natural pet care, you are aware that terms such as "underlying weakness" and "immune stimulation" are used, and a variety of recommendations for symptom control or elimination are made. **But, what if their recommendations fail in your case?** *What if other symptoms appear or general results are too mediocre for long-term wellness?* **What would be the next logical step to take to encourage the healing process?** *How could you know what to do next when you cannot tell if the product(s) and protocol(s) recommended failed to achieve the desired results, or was it the pet's own biological failure to utilize these tools... or both?* **How do you choose the right remedy of homeopathy versus herbs?** These are frustrating questions faced by all animal caregivers and difficult to answer without the right information.

With this knowledge you can now quickly recognize and address *patterns* of healing or imbalance *which indicate a specific change is needed* based on symptoms currently observed. The faster you address and successfully support the body's attempt at reversing disease, the less weakness you have to contend with and the quicker you will achieve optimum results. This also reduces the financial burden of long-term care and chronic symptom chasing.

The Secret Behind The LifeStyle™ Success

In over twenty years of research and consulting, I have come across one sure fact that has never been proven wrong: the higher the quality of therapeutic ingredients you can provide in a concentrated, easy-to-utilize state, the quicker, deeper and more long-term the results will be. Once I began working with specific brands of natural products and remedies, I realized I achieved greater responses and overall success. I clearly saw the step-by-step LifeStyle™ approach develop because of the consistent results I could observe that I attributed to these specific remedies and applications.

Unfortunately, not all companies can be trusted to maintain higher standards. This gives us unreliable results on which to base the progress of true healing. I suffered the consequences of this with three of the top companies I had been recommending for years! In addition, I found results varied greatly when clients chose products on their own or substituted ingredients and I didn't appreciate the results; I took my consulting work and the lives that were affected very seriously! They say things change by desperation or inspiration—I have experienced a little of both. This was a dilemma I solved by formulating AZMIRA HOLISTIC ANIMAL CARE® supplements, remedies and diets after a particularly unsettling experience regarding product reliability.

I was called in to consult on two stage-four feline leukemia cases. One was a two year old male who seemed virtually symptom-free other than a mouth lesion and mild weight loss, but his cancer (viral load) was spreading as aggressively as in the second case; an eight year old female in a very poor, anorexic state with organ failure and uncontrollable fevers. The owners were both given my feline leukemia protocol with recommended feeding and supplement list.

The male was dead within twelve weeks and the female lived an additional very healthy nine years after a seven month recovery period. I was confused as their initial appearances and test results were opposite of what I expected to happen given the exact same protocol and products. The male certainly seemed to have more strength left to fight with, but his owner chose to purchase whatever similar product was on sale or recommended by the natural food store clerk, including a dry herb rather than standardized extract which caused him to stop eating due to its overly bitter properties. By the time they realized their mistake, it was too late. The owner of the female followed my recommendations; including buying the brands and herb potency I specifically listed. It opened my eyes to the fact that the higher the quality and concentration of product ingredients, the better the product worked and could be relied upon for repeated results.

The most important thing is that your pet receives the proven tools needed to heal.

I have always left out any mention of my natural pet product line for fear of making a book or article sound like an infomercial. I feared that could minimize the importance of my message and preferred instead to write lists of ingredients the reader should look for. But this cannot address the quality, potency, proper dosages or any specific outcomes vital to optimum healing and a full recovery. I want to assure you that the proper tools and information regarding their use are available to you and your animals so you can focus on the most important thing: your companion needs your help and guidance to stay well. There is a proven way to easily accomplish this. My award-winning products have made a difference in the success of my protocols and will make a difference for you. It makes the LifeStyle™ approach even more accurate and easy-to-follow successfully. Therefore, for your benefit I will be highlighting the Azmira® Products specifically in the context of my proven protocols.

Many veterinarians and owners have shared that The Holistic Animal Care LifeStyle™ combined with Azmira® nutrition and supplementation have completely taken the mystery out of alternative care for them, making it more approachable and successful by creating an easy-to-follow plan with specific outcomes and protocols on which to build.

These three simple steps to symptom reversal and product recommendations have been identified through careful documentation of the thousands of animals I have followed, the owners' observations and veterinary follow-up. Please understand that it is important you do read the entire book and not skip ahead to the symptom-specific guide so you can become fully familiar with how to properly apply those recommendations. A clear pattern of disease and symptom reversal is there once you know what to look for.

For many years I have taught this pattern of disease in seminars and articles. I call it "dis-ease" to signify the truth behind all symptoms or conditions, be it emotional or physical—it is a matter of *imbalance* or dis-ease in the body due to some injurious agent. Each year I gained additional knowledge through research and received valuable feedback from owners, trainers, groomers, rescue shelters, breeders and veterinarians. I have improved on some pet care techniques, learned new symptom markers and recognized more of the nuances of the healing process. This information has veterinarians and caregivers successfully deciding the next course of action, as it can for you. With this information I have been able to update my chapter on specific symptom reversals providing you with a larger variety of symptom nuances to address, but please do first read the chapters on Understanding How Pets Get Sick and Steps One, Two and Three. Also read the chapter on addressing symptoms and using remedies. It will help you apply my symptom reversal recommendations to their fullest potential by explaining the importance of proper detoxification and nutrition, daily supplementation and individual remedy applications when needed.

I am honored to have this opportunity to share this knowledge with you and your loved ones. Thank you and I wish you the best LifeStyle™ has to offer.

Lisa Newman, ND, PhD.

CHAPTER ONE

THE NATURAL PET

Millions of years before humans appeared on the evolutionary path Canis familiaris and Felis catus were busy establishing themselves. Today's dog and cat breeds are the result of the intense domestication and genetic manipulation by humans which followed. Unfortunately, this manipulation continues today, resulting in many pets struggling with common physical or behavioral issues. The Egyptians—humans who perceived cats in a higher, almost spiritual light—first aggressively pursued the manipulation of an animal's defining characteristics, such as color and body type. Breeding for "looks" or other specific traits continues today. Rising in popularity today—more so than at any other time in our history—is the introduction of new breeds of cats, the result of specific genetic mutations. Luckily horses, ferrets and birds haven't been that terribly affected although they too have their genetic weaknesses.

Dogs have suffered worse fates as each breed has become popular, often during the eras which gave us the Cocker Spaniel, French Poodle, Doberman Pincher, and Boxer, or from movie roles that bestowed upon generations the honorable Collie, adorable Dalmatian, and protective German Shepherd. Each breed has carried with it genetic codes for looks, size and color, but mutated the genetic information for sound health and emotional stability. Unfortunately the mix breeds, once thought to be immune to genetic conditions, can also suffer the worst of code building fates. As a result, many pet owners are faced with common health or behavioral difficulties.

In-breeding and excessive genetic manipulation have also minimized our animals' natural curative abilities. This has left our companions very susceptible. Generations exposed to vaccinations, chemical baths, flea/tick potions, dips or sprays, medications, and most importantly, poor quality ingredients, artificial colors, preservatives and by-products found in most pet foods and treats, eventually take their toll as the next in line is born prone to these injurious agents.

Cancer is one of the most dreaded diseases, and premature aging is becoming all too common today, even in less genetically manipulated animals such as birds and horses, due to the excessive exposure to toxins during their lives. Cats—once capable of easily reaching the age of twenty-five—now are seen as "seniors" at the age of six. Dogs die even younger, only living to be eleven when they should reach fifteen, even twenty years old for small breeds. My horses average thirty years in life, my cats have lived well in to their twenties and my large breed Rottweilers lived to fifteen, one even sixteen years. Most importantly they lived very healthy lives, not lives ruled by dis-ease.

Unfortunately, although pre-mature aging and cancer garners more attention, they have often been preceded by a long history of symptoms. Whether such symptoms are considered isolated ones or the result of a specific disease or organ failure, over 95% of these symptoms are preventable with proper care. What's more maddening is the fact that the "advertised" age of senior dogs and cats is now six years of age whereas when I first started out it was nine and twelve years old. Why have the veterinarians lowered the age a pet is considered in its "senior" years rather than question why they are aging at a more rapid pace today?!

Concerned owners spend hundreds, if not thousands, of dollars each year suppressing various health or behavioral conditions, many of them chronic. Each cycle of symptoms mounts a new campaign of drugs, shampoos, creams, and supplements, including diet and training/handling changes. While many changes do *temporarily* suppress the discomfort of the symptom, the condition gradually gets worse. As the pet gets older, his or her resistance to disease and tolerance for our control weakens, and symptoms become more difficult to treat. This cycle—of suppression and a relapse of the symptoms once medication has stopped—is an all too familiar one for many pets and their caregivers. A holistic lifestyle approach through detoxification, diet, supplementation of nutrients and herbs, homeopathic remedies, exercise, communication (teaching without trauma) and proper grooming can play an important role in providing your animal with optimum health and emotional wellness.

CHAPTER TWO

NATURAL PET CARE

To better understand how the three simple steps of the Holistic Animal Care LifeStyle™ process can work for your companions, it is helpful to first understand what holistic care basically is. It is according to the laws of nature. Holistic means "whole"—addressing the entire body rather than its parts. Holistic care encompasses the whole body, including mind, spirit and even the environment in which it lives. The application of various modalities is done in a synergistic way to help stimulate, strengthen and support the body's own biological processes and natural defenses to premature aging and disease. This is used as a means of preventing— as well as reversing—biological imbalances which lead to health or behavioral problems.

Nutrition is fundamental to a natural pet care program such as the Holistic Animal Care LifeStyle™ program and can often be the deciding factor between emotional wellness, health and disease. Poor nutrition will quickly lead to an imbalance, cripple the body's curative abilities, cloud the mind and possibly create behavioral problems. Regardless of the amount of attention, drugs or natural remedies given to a pet, if the pet is not receiving adequate nutrition, he or she is lacking the basic tools with which to support wellness and a curative response when needed.

Nutrition is also the cornerstone of a modality known as NATUROPATHY. Defined by a medical dictionary as a "drugless system of therapy," naturopathy is a comprehensive approach which emphasizes supporting the body's physical attempts to eliminate disease. My work is based on naturopathic methods which follow a central idea that a major cause of disease is an excessive buildup of toxic materials (often due to improper

3

eating, environmental toxins and lack of exercise) which clog the eliminatory system. Various techniques are used to clean out (detoxify) the body and stimulate reversal of symptoms and disease. Besides the cleansing process, animals are put on supportive programs of high quality nutrition, proper food combining (to stimulate and aid digestion) and the judicious use of nutritional supplements, herbs and homeopathy. Prevention is always considered the best cure.

Basic to folk medicine and every culture since ancient times, herbs are probably the most fundamental of specific remedies to stimulate natural healing. I rely on them with great success. It is widely believed that people began using herbs after observing how animals in the wild will often instinctively select appropriate herbs when they are ill. In HERBOLOGY, emphasis is placed on the use of specific herbal leaves, roots, bark, flowers and seeds to assist the healing process by primarily helping the body to eliminate and detoxify, thus taking care of the underlying problem the symptoms are expressing. As compared to their pharmaceutical counterparts, herbs provide a slower and deeper action. They are quickly becoming very mainstream, as nutraceutical products (nutritional supplements) are lining shelves at drug stores these days.

Another modality, which provides an even slower and deeper action, is HOMEOPATHY. I have found that sometimes the use of nutrition or herbs is not sufficient. They will begin the cleansing process and support the body (by strengthening it so that it can go through the necessary curative process), but often it is the homeopathic remedy which stimulates the deeper level of healing or specific symptom reversal as needed. The real beauty of the homeopathic system lies in its safety and the simplicity of its basic principles, as well as the exhaustively researched criteria behind thousands of remedies used successfully for hundreds of years.

The German physician, Samuel Hahnemann, founded homeopathy on one basic unifying principle that has held true ever since it was originated in the late 1700's. Hahnemann's "provings" of homeopathy were based on **"like be cured by like"**— a substance that can mimic symptoms helps cure them as well. This principle revolutionized the understanding of symptoms and disease. Hahnemann noted certain similarities between symptoms produced by some diseases and by the very drugs used to treat them. From this he formed his LAW OF SIMILARS to identify that a disease could be cured by whatever medicine produces similar symptoms when given to a healthy person. Its beauty is that the treatment provided goes with, rather than against, the body's own efforts to regain health by restoring balance to the weakened system, be it digestive, eliminatory, immune, etc.

A simplified example of how homeopathy works is that of bee venom. We know that a bee sting will cause a certain topical reaction, including swelling, fluid accumulation, redness of the skin, pain, and soreness that is accentuated by the application of heat or pressure. Some sensitive animals will experience mental, physical and emotional symptoms such as apathy, stupor, listlessness, or the opposite, whining, restlessness and fearfulness. If a homeopathically prepared **dilute solution** of the venom (known as *Apis*) is given to a pet with these symptoms—even if they are caused by something other than a bee sting, like an allergic reaction—the condition will soon begin to clear up. The essential key is that the symptoms are quite similar to what the remedy, in its undiluted state, would create. Flower essences (balance emotional states) and tissue cells salts (support physiological processes) act similarly in stimulating the body's own natural healing and homeostasis. This all comes together to help the holistic pet strive within the LifeStyle™ naturopathic approach.

The Holistic Pet

I define the health of a holistically reared pet to be a state of balance existing on three interrelated levels: the physical, the emotional, and the environmental. A healthy pet experiences physical vitality and freedom from physiological malfunction, emotional clarity resulting in good behavior and happiness, and receives (as well as contributes) joy, love and security in their living environment.

This is the opposite of a chemically reared pet, who is often found to be in a state of imbalance or dis-ease. The consequences are an unhealthy pet who experiences lack of physical vitality. This animal suffers from chronic symptoms, premature aging due to physiological malfunction, and emotional stress resulting in negative behavior. Most often an unhealthy pet also lives in a physically toxic environment. It is impossible to have one organ system affected without it then affecting the others. Frequently, deep in a state of general imbalance, the body will be assaulted by certain substances that an otherwise healthy body would have no problems processing—allergens, viruses, bacteria, toxins—yet the unbalanced body crashes.

The Holistic Animal Care LifeStyle™ was developed to identify and address the needs of these pets. Every animal caregiver's primary goal should be to provide their companion with emotional and physical well-being—to prevent and reverse disease by supporting the body's natural curative process—rather than simply suppressing the signs of imbalance.

What's exciting about The Holistic Animal Care LifeStyle™ is the very fact that it is so simple and safe to use.

Treat the body well and the body will be well.

By providing your pet with ample love, play time (exercise), quality nutrition, proper supplementation, and holistic remedies when appropriate, your animal's body will remain in a healthy balance. If assaulted by certain substances which develop an imbalance, the body simply reestablishes its balance, preventing further degeneration.

CHAPTER THREE

Understanding How Pets Get Sick

In order to better understand why the three simple steps of the LifeStyle™ process works well in reversing dis-ease, it will be helpful for you to first understand how an animal gets sick. Once you help your pet to become healthy you can prevent dis-ease from happening again. If your pet is now fairly healthy; this knowledge will help you provide the tools for optimum health. Although a number of pets who are born genetically compromised develop certain conditions, the majority of pets are simply suffering the long-term consequences of chemical ingestion and exposure to an emotionally and/or physically toxic environment. This alters the primary biological functions in the body, places undue stress on vital organs and glands necessary for proper immune function and destroys healthy tissue. The result is a body out of balance, or dis-eased.

Unhealthy Pets Have Often Been Exposed To A Toxic LifeStyle™

- Standard commercial pet foods, artificially made treats—sweetened, salted, liver or yeast-based.

- Shotgun medications; when general antibiotics are given before a specific infection is identified and the indiscriminate use of "standard" medications such as steroids for allergies and inflammation.

- Excessive vaccinations *and* yearly boosters—especially when given during times of surgery or illness.

- Toxic cleaning supplies and pest control products (particularly flea collars or monthly heartworm, flea and tick preventative medications).

- Environmental pollution (without the benefit of regular detoxification).

- An emotionally and/or physically stressful living environment— past and present.

I would have to say that commercial pet diets and treats account for the largest assault on the body, and are the primary reason pets develop symptoms. I am not talking about food allergies here. It is my belief that the quality (or *lack of* good fresh quality) of the ingredient can do more harm, and more likely trigger a response, than the ingredient itself. Through the Holistic Animal Care LifeStyle™, the foundation of which is a clean, healthy diet, many pets are now eating a specific ingredient they previously tested positive for allergies to. Supplements are vital to the success of my protocols and the process of true healing but the standard use of by-products and meat sources unfit for human consumption severely compromises the pet's body's ability to digest and assimilate these nutrients well.

A Toxic Bowel Creates a Toxic Body

The use of artificial colors or flavors, chemical preservatives, nitrates and rancid animal fats also interfere with digestion, adding a double whammy to the body in conjunction with the poor quality ingredients already presented for digestion. Poorly digested matter becomes harder to eliminate, causing a backup of old fecal material in the bowel, which further prohibits assimilation of vital nutrients.

I have dubbed this the **screen door effect**. Here in the desert where I live, we love screen doors and the ventilation they provide. But we also struggle with blowing dirt, and on the few days of the season when we also get rain, my screen door can become caked with dirt. If I go out and brush it off right away there is not much of a problem, but if I wait a day or two the dirt can harden, especially if it rains again. Rain only adheres the top layers of dirt more firmly onto the previous ones and can create an adobe mud effect, where the dirt becomes so hard that it cannot be brushed away and actually begins to block the flow of air.

This is similar to what we have learned is happening inside a poorly maintained colon. Imagine the colon as the screen door to the body and nutrients are the air. As improperly digested matter moves into the colon and complete evacuation is not encouraged (mostly pets lack exercise, and can't always go outside to have a bowel movement when they have the urge), old fecal material begins to "collect". This material "lines" the walls of the colon, and chemicals (such as ethoxyquin, a commonly used pet food preservative that is moisture prohibitive) further create a lack of moisture and lubrication necessary for a properly evacuated stool. This lack of moisture is not only responsible for further drying up the fecal material and hardening it inside the colon, it finally produces those small, hard, dry stools that do pass.

Most companies try to convince you these stools only mean their food is more "digestible with less waste to pick up", but what do you think a medical doctor would say to you if you described your own stools as coming out like that?! Certainly, a better quality food will produce less stool volume (generally due to less fillers *first,* better digestibility *second*), but it should not be from lack of moisture in the stool. Think about it: a dry wad of tissue paper is so small, yet when wet it swells up to three times the dry size—even though the mass of tissue paper has not changed. The colon requires ample hydration to function properly. Please always provide fresh, filtered drinking water.

As old fecal material builds up inside the colon, the screen door effect comes into play. It becomes harder and harder for the body to clean out this material on its own. This interferes with the body's ability to absorb or "ventilate" nutrients from digested matter in the colon into the blood stream, for distribution among the body's hungry cells and energy-depleted organ systems. What is leaked into the bloodstream is the excessive waste stuck inside the colon. This begins the toxic reaction.

The harder the ingredients are to break down and process, and the more chemicals present, the more stress is placed on the body to function. As with anything, the harder it has to work, the quicker it breaks down and falls apart. More importantly is the fact that through improper digestion and assimilation, the body lacks the resources to utilize whatever nutrients are entering which are vital to proper biological processes such as immunity (resistance to physical and emotional stress). Improper digestion and assimilation also lead to a buildup of general waste (toxins) in the body, which places a huge burden upon the eliminatory organs. As the liver and kidneys become burdened, the body attempts to detoxify through the largest eliminatory organ it has, the skin. Hence the development of skin and coat problems normally associated with poor coat and skin condition, or allergies—the most common diagnosis. Additionally, the lymph system and endocrine system are over stimulated, possibly leading to the development of a deeper, more serious disease like reactive arthritis or cancer.

The next most common cause in unbalancing an animal's health is their exposure to chemicals and irritants in other, non-dietary, forms. This can be as simple as a chemical-based breath mint given as a treat or as complicated as your animal's annual vaccination boosters. Include artificially perfumed shampoo, medicated skin treatments, chemical flea or tick control products, household cleaning agents, and long-term medication. If you think of the body as a healthy balanced scale, and you keep adding these chemicals to one side maintaining the scale off-balance, eventually that side will hit bottom. But if you keep good nutrition replenished on one side and minimize the buildup of chemicals on the other, this scale stays in balance—the body stays healthy.

Therefore, it is important to also acknowledge other factors which may be imbalancing the body and interfering with homeostasis, so that they may be addressed as well. Structural imbalances are often a prime underlying cause of dis-ease. Old injuries or genetic malfunctions, such as rheumatoid arthritis, can place stress on certain organ systems. A build-up of calcium deposits and spinal inflammation may also put pressure on specific nerves involved with digestive organs, such as the stomach. This can interfere with the normal function of the stomach and lead to improper digestion and assimilation of nutrients. Often, addressing the structural problems will help finally reverse the "chronic" condition. Chiropractic adjustments, massage, acupressure and acupuncture can all be additional beneficial naturopathic tools in your fight against your animal's symptoms.

In looking at other issues which can also imbalance in the body, negative emotions and a stressful environment are often overlooked. Have you ever felt "butterflies in your stomach" and experienced a loose bowel due to a stressful situation? Pets who often experience extreme emotions (fear, nervousness, and tension) are also more likely to suffer from behavioral issues, digestive problems and glandular imbalances, which may exacerbate chronic symptoms. These extremes can be related to family changes such as relocating, members leaving or dying, divorce or new births, new jobs, etc.

The pituitary, adrenal and thyroid glands are very susceptible to hyperstimulation and exhaustion, due to chronic emotional stress. These are glands associated with the "fight or flight" reaction to negative stimulus, common to all living things. Therefore, it is not only important to provide a safe and nurturing environment for your pet's emotional well-being, but to use nutritional supplementation and remedies (especially flower essences) to re-balance the emotions. This combined approach can often be the key to a more complete physical healing.

When an animal's health is out of balance, waste builds up in the bloodstream and burden the eliminatory organs. A specific culprit, or injurious agent, in many conditions is urea, the normal waste product of meat protein metabolism. This accounts for the high number of pets who test positive for meat allergies. The poorer the quality of meat and the more difficult it is to digest, the more waste product is produced during its digestion. As urea buildup occurs in the body, a gout-like reaction may occur. Yeast is also frequently at fault in burdening the liver—as it can be difficult to break down—and is in everything!

Urea or yeast toxicity manifests itself in certain symptoms, most notably:

- Known or suspected allergies to yeast, beef, pork, meat, meat by-products or meat meal
- Ear infections, eye discharges and upper respiratory problems, including asthma
- The excessive licking and chewing of paws, resulting in lick granuloma
- Prickly heat-type rashes, itchy skin, with or without hot spots, pimples or pustules
- Slower healing of skin problems and excessive loss of hair or poor coat condition
- Foul smelling breath and/or stool (especially with mucous or off-colored), flatulence
- Increased fatty tumor, cyst or cancerous tumor production
- Poor digestion and assimilation of other nutrients, blood sugar instability—diabetes
- High levels of liver enzymes and eosinophils detected (represents a damaged liver)
- Decreased phosphates found in the urine due to kidney disease
- Liver, pancreatic, gallbladder and kidney dysfunction or failure
- Weakened immune responses, especially chronic infections or cancer

- Premature aging, with or without chronic arthritic or digestive symptoms

- Neurological issues, including seizures

- Aggression and other training or behavioral problems in certain pets

- Increased sensitivities to pollution, vaccinations and chemicals in general

- Parasitic infestation, especially fleas and ticks (feeding off of skin-eliminated waste)

As a side note on parasites, I have long experienced that for the protection against flea and tick infestations, **garlic is actually more powerful by itself** than yeast alone or in combination with yeast. In addition, a clean diet, resulting in fewer waste products to eliminate, greatly reduces the waste eliminated through the skin. This waste is the very thing that attracts a flea or tick to the body in the first place and then actually sustains (feeds) them! Old fecal material in the colon also attracts and feeds internal parasites such as worms.

As urea, metabolized yeast and other excessive wastes build up in the body and undue stress is placed upon vital organs, it is not uncommon for the body to begin experiencing system malfunctions. It is a vicious cycle and one clearly identifiable, if you know what to look for.

First the digestive system is affected; stomach and intestines struggle as it becomes even harder to break down ingredients, increasing metabolic waste circulating in the blood and organs, interfering with vital nutrient utilization needed to stimulate the body's own defenses. Finally the eliminatory system becomes congested and places undue stress upon the lymphatic and immune systems. *Chronic symptoms develop—and suppression is initiated.* Once medication and/or remedies are stopped, the symptoms return and the cycle eventually continues. Ultimately, there is organ and gland malfunction, possibly leading to premature aging and an early death. Frequently, it may seem to come out of nowhere. You might exclaim, "yesterday he was so healthy"—but it does not happen overnight. It takes time for the body to become so burdened—and the scale to be so out of balance that it "suddenly" hits bottom. There are always early warning signs.

Any pet suffering from poor health related to genetics, organ disorders and "allergies" or toxicity can truly benefit from The Holistic Animal Care LifeStyle™. Regardless of the symptoms and diagnosis, the underlying cause can be fundamentally the same. Hence, I encompass all three under the term, "sensitivities". A wholesome, toxin-free approach to diet and environment cannot only prevent a symptom, but help reverse it more quickly and effectively than the further application of chemicals.

When pets with chronic dis-ease are placed on an ongoing Holistic Animal Care LifeStyle™ program, the results can be miraculous. As each month passes and the body strengthens, it becomes less and less "sensitive" to toxins. The animal then exhibits less severe symptoms with each cycle—becoming easier to address each time, with acute symptoms reversing more quickly. **A holistic LifeStyle™ should be followed rather than relying on simple symptom suppression.** Once a better diet is in use, don't stop detoxification and supplementation as soon as symptoms have been suppressed. The body will become burdened again (having already shown a predisposition to this weakness) and will again respond to toxins or stress. Continue supporting the immune system to achieve symptom reversal and prevent reoccurrence. This can be very simple to do.

Even pets who are seen as "fit and healthy" can soon realize their fullest genetic potential. Until you have something to compare to you won't know the outcome. This is why my most loyal followers have been those owners who believed that their prior holistic approach was providing the best care possible. Once they quickly see the results of my unique process and products, they can better appreciate the difference it can make.

As you will learn, treating your pet's symptoms holistically in this systematic fashion is the quickest, most effective way to completely reverse an underlying condition. In those animals that have been genetically or environmentally predisposed to deeper dis-ease, natural pet care will, in the long run, serve to minimize degenerative possibilities and maximize their curative potential. Plus, it will save you money by eliminating the hit-or-miss approaches.

The Holistic Animal Care LifeStyle™ will help you take the three simple steps to identify your individual pet's needs and provide specific tools to help achieve wellness. Acute symptom reversal is often possible within days. Years of success have proven that even with chronic debilitating dis-ease, the judicious use of homeopathic, herbal and nutritional supplementation in a *continuing* course of treatment will definitely contribute to the strengthening of each animal's constitution and reduce, or eventually eliminate, their condition.

Quite possibly, you will find that the holistic LifeStyle™ choices I am recommending you consider may serve your needs better than the more conventional approach to symptom relief. I can guarantee that you will find a holistically-reared animal to have the greatest chance at being the healthiest and happiest pet you ever had.

Simply suppressing symptoms pharmaceutically cannot only be very frustrating but may lead to a premature death. Year after year of toxins attacking a body—barely protected by a struggling immune system—will only serve to weaken the body further in the long run. A sound nutritional program supported with ongoing detoxification, proper supplementation and rebalancing homeopathically or with herbs, while avoiding (or at least limiting) vaccination boosters, chemicals and drugs, are the best way to prevent or reverse poor health holistically!

CHAPTER FOUR

STEP ONE:
NUTRITION & DETOXIFICATION

The primary line of defense in preventing or treating symptoms is a sound nutritional program. The goal of Step One is to provide healthy food and promote improved nutrient utilization through detoxification to fuel a process of wellness (preventative or symptom-reversal). Your pet's natural diet should consist of fresh, high quality, easy to digest and assimilate ingredients. I will be focusing more on dogs and cats in this section but the same principles apply regardless of what type of diet—omnivore, herbivore or carnivore—your pet needs. Home cooking is optimal but might not be very practical; therefore, you must be very careful to seek out a quality commercial product.

Become an educated label reader. Look beyond catchy terms such as "natural", "organic", "healthy", "symptom-related diet" and "human-grade quality," and ask the manufacturer directly to prove their quality and guarantee their formula since there is no true authority in the pet food industry. According to AAFCO's (American Association of Feed Control Officers) 2004 handbook, **thrown-out restaurant tallow** (*fats;* page245) or **food wastes** (*miscellaneous;* page 321) and **hydrolyzed hair** (*animal products;* page 256) is fine, so is **shoe leather** (*animal products;* page 259) as appropriate pet food ingredients—not to mention **dried animal wastes** (*recycled animal waste products;* page 328-30!) and **unborn calf carcasses** (*animal products;* page 258). These unhealthy ingredients can be legally identified on the product label in misleading terms such as "meat by-products" and not by their actual names! They do not think quality matters as they also advocate using diseased or decayed flesh, instead

15

AAFCO considers most herbs as "unapproved" pet food ingredients.... I beg to differ with their logic, and I think you will too, once you see the facts. In this industry, as in many others, it comes down to using the cheapest ingredients you can get away with and lobbying to keep others, who are raising the bar, stifled.

FADS: *False Advice Delivers Sorrow*

Beware of "lite" diets—they may actually cause weight gain in the long run. I have never formulated one for Azmira® since there is no need for a reduced calorie diet, only a wholesome one fed in controlled quantities. Symptom-specific diets are simply a profitable marketing tool at best and a toxic food at worst. Commonly used fillers such as ground peanut hulls may be filling, but void of nutrients. They can be damaging to the sensitive lining of the digestive tract. Peanuts are also a crop which is heavily sprayed with pesticides, therefore the hull is very toxic.

In a reduced calorie diet, nutrients may be lacking or dietary fiber may interfere with nutrient assimilation. The brain decides if there is enough nutrition available to the body regardless of the diet's "quality." Calories are stored instead of burning them, to ward off possible starvation, when this fuel is lacking. A properly balanced, quality diet which is fed in controlled (not reduced) caloric quantity and provides easy-to-assimilate nutrients will naturally bring your pet to the proper weight.

Another gimmick to watch out for is formulas which address one life stage over another. This is only the repackaging of very similar formulas with the plan to have the average household purchase more than one bag at a time since most families have pets of varying ages (i.e. adult and senior). In fact, each life-stage requires the *same ingredients* only *different calorie requirements and protein levels.* The same can be accomplished with the same formula while varying the amount fed on a daily basis. For instance: the senior pet will consume approximately twenty percent less food than an adult animal of the same weight level, and a puppy will consume twenty percent more protein (meat) than an adult. This is easily accomplished through portion control, and the addition of canned meat to the dry formula.

One thing I also recommend is that you beware of feeding raw meats. Although diets such as B.A.R.F. (bones and raw foods) are now becoming the "in" thing, I have found in more cases than I would care to see, a deterioration of the pet's condition, rather than support. I believe this is due to the fact that animals evolve to fit their environment... and our pets have been so domesticated for so long that they have "evolved" into *cooked* food eaters and lost the ability (of the wild) to digest raw meat tissue, bone, hide, feathers, etc. The argument for B.A.R.F. is that raw foods contain live enzymes that are killed during cooking. This is true. But what I find interesting with this argument is the fact that digestive enzymes are most often recommended for B.A.R.F. diets! Why is this if the live enzymes in raw meats are most beneficial? Even with the use of digestive enzymes, I still see most pets struggle to digest raw animal tissue. The simple fact of the matter is that lightly cooking (which *will not* destroy *all* enzymes and nutrients) helps begin to break down meat so that it is easier for the digestive tract to handle.

Frequently, raw ingredients, especially chicken and fish, which have not been properly handled, can pass E-Coli or parasites to the pet—which then suffers terrible gastrointestinal distress. Raw bones pose additional problems. James J. O'Heare, Ph.D., in his 2005 book, *Raw Meat Diets for Cats and Dogs?*, brings many good arguments to light. This well researched work clearly identifies the dangers of infestation (E-Coli, etc.) and choking on raw bones as primary concerns. He provides many studies, including my own, that have been conducted to prove and disprove the benefits. Conclusions are drawn from these facts.

Seek Out Easily Assimilated Nutrition:
available fuel for the body

Remember to feed only Grade A or B meats (human grade) and avoid the four-D meats (dead, dying, diseased, or disabled animals not fit for human consumption). The state these meats are in is one of decomposition and their original nutritional value as viable protein has diminished considerably. Four-D meats are the most commonly used in pet foods, including those from "organically raised" animals *who now certify* as four-D; regardless of life care, the condition the meat is in is more important than it's history. I prefer to feed traditionally raised, *human-grade fresh whole muscle* meat instead of naturally raised *but sold as four-D* meats.

Even worse is some companies' practice of claiming organic yet, *although true,* only trim pieces (meat by-products) are used. This provides much less nutrition than whole muscle meat protein so they have to add, of course, "organic" grain *by-products*. Think about it; the expense of natural beef or chicken makes using the high quality whole muscle meat less cost-effective. I checked into it when I wanted to make an organic pet food and my finished product would have cost the consumer, in 1997, twenty-five dollars for a four pound bag! Not many would pay that much but they will pay more for perceived quality in "naturally-raised" meat and "organic" ingredients. These manufacturers use the organic certified sources *but at the discounted price rancid, non-edible ingredients cost,* thus making a food at the same cost as the other lower priced pet foods but charging 25% more at retail! Besides, for now, AAFCO says it is illegal to list the word "organic" on a pet food bag although some companies are getting away with it. It is all about the marketing and what they can put over on the unsuspecting public.

Not only is the consumer duped but the pet is robbed of vital nutrition and when something happens, like cancer, no one suspects the diet because it is "organic" and "natural." But the truth is that the crap they put in it did not help keep the animal well. Period. I do not care that there are no chemicals or preservatives added; vital nutrition is missing. I am offended both as a consumer and as a pioneering natural pet food manufacturer to watch the marketing campaigns explode in this industry that just hide the truth: stock profits are more important than real nutrition. It also says that profits are more important than your animal's life.

Grain by-products are also a big problem in commercial pet products that rob the diet (and the body) of available nutrition. Wheat millings, brewer's rice (left over from the brewing process), and flours are not only devoid of nutritional value and inexpensive fillers, but they can severely compromise your pet's health. Often these grains are purchased rancid and moldy (this is "pet-grade" for an additional cost savings), adding the possibility of a toxic reaction. Several foods have been recalled due to moldy grain... why does this occur if they <u>are</u> using the highest human quality? It shouldn't! As in many foods, both for humans and pets, there is an "expectable" level of "contamination" allowed in the finished product. Many companies take advantage of this loop hole. Unfortunately, some pets can not tolerate these levels and still become ill or die. Besides, for many manufacturers, it is too tempting to the bottom line not to use the cheaper pet-grade despite what their marketing might say. Grade 1 or 2 grains (all human grades) should <u>only</u> be used, *preferably whole ground,* to assure their nutritional goodness remains intact. Most of the available nutrition is in the parts of the grain that are missing from the by-products.

Key Ingredients for a Healthy Manufactured Diet

- **Fresh, wholesome ingredients** are important to your pet's health and the diet's flavor. There should not be an unpleasant odor when the bag is first opened or within forty-five days of feeding from the same bag. *If there is an unpleasant odor, this indicates that* *rancid or moldy grains, and/or fat and decaying or putrid meats were used to manufacture the product.* Fresh, healthy food smells and tastes like recently prepared meals. Many owners believe their animals have lost their appetite for a particular product, when in fact, the pet turns away after being offered the food for a few weeks because the diet was not very tasty to begin with and now is simply inedible to the pet's palate. The owner changes brands which work initially, until that particular product is no longer fresh and tasty.

- **Balanced, combined ingredients** of proteins, fats and carbohydrate sources seems to suit most pets better than single source ingredients—contrary to popular belief.

- **Identifiable *and digestible* animal meat protein or fat sources** such as beef, beef meal, lamb, lamb meal, lamb fat, chicken, chicken meal or chicken fat, turkey, ostrich, etc. Never feed a diet with vague ingredient terms like "meats", "poultry" or "animal fats"—which can include anything including euthanized birds, dogs and cats.

- **Quality sources of dietary fat** are vital for energy and good coats. Vegetable or fish oils should be used for dogs, these are easier to digest than animal fats—true even for high energy and sporting dogs. On the other hand, cats require high energy fats, such as fresh chicken or lamb fat, due to their unique metabolism.

- **USDA Grade A or B animal meat protein sources** that are preferably raised without growth hormones or recently given antibiotics. Organic meat is not cost-effective unless trim with bone pieces are used which lowers the nutritional value of the diet's protein content.

- **Concentrated protein sources known as "meal"** (as in **"lamb meal"** or **"beef meal"**) are preferred over whole meats (listed only as "lamb" or "beef"). *This is not to be confused with "by-product meal" (see list of ingredients to avoid).*

The term "meal" simply refers to the process of removing up to 80%, but no less than 45%, of the ingredient's natural water content, so there is more *meat protein* for your money, since water only adds to the ingredient's weight (by which it is listed—first, second, etc. by the heaviest one first—on the ingredients' label).

For instance, it is very deceiving to find chicken listed first, when the majority of protein is coming from grains, not animal protein!

The third ingredient, corn gluten meal, might be the cheaper protein ingredient (being a grain rather than an animal meat source), and the majority of *protein actually* available. It greatly reduces the cost of ingredients due to the actual amount of animal protein used in the formula. One pound of meal is equal to approximately three pounds of whole meat, and there is an additional charge to dehydrate it down—therefore many companies use the meat to draw you to the label, but use another cheaper ingredient for the actual protein—one that could be triggering allergies or poor digestion. This is true for all chicken, turkey, rabbit, fish and other animal meat protein sources used in commercial pet foods.

Another deception by some companies is to scare you into thinking that "rendered" meat in competitors' brands are bad. All "meal" is not by-products and "rendered" only refers to a process. Rendering can refer to dehydrating the fresh whole meat into meal and powdering it for mixing into the final batch.

- **USDA Grade 1 or 2 whole grains,** preferably free of chemical pesticides or herbicides. Organic grains are also not cost-effective to be used in commercial pet foods, so if your pet's food claims "organic", demand written certification plus look for whole ground rather than flours, etc. "Pesticide-free" is available or "washed" grains are possible. For home cooking, go for the best organic ingredients you can afford!

- **Whole ground grains.** Avoid "flours," "mill runs" or "by-products." Grains should be fed for optimum nutritional value and additional healthy fiber.

- **Vegetable and fruit fiber** should be present, such as carrots and apples for proper digestion, natural flavoring and trace nutrients. Fiber in general is important for proper elimination, and fiber (additionally provided in whole grains) might as well be full of vital nutrients as well! Potatoes are NOT a suitable or nutritional source of fiber.

- **Priced appropriately**—*remember that you do generally get what you pay for,* but you must be sure that you are getting your money's worth. You could be paying for an expensive advertising campaign, not food value.

If the food cost $10 retail for a 40 lb. bag, and the cost of making/ marketing the food is as follows—printed *paper* bag costs $ .85, shipping the product to the distributor costs $1.00, advertising and handling costs $.75, a $2.50 profit for the manufacturer, a $1.25 profit for the wholesaler and a $2.25 profit for the retailer you are buying the food from—then how much do you think was actually spent on the ingredients to begin with! Also, take into consideration how much is needed to sustain your pet. In addition, the cheaper foods are actually more expensive, due to the fact that you have to feed so much more than a better quality diet made with less filler.

- **Product should be fresh when purchased.** *If you bought fresh-baked bread yesterday, it would be wonderful to eat... but would you still be eating it two weeks later?!* Be sure to check the date of manufacture—regardless of the expiration date—never feed food (especially a naturally preserved diet) that is older than four months, unless it is packaged in a completely sealed, airtight, <u>barrier</u> bag. The food may be considered "fresh" by the manufacturer, but how fresh is it really? Paper bags, most commonly used, allow air to flow through the kibble exposing it to oxygen which turns the food rancid quickly. The plastic liner on paper bags is only there to keep the food's oils from leaking through the paper.

Azmira® was one of the first companies to use a revolutionary barrier bag, laboratory proven to maintain optimum freshness for over one year when unopened. Once opened, with the bag folded and clipped, food remains fresh for almost two months. Some companies put their kibble in a small barrier bag for marketing but their larger size bags are made of paper, so be sure to check for the difference! Stale food not only does not taste so great, it has lost most of its nutritional value through oxidation regardless of its original high human-grade quality! Never purchase more than you can feed in six weeks or you will be feeding empty calories.

Ingredients to AVOID In a Healthy Diet

- **Chemical preservatives,** such as the rubber stabilizer and herbicide **Ethoxyquin,** which is similar to Agent Orange, have been linked to birth defects, cancer and other immune weaknesses. Over the past fifteen years, due to a groundswell of consumer protest, Ethoxyquin is now being replaced by many manufacturers with ascorbic acid, vitamin E and rosemary extract to stabilize fats and meats. **BHA and/or BHT** are also being considered for replacement by many manufacturers. **Propylene Glycol**, a relative of antifreeze, is often suspect in kidney disease but is still used as a plasticizer and sweetener, especially in "moist" kibble diets. **Nitrates**, unfortunately, are still commonly used in smoked treats, even "natural" ones, and other foods but are suspected in creating health issues including digestive upsets.

- **Artificial and/or unnecessary flavors or colors.** *Why put propylene glycol, sugar or salt in a pet's diet?* When food is fresh and flavorful, sweeteners should not be needed to entice appetite and salt should never be used to cover up rancid smells. In addition, if pets are color-blind, why do their individual kibble pieces need to be bright green, red and yellow?

- **Foul smelling foods** must be avoided at all cost. If it smells like traditional pet food (you know that smell: even in just-opened, fresh bags it smells rancid) then it can be harmful to ingest over your pet's lifetime. When garbage goes in, garbage must come out; this is what is behind so many general symptoms.

- **Greasy food** that leaves smelly oil on the bag or sheen on canned formulas means it is heavy in **animal fats or tallow** (rendered carcasses and recycled cooking grease from restaurants). These are difficult to digest—and most often rancid prior to manufacturing. This also accounts for that rancid "pet food" smell, even in "fresh" bags.

- **Animal by-products** *such as "beef by-product," "lamb by-product," "chicken by-product"* (by-products are a mixture of the whole carcass including cancerous tumors, hide, hooves, beaks, feathers, and fur) are used as protein sources. Their mysterious cousins—*"meat" or "meat by-products"* (a mixture of whatever mammals, including roadkill, swamp rats, euthanized dogs and cats, were ground up together), *"fish by-product"* and *"poultry by-products"* (a mixture of whatever ocean creatures and feathered animals, including pigeons, who got ground up together). *Need I say more?*

- **Grain by-products** such as *"mill runs," "flours," "middlings," "husks," "bits,"* and *"parts"* should be avoided at all costs. Not only are they void of nutrients (having had all the nutritionally rich parts already removed), they may actually be too harsh on the digestive and eliminatory tracts, causing more irritation as the body attempts to process their fibrous substances. These grain by-products are simply cheap fillers and can additionally be used as a protein source (although non-digestible and therefore, non-assimilated!) to increase the finished product's weight and mass.

- **Soybeans, onions, olive oil and chocolate in your dog's diet are especially difficult to utilize;** for instance, dogs cannot digest soy. The canine digestive tract lacks an amino acid necessary for the utilization of protein and fatty acids in soybeans. Tofu, the curd, and cold-pressed soybean oils are already processed through an enzyme or extraction process and can be tolerated by most dogs—but many foods, supplements and treats still contain soybean (whole, ground or flaked) which can trigger bloat, an often fatal reaction. Be sure to check each label; soy is a cheap filler and a poor protein source for dogs. Cats fare better on soybean since they can readily digest it. Dogs also can not digest onions which cause an anemic condition and possible death while olive oil can interrupt daily digestion, irritating the stomach, the gallbladder and pancreas. Dark chocolate contains compounds which can kill.

- **Fillers** such as powdered *"cellulose", "cellulose fiber"* (can include recycled newspaper, sawdust and cardboard), *"plant cellulose"* (usually identifies ground peanut or soybean hulls which are very damaging to sensitive colon tissues), *"beet pulp"* or *"grain by-products"* also have no nutritional value but add cheap bulk and weight to the finished product.

- **Yeast,** long touted for flea control and a shiny coat, is used as a cheap source of B-vitamins, amino acids and some nutrients, natural flavor and color, but yeast contributes to symptoms by burdening the liver and interfering in proper digestion.

- **Sugar** is added to most commercial diets and treats. Known as *"sucrose", "beet pulp", "molasses", "cane syrup", "fruit solids"* and of course, *"sugar."* It is a very cheap and heavy filler (reducing the need for additional weight in protein-rich meats) which literally can addict a pet to its food! Additional sugar in the diet is the primary trigger of weight problems, diabetic conditions and behavioral problems in pets today. Do not be fooled by the latest marketing gimmick: beet pulp "with the sugar removed" still contains sugar. Certainly it is less concentrated but there is still sugar left in the fiber—enough to create a sugar reaction in most pets.

Changing Foods

People are often concerned that changing their pet's diet will only result in digestive upsets... true, if you are changing between one poor quality and chemical-based diet to another! When switching to a healthier, more natural diet there should be no irritating or toxic ingredients to upset the balance. In most cases the biggest problems are soft stool and gas, due to the fact that you probably are over-feeding the new diet, especially one that is nutrient dense with no fillers.

One cup of a grocery store food is full of filler, often 70% or more! A better brand of grocery type foods or even pet shop or prescription diets can be just as bad, or may have less filler but other types of by-products which may alter the volume of nutrients available in that one cup. When switching to a higher quality food, there can be less filler involved. Therefore, feeding the same quantities (cup for cup) would result in over-feeding of the better brand and gastric upset. Your best bet is to carefully read and follow the manufacturer's specific recommendations for the food you are now feeding and then watch your pets carefully for the first few weeks to see how they react.

Over-feeding often occurs when people begin home cooking for their pets. I have worked with four basic home-cooked recipes over the years which I have found to be a great foundation for all diet needs and life stages after six months of age. I have several suggestions on healthy ingredients to create variety as pets can become bored with their food flavors. The suggestions are given in order of best choices first (ie. barley is better for dogs than brown rice) that should be fed more frequently. Meals should be served slightly warmed and never microwave your pet's food, as it reduces food's nutritional value. Mixing a little hot water into the cold food will warm it up and provide additional fluids for your pet's consumption.

I have included vegetarian menus although I do not recommended that you feed a dog or cat a vegetarian diet often or long-term. They require meat in their diet. Do not use it for weight-loss; the body needs meat for protein to maintain muscle while encouraging the loss of fat. It is appropriate for semi-fasting (meat elimination for one day), crisis feeding, blood sugar management and allergy identification/elimination only!

These daily recommendations are for an average twenty-five pound dog or ten pound cat with (choices) of ingredients:

Basic Meat, Grain and Vegetable Meal for Dogs

Yields approximately 2 ⅔ cups

Ingredients:　1 ¾ cups cooked grains (barley, millet, oats, brown rice, please, no white rice!)
⅓ cup lean, slightly cooked meat (beef, lamb, rabbit,

turkey, chicken)
½ cup cooked beans (lentils, kidney, black, pinto, lima)
¼ cup raw, grated carrots and beets which are great
detoxifiers (no potatoes)
2 teaspoons oil (sesame seed, canola, safflower,
sunflower—no olive oil)
1 or 2 tablespoons fresh raw, minced garlic (no onions!)

Directions: Cook meat in oil. After mixing all the cooked grains, meat
and beans together, add the remaining ingredients. Mix well.

Vegetarian Meal for Dogs

Yields approximately 3 ⅓ cups

Ingredients: 2 cups cooked grains (see list above, add amaranth for
exceptional protein source)
4 ounces firm Tofu (drained, crumbled and seared in oil)
2 teaspoons of oil (see above list)
1 medium fertile egg
½ cup fresh raw vegetables (as listed above)
1 or 2 tablespoons fresh raw, minced garlic (no onions!)

Directions: Scramble together the seared tofu and egg in oil along with
any seasonings (no salt) or natural flavors (try powdered
vegetable broth). Add to cooked grains and other
ingredients. Mix well.

Basic Meat, Grain and Vegetable Meal for Cats

Yields approximately 1 cup

Ingredients: ⅓ cup cooked grains (barley, millet, oats, brown rice,
please, no white rice!)
¼ cup lean, slightly cooked meat (lamb, turkey, chicken,
salmon, tuna, beef)
2 medium fertile eggs
1 tablespoon minced raw sprouts or grated carrots and beets
2 teaspoons oil (virgin olive oil, sesame seed, canola)
½ teaspoon fresh raw, minced garlic

Directions: Scramble eggs and meat in oil, add to cooked grains and then
the remaining ingredients. Mix well.

NOTE: *For long-term use, add a powdered taurine supplement,
using one-eighth the recommended human dose. Taurine is*

an essential amino acid which is found in meat but is lowered through cooking. Lamb contains the highest concentration of taurine, enough to sustain a cat without supplementing. This diet is suitable for ferrets, with the addition of double the meat and oil. Be sure to provide dry kibble, fresh vegetables and fruit as treats.

Vegetarian Meal for Cats

Yields approximately 1 cup

Ingredients: ⅓ cup cooked grains (see list above, add amaranth for exceptional protein source)
½ cup creamed small curd cottage cheese
2 teaspoon of oil (see above list)
1 medium fertile egg
1 tablespoon minced fresh raw vegetables (as listed above)
½ or 1 teaspoon fresh raw, minced garlic (no onions!)

Directions: Scramble the egg in 2 teaspoons of oil. Do not add seasonings. Add to cooked grains then other ingredients and the cottage cheese last. Mix well.

NOTE: *If absolutely needed for long-term use, add a powdered taurine supplement, using one-forth the recommended human dose.*

By serving clean, wholesome foods you should have no problem making the switch to a more natural diet for your pets other than the possibility of over-feeding. Switching your pet's food is a big step towards providing optimum fuel for daily prevention, as well as reversal, of dis-ease.

Proper Feeding Guidelines

How you feed your companion is as important as what you feed—in preventing dis-ease. Dogs and cats fed only one meal per day often develop weight or digestive problems. The one meal puts too much stress on the digestive tract—rather than half the amount, twice per day—which would allow the body to more thoroughly digest and assimilate the food. For overweight, sick or senior animals, smaller, frequent meals fuel the metabolism which helps digestion and assimilation and promote proper weight maintenance.

FEEDING INSTRUCTIONS

DOGS

I do not recommend free style feeding, where your dog has unlimited access to food. Not only can they overeat, you will be less likely to notice as soon, if feeding behavior changes. Check weekly that your dog is assimilating well and sustains weight. This is done by checking stools and feeling for the ribs. A good weight is when you can feel the ribs but can't see them.

Feed puppies:	4 meals per day from weaning to four months or free-feed
Growing Puppies:	Feed 3 meals per day until nine months of age
Adult dogs:	Should be fed twice per day after nine months of age
Senior/Sick dogs:	3 meals per day, or more as required
Over/under weight dogs:	Feed according to *desired* weight, give in two to four smaller meals. The more frequent the meals, the faster a dog's metabolism will balance itself.

CATS
these recommendations apply to ferrets as well

I do recommend free style feeding where your cat has unlimited access to food. Many cats prefer to feed at their leisure. But beware, they can overeat, and you will be less likely to notice as soon, if feeding behavior changes. So, only put out a day's worth at a time. Check weekly that your cat is assimilating well and sustains normal weight. Some practitioners warn against free-feeding stating that cats will be tempted to overeat each time they pass their dish or at least produce digestive enzymes in response to "smelling" the food, which could lead to digestive upsets. I have never found this to be true as most cats do not walk by their feeding dish unless they are ready to eat—unless the dish is central to all activities!

Feed kitttens:	4 meals per day from weaning to three months or free-feed
Growing kittens:	Feed 3 meals per day until six months of age or free-feed
Adult cats:	Should be fed twice per day or free-feed

Senior/Sick cats	3 meals per day, or more as required
Over/under weight cats:	Feed according to *desired* weight, give in two to four smaller meals. The more frequent the meals, the faster a cats' metabolism will balance itself.

Choose Your Pet's Feeding and Water Dishes Carefully

Use ceramic, glass or stainless steel feeding dishes and water bowls. They are less likely to develop bacteria or viral infections since they don't scratch like plastic. Aluminum dishes can actually give a pet aluminum poisoning, as they ingest tiny slivers off the bowl, chewed off during eating or scraped off during mixing the meal with a utensil.

Remember to provide plenty of fresh, filtered water—never tap which is chlorinated and may contain contaminants. Be sure that it is kept cool and can not be tipped. Do not allow an outside water bucket to fill with debris. Beware of buckets becoming iced over in your barn or stalls. This will prohibit the horse or farm animal from drinking long into the day, enough to dehydrate them, even in cooler conditions. Dehydration can easily happen, even in winter!

Store Your Pet's Food Properly for Retaining Optimum Nutrient Value

Use the original barrier package the food was sold in to maintain freshness, which maintains nutrient viability. This bag can be resealed by folding down the flap and clipping it shut, it can then also be placed inside another container for storage. Barrier packaging is also a great deterrent to ants and mice when properly resealed. If needed, for foods in paper or plastic-lined bags, use only ceramic, glass or stainless steel storage containers—they are less likely to react with the kibble and promote rancidity. Placing kibble directly inside a plastic tub, even food-grade plastic, encourages oxygenation and the loss of nutrients. Some plastic trash cans will leach chemicals into the food that were used in plastic manufacturing, such as formaldehyde and PCB's. Using an aluminum can will expose your pet to aluminum toxicity and is the quickest way to destroy your pet's diet. Your pet's food's freshness is as important as its quality of ingredients.

DETOXIFICATION encourages improved nutrient utilization

The goal of Step One is to clean up your pet's diet and promote detoxification to kick off a successful preventative or rehabilitative program. This improves your animal's immune system's ability to keep itself well and ward off premature aging and dis-ease by being able to utilize nutrition properly.

It can not be emphasized enough that one of the first steps to take—towards establishing a successful Holistic Animal Care LifeStyle™ program—is proper detoxification. Detoxification prepares the body to better digest and assimilate the vital nutrients necessary to help stimulate healing and strengthening. Regardless of what types of wonderful new products you feed your pet, if they cannot properly utilize a product's nutritive or therapeutic properties, then the end results will be disappointing. In fact, without proper detoxification, you are severely limiting the body's overall curative potential.

Once the initial detoxification process has occurred and better nutrient utilization is realized, usually within the first six to eight weeks, general condition reversal has often occurred. **It is not uncommon in over fifty percent of cases presented to see that detoxification and dietary changes of Step One alone quickly reversed general symptoms.**

Eighty percent of pets, including those with deeper, hard to reverse conditions, will continue to improve with the addition of nutritional supplements described in Step Two. An additional fifteen percent discussed in Step Three, will need homeopathic and herbal remedies to help trigger and support the pet's ability to heal or manage symptoms. Five percent of chronically ill animals will also need medication, but the detoxification, nutritional and herbal products, plus symptom support recommendations behind the LifeStyle™ will minimize side effects and improve results.

There are two safe and effective ways to gently trigger, or induce, the body's eliminatory systems—including the kidneys, liver, lungs, skin and lymph system—to process waste removal on a deeper level than is required for daily maintenance. By utilizing one or both of these methods, you will be giving your animal a jump-start on not only preventing symptoms, but reversing and possibly completely eliminating dis-ease.

Induced Detoxification Method One: Fasting

Fasting is the method most people have associated with the process of detoxification in natural healing. Fasting is much more than simply withholding food. It is the process of fasting which works at gently cleansing and rebalancing the body. Breaking the fast properly is as important as the fasting period itself.

Begin by imposing a short twenty-four hour period of fasting to promote detoxification of the digestive system and rebalancing of the eliminatory organs and blood cells. Many people associate fasting with starving their dog or cat; this couldn't be further from the truth. Fasting can save your dog or cat's life! Horses, ferrets and birds are another thing: I do not recommend fasting as their metabolisms require daily calories to maintain their metabolic needs. In fact, it is a serious thing when a bird or horse stops eating.

Fasting benefits the dog or cat exceptionally well by encouraging the body to detoxify and re-balance. The fasting methods we will explore are very safe and gentle. The pleading, begging look their pet might give them at dinner time seems to bother people the most. Twenty five percent of that look may be hunger-related, but the other seventy five percent is definitely control-related. Pets, particularly begging dogs, are masters at controlling their masters.

To avoid the pleading look during fasting, do something fun with your pet, at their usual dinner time. Bring home a new toy (but not out of guilt!) or take your friend out for a fifteen minute walk. These activities will serve dual purposes. Not only will they occupy you and your pet's thoughts but will provide much-needed exercise. If you still feel guilty, just remind yourself that they are *begging for their life,* and I do not mean that is because they are starving to death!

Always check with your veterinarian first before starting a fasting program. Be sure that there are no <u>medical</u> reasons that she or he may feel it is not wise to fast your pet at this time. Possibly you are also treating your pet for diabetes and must maintain their blood sugar with food as well as insulin, or your veterinarian feels that your pet is too weak in general to fast due to a recent bout of minor infections (which actually is the perfect time to fast). Although I have successfully fasted many animals in exactly these circumstances, it is always wise to rely on a trusted medical opinion, especially if you have a veterinarian who understands and supports your goals of providing your pet with a holistic LifeStyle™. For more information on approaching your veterinarian about supporting you in working more holistically, see the chapter titled **HOW TO BE YOUR VET'S BEST FRIEND.**

Fasting Is So Important

Anyone who has tried to clean with a dirty sponge can relate to the fact that a dirty sponge will not absorb any more impurities, leaving the counter just as dirty. Changing to a naturopathic program with a colon and blood stream full of debris will only negate the benefits of the supplements and herbs which won't be as easily absorbed and will have to fight all this immune suppressing waste. A short fast, especially combined with homeopathic support, can make a world of difference. See "Induced Detoxification Method Two: HOMEOPATHIC REMEDIES" for more information.

Inducing detoxification through fasting is a vital part of Step One: old fecal material is expelled from the colon while vital eliminatory organs, such as the kidneys and liver, and blood cells in general, are given a break from processing daily waste, thus allowing for a deeper processing of backed-up toxins. This results in an improved digestive and eliminatory system, necessary for the intake of both nutrients and therapeutic substances (as found in herbs), which will help strengthen the immune system and build resistance to injurious agents. The reduction of toxins in the body also improves the overall condition of the pet, often enough to reverse most symptoms on its own. It is common, following a short fast that the more obvious symptoms immediately begin to improve.

There are two ways to fast for induced detoxification which I highly recommend and perfected over time making the process simpler. The biggest difference between the two is the condition which your animal is in prior to starting the curative process. The standard fast can be used with all pets while the modified fast works best with pets with special needs such as maintaining blood sugar levels or when warding off further starvation.

Standard Fasting Protocol

The standard method is for pets with acute or chronic symptoms—that are otherwise in good health—and can pretty much adhere to a straight fast. Age makes no difference, as I have seen fasting successfully return balance to a struggling one week-old puppy or a fourteen year-old dog. The standard fasting process is pretty straightforward; assuming that your pet is fairly healthy to begin with—you may have to adjust the process according to your individual pet's needs. This can include using carrot or apple juice, diluted one-to-one with purified water, to help maintain blood sugar and stamina for very young, ill or weakened animals. Use one ounce dilution per ten pounds of pet, every four hours.

Day One

- Feed breakfast as you normally would on the morning you are to begin the fast. Simply eliminate the evening meal altogether.

- Use Azmira®'s homeopathic **D'Toxifier** if you wish to combine this with the fast for superior results.

- Be sure to provide plenty of fresh drinking water and non-acidic fruit juices.

- Provide fun-filled activity in fresh air and sunshine twice during the day of fasting, followed by a damp terry cloth rub down.

- Be sure not to overtire or stress-out your pet. Allow them to sleep undisturbed as they will sleep more during detoxification to preserve energy for the process.

Day Two

- The following morning (after twenty-four hours of fasting) you'll feed half the normal quantity of breakfast. To make this process really special, break the fast with **cooked oatmeal** (excellent at absorbing impurities in the digestive tract) instead of the regular diet, at 1/8 cup cooked oatmeal per ten pounds. A teaspoon or two of **raw honey**, encapsulated Garlic Daily Aid (raw garlic is too harsh) and some type of anti-inflammatory such as Yucca Intensive, both from Azmira®, can be very soothing and cleansing to the digestive system after fasting. A little milk or tuna water can be added for flavor.

- Again provide exercise in the fresh air and sunshine, twice during the day of breaking the fast, followed by a damp terry cloth rub down.

- Remember plenty of pure spring or filtered water, needed to flush out wastes. Add a few tablespoons of juice to four ounces of water, which will encourage drinking, and give an ounce per ten pounds of body weight four times that day to be sure pet has consumed adequate fluids.

- Be sure not to overtire or stress out your pet. This will rob energy from the curative process and slow intestinal cleansing.

- For dinner, simply return to the normal quantity (and hopefully, better quality) of food. If the animal has a particularly sensitive stomach then feed a second meal of oatmeal, increasing it to suit the pet's appetite. Canned food can be combined with oatmeal as well.

Supplements should also be introduced or added back into the diet at this time. To help maintain general health and well-being this is a good fasting protocol for weekly use. I have regularly fasted my own dogs on Mondays and they have come to look forward to that time. There is never any begging, and they don't even come to the kitchen Monday evening—knowing they won't be eating but rather, they always seem to find time for a game of chase just then. I do not fast my cats except in the early spring (for yearly deworming and detoxification), unless they are sick or choose to themselves. Since cats have a higher metabolism, daily calories are always needed.

Modified Fasting Protocol

- For pets with special needs, cutting back 25% to 50% of their standard meal—with the addition of Azmira®'s daily foundation nutritional supplements, herbal extracts (with detoxifying properties) such as Immuno Stim'R and Skin & Liv-A-Plex, and non-acidic vegetable and fruit juices (apple juice is best)—will also serve to stimulate a deeper elimination, without upsetting their metabolism. Use Azmira®'s homeopathic **D'Toxifier** if you wish to combine this with the modified fast for superior results.

- Break this fast with oatmeal, as you would the standard fast.

You will quickly find what suits you and your own animal's needs regarding a standard or modified fast and the regularity of a weekly or seasonal fast. Remember that exercise is very important at all times. This is especially true during cleansing, to help move toxins out of the body by stimulating the eliminatory organs further and oxygenating the blood. The terry cloth rub down helps to stimulate the skin (the largest eliminatory organ) and to aid it while it continues to process waste from the body's detoxification.

If an odor is present on a dog's skin during fasting, simply add a quarter cup of baking soda to one gallon of warm, purified water and rinse off the body with this solution only, followed with towel drying. You can wipe down a cat with this solution and towel dry for similar results. The baking soda will help neutralize these odors and balance the skin's pH, reducing itching. Avoid using tap water as it contains chlorine, which will be absorbed back into the skin… very counterproductive to a successful detoxification and a known skin irritant that will increase itching! If tap water is the only available water, then boil it for fifteen minutes to help "burn off" the chlorine. Be sure to let it cool down before using.

For severe cases especially when infection is present; adding a whole, cut up lemon boiled in the above water for twenty minutes (then strained), turns the baking soda rinse into a powerful deodorizer and a wonderfully healing skin tonic which acts as a disinfectant.

Helpful Supplements for Acute Detoxification Needs and Preventative Use

Top detoxifying herbs, vegetables and fruits gentle enough to use during and after a fast

*these herbs are found in Azmira®'s Daily Boost

- **Apples and apple juice** provides needed energy while supporting detoxification.

- **Beets,** especially the raw juice, provides several supportive nutrients and a naturally sweet flavor. This is different than the beet-pulp filler used in pet food as the sugars are not concentrated, nor the fiber compromised of nutrients from processing.

- **Burdock Root** helps remove catabolic waste from cellular activity.

- **Carrots** are trace mineral-rich, high in vitamins, alkalize the body and provide excellent juice for maintaining the fast and flavorful fiber when breaking a fast.

- **Celery** is trace mineral rich, high in vitamins, alkalizing for the body and flavorful to pets. While breaking a fast this makes a great snack for your dog.

- **Dandelion*** is an effective blood purifier and general organ cleanser.

- **Garlic** is a high-powered antibacterial, anti-viral, anti-fungal, and anti-parasitic herb, available in Azmira®'s Garlic Daily Aid.

- **Ginger** after the fast can help the digestive system, reduce gas, and aids hypertension.

- **Kombu** is a sea vegetable which alkalizes the body and purifies the blood of fats. A soup can be made by keeping 1 cup water at a low boil and cooking one leaf for ten minutes then turning off the stove and allowing the leaf to cool in the water before removing. Give as you would other juices or can be used in oatmeal mixture.

- **Milk Thistle*** is good for liver cleansing and detoxification support.

- **Papaya juice** during the break rebalances and aids digestion and helps flush wastes. Dried papaya is also another treat source that is both flavorful and healthy but used sparingly as it is very sugary and plaque producing on the teeth.

- **Parsley** is trace mineral rich, oxygenating to the blood, helps detoxify odors. Some pets love to eat this as they would grass. A few sprigs are okay during the fast. Some cats and dogs like parsley as a treat.

- **Parsnips** are a wonderful support when detoxifying the kidneys.

- **Spirulina's** high chlorophyll content aids enzyme production and digestion. Powder can be added to the oatmeal for exceptional continued detoxification.

- **Spinach** is an excellent source of nutrients and trace minerals.

- **Sprouts** of all kinds are beneficial to the daily detoxification process.

- Azmira®'s Yucca Intensive is a natural anti-inflammatory that supports circulation and liver and kidney detoxification while reducing discomfort from irritated intestinal tracts.

Avoid harsh or highly acidic vegetables like tomatoes and onions (which can be deadly to dogs), or difficult-to-digest ingredients like cabbage which produces gas. Also avoid the use of harsh fibers such as psyllium, which when used as a sole means of fiber can further irritate and damage sensitive intestinal tissues, at times, leading to blood in the stool. Although a good ingredient for producing bulk and encouraging elimination—the negative side effects of psyllium outweigh the benefits—during detoxification. To help produce healthy stools Azmira® has NaturFiber, a combination of fruits and vegetable fibers along with psyllium, which is great to introduce while breaking the fast. It produces bulk, moves more "stored" waste out of the colon and has Chinese mushrooms for restoring intestinal health.

Induced Detoxification Method Two:
HOMEOPATHIC REMEDIES

To further encourage complete elimination, regardless of which fasting protocol you choose, it is best to combine fasting with homeopathic detoxification. In the event that you are not comfortable with fasting, or that your pet cannot be fasted for medical reasons, homeopathic detoxification works just as well by itself and is very safe in all cases, with all animals. The one drawback is that homeopathic detoxification can take almost twice as long to achieve the end result when used alone, as when combined with fasting. The best detoxification protocol, when initiating a LifeStyle™ change, is to apply homeopathic remedies during the fasting period. For other instances of general detoxification during the LifeStyle™ process, apply as needed with or without fasting.

Arsenicum or **Nux Vomica**—often the first remedies of choice of homeopaths in establishing equilibrium of biological functions and to counteract many chronic effects—do such in terms of stimulating and balancing the overall body during detoxification. They help to counter nausea, irritability, digestive disturbances and portal congestion sometimes associated with the curative process, and in my opinion one should always be included, regardless of what other remedies are chosen. The best homeopathic combinations for detoxification on the market today include one of these. I have even reversed many acute toxic reactions (including pesticide poisonings) with the use of **Arsenicum** alone and used **Nux Vomica** for digestive upsets of all types, especially those from poor diets. Azmira®'s homeopathic D'Toxifier includes *Arsenicum* and other remedies which can stimulate the curative process, detoxifying vital organs, improving nutrient assimilation, rebalancing glands and strengthening the body's ability to heal itself.

During the detoxification process it is best to work with the lower potencies, **X**'s to low **C**'s. Homeopathic detoxification should be used daily for no less than two weeks, preferably six to eight weeks. *This is during the cycle the body naturally follows when it replaces old, worn out and diseased cells with new, nutrient-fueled, healthy cells.* Give one daily dose at bedtime for most cases, or one dose upon rising and again at bedtime for more chronic cases. It is recommended you work within Nature's own nighttime cycle of rest, with elimination upon waking at the end of the cycle. At this time, first thing in the morning, a walk helps void the bowels and bladder during the final stage of elimination. This cycle encourages optimum detoxification. During the rest period the body

rallies its resources for the detoxification process, since this energy is not being demanded by other systems for healing.

After the initial detoxification process, a maintenance program can be initiated on a weekly basis. Maintenance means a single weekly dose at bedtime to help process current waste build-up, stimulate proper kidney and liver functions and support general good health. It does not mean that homeopathic detoxification should be used in lieu of proper feeding, supplementing and care, but definitely as a support to proper biological functions such as digestion and elimination. See Working with Homeopathic Remedies and **Chapter Ten: Symptoms A to Z** for symptom-specific solutions and remedy suggestions.

Auto-induced Detoxification Process

Detoxification Can Be Brought on by the Animal's Own Internal Abilities

There is another process of detoxification which is a natural biological mechanism and has the same results although it is auto-induced. Instead of the caregiver applying fasting or remedies—the body can stimulate its own curative abilities in the face of an injurious agent, for instance a chemical. When the body senses the presence of a toxic substance, diseased cell or an imbalance of metabolic waste it mounts a defense starting with detoxification. This natural mechanism promotes the destruction of old, worn out cells and the removal of waste through cellular respiration and elimination—often through the skin, digestive or urinary systems. This can create a so-called symptom, but it is actually only a condition of the detoxification process and quickly clears up on its own given that the body is well fueled. The body can then continue this self-initiated curative response; rebalancing and strengthening to eliminate the injurious agent and to reverse the symptom uninterrupted.

Helpful Hints to Aid General Detoxification and the Curative Process

- **Provide plenty of purified water,** as water is needed to facilitate the flushing of wastes being eliminated. Avoid using tap water containing chlorine and chemicals (which may be too harsh for the kidneys to handle) or distilled water which may facilitate too quick of a detoxification. Be sure that drinking water is always free of metals and mineral sediments.

- **Groom daily,** to help brush away toxins being eliminated through the skin. This also stimulates circulation, further aiding elimination and removal of old, dead skin to stimulate the growth of new, healthier coats. Wash away any ear infections with Azmira®'s herbal Rejuva Spray (follow instructions on the bottle). Wipe away penile or vaginal discharges to avoid developing infections and if needed, wash daily with a small amount of Azmira®'s Organic Shampoo. This includes infected sores or hot spots on the body which can then be sprayed with Rejuva Spray. Use Rejuva Spray and/or Azmira®'s homeopathic Rejuva Gel on impacted anal glands and tissue irritation. Don't forget to use the baking soda wash I described earlier for body odor.

- **Maintain a calm environment** to encourage rest needed to build resources for detoxification and rejuvenation (strengthening). For highly strung pets utilize Azmira®'s R&R Essence to minimize emotional stress and Calm & Relax to physically rest the body and promote sleep needed for healing.

- **Provide daily exercise in fresh air and sunshine** to encourage circulation and cellular respiration, which supports the removal of deeper toxins. This also improves your pet's attitude, which supports healing and is a wonderful way to maintain wellness and encourage the daily curative process when used as part of The Holistic Animal Care LifeStyle™.

- **Respect your pets quiet times and needs** even if they seem to be withdrawing a bit from the family. It is normal for pets going through detoxification to sleep more, refuse to eat a meal or two (continuing the fasting process on their own when needed), become irritable or nervous, and seek out warmer or cooler areas to hang out in depending on their needs. Do not force-feed during this time.

- **Avoid the use of all chemicals and drugs** (that are not absolutely necessary for sustaining life). They will severely interfere in the detoxification process and may even be more harmful to your pet during this time. As the curative process moves deeper into the constitution, the body may react even more than usual to these substances... possibly causing an adverse reaction!

- **Avoid giving a vaccine booster** within six weeks prior to, or after, this type of deeper detoxification. As with other chemicals, the body may have a harder time detoxifying shortly after a

vaccination, or may react even more than usual to it, following deeper cellular cleansing.

- **Address symptom aggravations gently** through the use of nutritional supplementation, homeopathy, flower essences or herbs. This will allow the cleansing process to continue while keeping the symptoms from becoming too uncomfortable for you or your pet to experience.

- **Keep track of your pets progress** to help you better understand the process they are actually going through. If you jot down a few notes each day, you will be less likely to scare yourself into thinking that it has been "days" since your animal last ate… when in fact it might have only been two meals.

On the one hand, if a discharge started three days ago and was clear but now has turned yellow, you will need to add natural antibiotics such as Garlic Daily Aid, Blood & Lymph D'Tox and/or Goldenseal Extract to fight off any possible infections that may have begun. Then you will want to keep track of how many days the discharge stays yellow, or how quickly it responded to the garlic, etc. so that you may seek out other support if needed. On the other hand, if you noted that a chronic discharge took two weeks to clear up, then returned in three weeks, but only took four days to clear up that time and did not return for two months the next time… then you begin to see a pattern which indicates you are on the right track with your protocol!

Each time the body experiences a curative response or healing crisis, *which has not been suppressed* but rather supported, it strengthens; chronic symptoms return (cycle) less frequently and less aggressively until eventually the symptoms are reversed and eliminated completely.

What to Expect during Detoxification and Rebalancing

Detoxification is the process of dumping waste; therefore, waste will present itself during the process and must be addressed. This includes, but is not limited to, the aggravation of the very symptoms you are possibly trying to address by starting this cleansing process. Other symptoms of detoxification can be diarrhea, flatulence, rashes and/ or pimples. Fever (indicating the body is destroying old, toxic cells), crystals and debris in the urine (the urinary system is cleansing) or slightly bloody stools (the digestive tract is eliminating old fecal material) can also occur in the more compromised animals.

This is a good sign! Commonly referred to as a **curative response,** this is a clear indicator that the body has indeed been stimulated into cleansing by whatever detoxification protocol you are following. When this occurs, the first impulse many people have is to run to the veterinarian to get a drug to suppress the resulting symptoms. This is the worst thing that can be done at this time.

In striving to reach your pet's curative potential, it is vital to the process that symptoms be supported rather than suppressed. More so than at any other time, suppression of these symptoms, even through the use of natural remedies rather than drugs, will only force the underlying imbalance even deeper. But the use of chemicals and medications— especially steroids and antibiotics at this point—will also severely burden the body and throw a huge wrench in the works! At the very least, people have prematurely terminated the cleansing process, unnecessarily fearing the return or worsening of their pet's symptoms.

Though symptoms may now have been suppressed, prematurely ending the cleansing process altogether only means that you and your pet will eventually have to go through the process again if you can ever hope for true healing. It is best to address the symptom as gently (naturally) as can be, while continuing the detoxification process. Many things can be done to help minimize the extent of symptom aggravation (curative response) your pet goes through, without suppressing the cleansing and strengthening process.

Please note that aggravations <u>do not</u> have to occur for the body to be properly detoxifying. It is more common for the process to happen relatively easily for most pets, regardless of their previous conditions!

On the one hand, pets who seemed to be in balance and healthy prior to detoxification can exhibit the worst symptoms... from an imbalance *years ago* that was suppressed *back then*. The bottom line is that you must be aware of your own pet's individual process and support that— regardless of any preconceived notions you may have regarding what the process *should be* like. Simply address the symptom(s) as you see them, continuing to process towards wellness. If warranted, detoxification can be suppressed by simply ending the remedies and the fasting period.

To help you gauge the severity of your pet's symptoms or condition before or during detoxification and when going through the curative process in general, I have described the difference between a curative response and a healing crisis, the latter possibly requiring veterinary intervention, so you can best choose which protocols to follow and when.

In addition, throughout **Chapter Ten: Symptoms A to Z,** I share additional homeopathic remedies I recommend for the nuances of specific symptoms, such as for diarrhea or pimples, to aid in that symptom's specific detoxification and reversal process. For instance, one cat may have mucous-based diarrhea whereas another has watery diarrhea. A variety of general symptoms can respond to the same remedy, such as *Arsenicum,* but the closer you can match the homeopathic stimulation needed by the individual animal, the quicker the results will be. Therefore, one or several individual remedies may be chosen based on your pet's specific needs, or symptom nuances. You may have so many weaknesses to contend with that you are not familiar with, that you may find one of the many combination products commercially available works just as well. This can be preferred as they address the changing symptom nuances as the curative response progresses, without your having to be on top of every little change daily. For instance, mucous-based diarrhea turning to a watery stage as the colon rebalances itself. The beauty of homeopathy is that if the body does not need a remedy it will simply ignore it. The remedy will not interfere with normal wellbeing.

Once detoxification is begun, if you are not already doing so, go for the best quality nutritional food products you can afford. Think of it as an insurance policy against poor health and future veterinary care expenses. Make sure the food has proven itself and read the label! Even with the best quality and balanced diet of commercial, home-cooked or raw meats, nutritional supplementation is necessary to provide many nutrients now missing from our food chain. For instance, some research indicates that fifty years ago spinach had up to 80% more nutritional value than today! This is true (in varying degrees) for other vegetables, grains and fruits... as well as meats from animals fed "off the land." This is because our earth has been stripped of many of the naturally occurring micronutrients found in soil, which were taken up into the plant living off of it. Years of over-farming, using toxic chemicals or fertilizers and environmental pollution (such as acid rain), has taken its toll.

Even organic farming methods cannot guarantee that the produce will be more nutritious, as it may take approximately fifty years to completely return these nutrients back into the ground through organic fertilizing practices! Therefore, it is important that we supplement our animals' (and our own) diets to assure that we are all receiving the fundamental nutrients required. Even pet foods which are "nutritionally complete" according to AAFCO aren't complete according to what is truly needed for basic good health. For instance, they allow X amount of protein per cup of food, but that protein does not have to be *digestible;* therefore, it cannot be assimilated as protein! The same holds true for certain sources of vitamin A or calcium, just to name a few!

Therefore, proper nutrition not only includes quality, easy to digest foods such as award-winning Azmira® Nutritional Products, but the appropriate supplementation to support optimum wellness, as well as stimulating your pet's curative potential, when needed, for symptom reversal.

CHAPTER FIVE

STEP TWO:
THE FUEL TO HEAL

Regardless of how good the diet which you are feeding is, I recommend supplementing with a well-balanced vitamin and mineral supplement, additional vitamin C adjusted as needed, and a daily dose of garlic extract (for nutritional sulfur to aid in tissue repair plus its tremendous antiparasitic, antiseptic and anticancer benefits are great for preventative health care). Consider these concentrated nutrients as the "fuel" used by the body to run on. Whereas the detoxification process is similar to draining the crank case to eliminate oil sludge, proper nutrition's aim is to provide clean oil to run the engine well. It takes specific fuel to get the body from point A to point B. The use of these additional nutrients makes it easier to target and reverse certain weaknesses or symptoms, something no single pet food could ever provide to meet each pet's needs.

Seek Out a High Quality, High Potency Daily Multiple

A daily "multiple" such as Azmira®'s Mega Pet Daily has several advantages over choosing six or eight individual nutrients. Primarily, it is cheaper to use a multiple. A complete and well-rounded supplement will also provide all the nutrients required for the proper utilization of its other nutrients—for instance, zinc combined with vitamin A. Without zinc, vitamin A has limited absorbability. More clients than I can remember fed a vitamin A supplement on their holistic vet's recommendation, which did not provide a source of zinc! Besides, the stress of feeding a dozen pills per meal, especially if the pet won't eat supplements in their food but needs to be pilled, versus one or two at a time, can create more harm than the nutrients can combat.

Understanding The Importance of Individual Nutrients

VITAMINS

Vitamins are the *spark plugs of life,* providing fundamental activity on a cellular level, often as co-enzymes to regulate metabolic processes. They are necessary for growth, vitality, resistance to disease, responding to allergens and toxins, and for healthy aging in general. The feline or canine body cannot synthesize the majority of vitamins; they must be assimilated through the diet. Unfortunately due to depleted soil systems and chemical-based farming, food today is too vitamin-poor to sustain proper levels of nutrients; therefore, nutrients must be supplemented to assure optimum health.

Vitamins are categorized as *fat* or *water*-soluble, describing the method by which the body dissolves the vitamin and transfers it through the intestinal wall. Dietary fatty acids and bile, produced by the gall bladder, are important for the absorption of fat-soluble vitamins, while water-soluble vitamins simply require water and are more rapidly absorbed.

Several factors can interfere with this process, including organ dysfunction. A lack of fatty acids in the diet, or liver impairment, will trigger a deficiency in vitamins A, D, E, and K, which must first be dissolved in fats before slowly being assimilated. Vitamins A and E, in particular, are easily stored as fat soluble vitamins in general, which may become too abundant in the blood and trigger nutritional imbalance.

Water-soluble vitamins B-complex and C are quickly assimilated and excreted, rapidly cycling throughout the blood and tissues, rendering them safe, even in higher dosages. Because they are synergistically vital to so many biochemical processes, the absence of one vitamin will often disrupt an entire metabolic process. These vitamins are also more fragile when exposed to air than fat-soluble ones, and improper manufacturing or storage may lead to lowered efficacy. This is why I developed Azmira®'s Mega Pet Daily; to provide a daily dose of powdered vitamins and minerals balanced for the average wellness protocol and stored in a capsule. Caplets and chewable tablets have a manufacturing process which compromises the stability of the nutrients, rendering them less potent. Opened powders in a jar lose their potency faster than any other form and are easy to over or under dose. A capsule provides two easy methods of delivery: as a direct pilling or opened and mixed into meals.

Vitamin Deficiency Disorders

Because of the synergistic nature in which the body utilizes vitamins, and the vital role they play in primary biochemical processes, depletion of a single vitamin can create an imbalance. Reduced levels of vitamins A and C may affect liver function, compromise tissue integrity (skin, organs, muscles, tendons and ligaments), restrict antibody formation and limit white blood cell function—rendering the body susceptible to infection and cancer. B-complex deficiencies can lead to fatigue, anxiety, aggression, seizures, and muscular weakness, as well as a host of other chronic symptoms.

Symptom Origin	*Potential Vitamin Deficiency*
Nervous System	B1, B3, B6, B12, Folic Acid and E
Immune System	A, B6, B12, E, B1, B2, B3, C and K
Skin & Tissue	A, K, B2, B3, B6, Biotin, E, and C
Bones & Joints	A, C, D and E
Blood (anemia)	E, B2, B12, Biotin and Folic Acid
Heart & Blood Vessels	E, B1, B3 and C
Intestines	B1, B3, B6, C and E
Eyes & Ears	A, D, K, B1, B2, B3, C and E

MINERALS

Minerals are *the building blocks of cellular activity.* They cannot be synthesized by the body and must be supplemented to assure proper assimilation of other nutrients. Minerals assure the body wide use of vitamins, enzymes, hormones, and other bio-chemicals needed for optimum health. They keep the body pH-balanced, promote proper digestion and assimilation and are vital to bone formation. Improper bio-availability of many minerals, particularly calcium and magnesium, can lead to storage—rather than utilization—resulting in calcification of joints and kidney tissues, including stones. As a matter of fact, I have supported the reversal of chronic kidney or bladder stones in thousands of pets with the introduction of a high potency, bio-available mineral supplement. Minerals regulate several biological processes such as osmosis (cellular fluid exchange), metabolic functions and detoxification, electrical activity in the nervous system and in the heart (govern regulated contractions). Minerals fuel the muscles and transport oxygen throughout the body for energy. Trace minerals, often lacking in pet products, are vital to healing in general.

Augmentation with a high quality mineral supplement is vital to the prevention or reversal of dis-ease. *Chelated* or *proteinated minerals,* those *attached* to an amino acid for superior transportation and assimilation, provide fundamental nutrients often lacking from dietary sources—as other forms can be difficult for the body to absorb. Today, there is much substantiating evidence of higher tissue saturation with protein-bound minerals versus simply inorganic sources.

Colloidal minerals are minute mineral particles which have been suspended in ionized water for rapid absorption. For many decades, colloidal silver has safely and effectively been widely used as an antiseptic and antiparasitic. Colloidal gold helps stimulate immune function. Colloidal processing of other, more commonly known minerals renders the same bio-effects more rapidly than their encapsulated cousins—but at a severely reduced potency—which may only be good in supporting the utilization of full molecule-based minerals. I do not recommend the use of colloidal or dietary minerals (food-based) as your sole or principle source.

According to **AAFCO** (American Association of Feed Control Officials), basic levels of the *essential* minerals needed daily to sustain a particular life stage must be included in all commercial pet food recipes. These levels are *fundamental*, and, in my opinion, not enough to maintain *optimum* health and vitality. You simply cannot get enough inorganic sources into the pet or afford to additionally supplement during the manufacturing of the food to reach these levels. Choose a food with chelated minerals—so that you have more bio-available nutrients with less toxicity—as a good foundation, and additionally supplement with a proper formulation of your pet's individual needs.

A word of caution: minerals are extremely hearty elements, which in striking contrast to vitamins, could more easily become toxic to the body, creating as much disorder as a mineral deficiency could. Many inorganic sources, most commonly used in pet products and diets, are very difficult to absorb but the body regulates it well (working harder than it should have to), avoiding overdose. Even with higher quality, more bio-available minerals, it would take an incredibly exaggerated daily ingestion of ingredients to reach severely toxic levels, but you should regulate their intake in any event. This is why a quality multiple vitamin and mineral supplement like **Mega Pet Daily** is important to eliminate the guess work in properly combining nutrients for optimum results.

When supplementing your pet for daily maintenance, preventive or rehabilitative reasons, it is important that you familiarize yourself with all the ingredients of all the products you are using! Many products, including treats, supplements and diets, contain phosphorous, calcium or magnesium (also listed as bone meal, oyster shells, ash, etc.), which in abundance could become toxic and throw the body out of balance.

Be sure that you are not *doubling up* on the same minerals. Not only is it unhealthy for your pet; it is a waste of money. Choose a good quality multiple supplement and only add to this if one particular nutrient is needed over the others for a therapeutic response. A prime example is when anemia results from a lack of iron, promoting a need to *temporarily* supplement the animal for a few weeks until reversal of symptoms and maintenance can be continued with a lowered dose. Iron can easily become toxic, so be sure that you properly monitor doses.

Once you understand this importance you will appreciate the ease of using the Azmira® Nutritional Supplements. There is no over-dosing if you follow the recommendations. Each individual nutritional supplement (ie. Azmira®'s **Super C 2000** or **B-Complex 50**) is formulated to augment the levels in **Mega Pet Daily,** to be used as needed for each individual's needs. Why should you feed 4,000 mg. of vitamin C when your dog only needs 2,000 mg.? Or vice versa?!

Mineral Deficiency

Symptom Origin	*Potential Mineral Deficiency*
Nervous System	Calcium, Potassium, Iron, Zinc, Sulphur, Molybdenum
Immune System	Zinc, Selenium, Chromium, Copper, Germanium, Iron
Skin & Tissues	Potassium, Sulphur, Copper, Iodine, Selenium
Bones & Joints	Calcium, Boron, Manganese, Phosphorous
Blood (anemia)	Iron, Copper, Zinc, Calcium, Potassium, Molybdenum
Heart & Blood Vessels	Chromium, Magnesium, Selenium, Cobalt, Calcium
Intestines	Iodine, Phosphorous, Selenium, Sulphur, Calcium
Eye & Ears	Iron, Zinc, Potassium, Sulphur, Selenium, Chromium

Food source supplements (from sea vegetation, oranges, carrots, etc.) are good nutrient sources for the general maintenance of healthy pets, but not potent enough to prevent or reverse significant dis-ease in a genetically compromised or chronically ill animal. Many of today's breeds are so predisposed to arthritis, allergies, cancer, etc. that therapeutic levels should be used for maintenance of healthy pets as well. Be sure that you provide at least minimum daily requirements of vital nutrients, in case, for whatever reason, your pet might not assimilate their food completely. It is additional insurance. I recommend these nutrients daily, based on a 50 lb. dog. Double this dose to cover a large breed dog and horses, for whom a little goes a long way. For small dogs, ferrets or cats, simply use half this amount. For birds, use just a sprinkle on their seed. These are the nutrients found in one capsule of Azmira®'s **Mega Pet Daily:**

- **Vitamin A** for a strong immune system, eyes, tissue repairs **5,000 mg.**
- **Beta Carotene** supports vitamin A assimilation **2,500 mg.**
- **Vitamin B1** for energy and emotional well-being **50 mg.**
- **Vitamin B2** necessary for fat and carbohydrate metabolism **50 mg.**
- **Vitamin B6** for red blood cell production, protein metabolism **50 mg.**
- **Vitamin B12** aids in calcium absorption; anti-inflammatory **50 mcg.**
- **Niacin** promotes healthy skin and nerves; supports digestion **50 mg.**
- **Pantothenic Acid** is an anti-oxidant vital to adrenal activity **50 mg.**
- **Folic Acid** is necessary for DNA; enzyme efficiency and blood **200 mcg.**
- **Choline** is a vital neurotransmitter; works with Inositol to emulsify fats **50 mg.**
- **Inositol** lowers fatty deposits on the liver; controls cholesterol **50 mg.**
- **PABA** protects skin from sun-related cancer; supports coat color **50 mg.**
- **Biotin** aids metabolism of fatty acids, amino acids; makes antibodies **50 mcg.**

- **Vitamin C**—minimum required amount to help utilize other nutrients **125 mg.**
- **Calcium** is needed for strong bones and teeth; reduces muscular stress **25 mg.**
- **Phosphorous** supports structure, oxygen to the brain, maintains pH **10 mg.**
- **Magnesium** is critical for bones, nerve and muscle function **3.5 mg.**
- **Potassium** supports electrolyte and pH balance; neurotransmitter **5 mg.**
- **Iron** combines with copper and proteins to form red blood cells **9 mg.**
- **Manganese** nourishes the brain, nerves; supports SOD / antioxidant **3 mg.**
- **Zinc** is a co-enzyme of SOD—protects against free radicals / cancer **8 mg.**
- **Iodine** is vital to proper thyroid function and proper metabolism **75 mcg.**
- **Copper** is for inflammatory response, bone mineralization, coat color **125 mcg.**
- **Glutamic Acid** supports nerve health; metabolizes fats and sugars **12 mg.**
- **Selenium & Chromium** each, are immune-stimulating minerals **12 mcg.**

The Super C 2000 Connection

I cannot say enough in support of good old vitamin C. If you stranded me on an island and offered the choice of one supplement, I would ask for Azmira®'s Super C 2000 without any hesitation. What a miracle nutrient! I am a firm believer in therapeutic doses and personally take 4000 mg. to 8000 mg. a day. Only garlic and honey can come close to being as well rounded and beneficial.

Vitamin C, or ascorbic acid, is one of nature's most powerful vitamins. As an anti-oxidant it protects food, vitamins and body tissue from disorder caused by free radicals, pollution and poisons. This essential co-enzyme produces cellular and tissue membranes, steroidal hormones, collagen, and pigment cells. It supports adrenal function and iron absorption. Ascorbic acid helps repair and strengthen collagen (skin, ligaments and tendons) and provides additional antioxidant properties to protect sensitive organs and membranes, in particular, against allergens, as well as viral, bacterial and yeast infections. At the same time it reduces cellular damage due to carcinogenic substances which may trigger cancer.

As a water-soluble vitamin, it is readily excreted by the body and must be replenished regularly. Small amounts may be stored in the adrenal glands, and animals, unlike humans, can actually synthesize their own vitamin C, although it is in insignificant daily amounts (approximately 45 mg. to 65 mg. per day), requiring additional sources. Citrus fruit digestion is difficult for most pets, so nutritional supplementation is optimal.

Maintenance is easily accomplished, and therapeutic levels can be obtained by dosing to bowel tolerance—until the point of loose stool, then backing down 250 mg. (cats and small dogs) or 500 mg. (medium to large dogs) at a time until stool is again normal. Some animals, cats in particular, may experience some other types of digestive upsets. The use of a buffered vitamin C is beneficial and well tolerated. I have found that a *calcium bicarbonate* buffer works very well in a majority of pets, and may actually be similar to what pets naturally produce on their own, making the body more receptive to the ascorbic acid. Another fine product, Ester-C®, was created by chelation (attached C to amino acids for quick absorption) and can be better tolerated and up to four times more bio-available than ascorbic acid or citrus-based vitamin C sources alone. We found however that Azmira®'s Super C 2000, fed in two divided daily doses, also increases the absorption rate but at a significant savings.

Bioflavonoids (vitamin C complex) are necessary to promote proper vitamin C function. Bioflavonoids, including *hesperidin* and *rutin,* prevent problems with the cardiovascular system, primarily reversing hardening of the arteries and weak capillary or vein strength. Most importantly, they help fight cataract formation, a serious eyesight problem in pets today. These nutrients are provided through Mega Pet Daily. This is a good example of how the Lifestyle™ foundation supplements work synergistically.

Recommended Daily Vitamin C Dose: Cats, ferrets & small dogs— 500 to 1000 mg.; Dogs—2000 to 6000 mg.: Horses—2000 mg. to 6000 mg. *Natural Food Sources:* Citrus fruits (which are difficult for most pets to digest), parsley, green peppers, Brussels sprouts and broccoli (also difficult to digest which is why supplementation is necessary).

Additional synergistic nutrients: B-complex vitamins, particularly B6, B12, Folic Acid, and Pantothenic Acid; Vitamin K; *C protects vitamin A and E s*upports testosterone production and the regulation of other hormones, especially adrenalin.

Demands for increased vitamin C blood levels: Physically or emotionally toxic lifestyle and environment; allergies, arthritis and other chronic disorders, including paralysis, epilepsy and cancer, exposure to environmental pollutants, chemicals, vaccinations and drug therapy; body and tissue growth, repair and strengthening; dietary animal protein metabolism.

Depletion of blood levels: Aspirin, prednisone, bute, excessive steroidal hormones, diuretics, antibiotics, anticoagulants, and antidepressant or anticonvulsant drugs used to treat seizure and behavioral disorders.

Deficiency: Degenerative weakness in intercellular tissues, rendering the body susceptible to infection and deterioration (premature aging); cellular mutation, leads to cancerous tissues; edema (tissue swelling, bruising and hemorrhaging indicates capillary weakness), chronic skin, bone or joint conditions, eye and ear weakness or discharge; heart conditions, dental problems, including gingivitis and rotting teeth, are also associated with vitamin C deficiency.

Overdose: None; although vitamin C will create digestive upsets or loose stool when tissue saturation is reached.

Rounding Out The Holistic Animal Care LifeStyle™ Nutritional Foundation

Azmira®'s Garlic Daily Aid provides the compound allicin through a broad-spectrum food loaded with therapeutic benefits, especially in its purest state, raw extract. Its antiparasitic, antibacterial, antiviral, anti-carcinogenic, antifungal and antiseptic properties are well documented. Garlic has been a staple in holistic health protocols for centuries. It promotes digestion and assimilation, and stimulates circulation, nutrient utilization and cellular elimination. Naturally occurring thiamine (vitamin B1) promotes natural pest control by repelling external pests such as flies, fleas, and ticks.

Recommended Daily Dose: Cats & small dogs—500 to 1000 mg.; Dogs—2000 to 4000 mg. : Horses—2000 to 4000 mg. This is the equivalent of consuming up to 40 cloves of fresh garlic per day! Your pet cannot stomach eating this much raw garlic, which is why I developed Garlic Daily Aid. Each small gel cap contains 1000 mg. of high quality garlic extract.

Demands for increased allicin levels: Physically or emotionally toxic environment with chronic symptoms, including allergies, arthritis, premature aging and, especially, cancerous growths; parasitic infestation; yeast, fungal, bacterial or viral infections; exposure to environmental irritants; skin tags, warts, fatty tumors and "growths." Most health issues can be more easily prevented *and reversed* through daily allicin supplementation, which supports the production of antibodies, tissue regeneration, blood oxygenation and cellular detoxification.

Depletion of blood levels: Prednisone, vaccinations, diuretics, antibiotics, anticoagulants, insulin, chemical worming, pesticides, infestation or infection.

Deficiency: General degenerative weakness with premature aging and immune dysfunction; cellular mutation from toxic build-up leads to cancerous tissues; chronic digestive weakness (IBS, liver or intestinal issues) with poor assimilation; skin conditions, joint inflammation, chronic infections or infestations, bad breath, lethargy, low birth weight, high blood pressure and cholesterol levels are also associated with allicin deficiency.

Overdose: None that I can find; some concern exists that garlic has the same compounds as onions and therefore are as deadly to dogs as onions. This is a fallacy, as garlic is different enough from onions to have been used successfully for centuries in herbal veterinary medicine with dogs, cats, ferrets, horses and other farm animals. I have fed and supplemented with garlic for over twenty-five years and will continue to do so despite the hysteria recently unleashed on the public. I have seen too many of these propaganda campaigns to know that the proof is in the outcome. Garlic has made quite a difference in the lives of animals I have documented and the thousands that have used Azmira®'s **Garlic Daily Aid**. Certainly, over eating garlic will create terrible stomach aches and gas with a bad case of foul smelling diarrhea (from extreme intestinal detoxification!). I am advocating reasonable, proven doses.

A Strong Recommendation

As I have described, **Mega Pet Daily, Super C 2000** and **Garlic Daily Aid** are what I refer to as my *foundation supplements*. These are, in my opinion based on twenty-plus years of experience, the most important nutrients you can provide daily for optimum health. However, in the past few years I have added another product to my daily supplement routine for all my animals at home—dogs, cats, horses and donkeys—with great success.

Azmira®'s **Daily Boost** is a formulation of adaptogenic *herbs*, those well suited for daily wellness. These herbs promote optimum digestibility and liver and gall bladder function while reducing colon irritation and flatulence. They are a blood tonic and blood sugar stabilizer. They also provide detoxification and antifungal properties which build resistance to allergens and dis-ease. Only a sprinkle a day of this product helps the body utilize the foundation supplements to their fullest potential. The expense is minimal—but the returns are priceless.

WATER

I also mention water here with the foundation supplements I recommend, as water is the most essential nutrient for living and fueling healing. Solid food can be withheld for days and sometimes weeks at a time, but *dehydration* (lack of moisture in the body) will quickly shut down mucous membranes lining the digestive tract, prohibiting fundamental nutrient or energy supplies to the bloodstream, vital organs and biological processes.

Demands: Physical stress, fever, weather changes, medications, vaccinations, diarrhea, liver or kidney damage, diabetes and hormonal imbalance can easily trigger dehydration. Water is necessary for proper digestive function; it encourages movement of chewed food into the digestive tract, provides a *carrier* for digestive enzymes and nutrient assimilation through osmosis, and supports detoxification and elimination. Adequate water must be present in order to form and properly evacuate all fecal material and urine. The use of chemical preservatives leads to those small hard stools the pet food companies try to spin as meaning more food is absorbed when wasted bulk is not present. Consider instead that the lack of moisture in the intestinal tract (the side effect of reducing moisture in the food for packaging stabilization) creates toxic build-up (producing fewer stools) and decreases nutrient assimilation.

All Bio-Chemical Functions Are First Fueled By Water

- digestive enzyme production
- cellular and energy metabolism
- hormone production
- fertility (organs and material)
- tissue repairs (a major factor in healthy bone, muscles, ligaments, heart, lungs, skin, tear ducts, glands & organs)
- proper brain function
- a sense of well-being

Deficiency: When you squeeze, with your thumb and forefinger, the skin on the back of a ferrets or cat's neck, the muzzle of a dog or the neck of a horse, and the skin requires more than two seconds to snap back, then dehydration is evident. *Edema* is the opposite of dehydration—where storage of moisture in the body can be the result of trauma to the body or biochemical dysfunction (the body is not utilizing water properly)—resulting in a puffy, tight or dimpled appearance to the skin and an imbalance in the elimination of toxins. Water intake is required to flush the edema from the injured tissues. *Dropsy* (the pot-bellied look), or *gout* (a protein metabolism dysfunction which results in joints suffering from urea toxicity), can occur when fluid is seeping from the digestive tract, the liver or kidneys, collecting at the belly and feet which are the lowest points in the body. Again, water is needed to flush the damaged tissues.

Recommended Daily Dose: Fresh, cool, purified drinking water should be made available in *unlimited* quantities. Drinking bowl should be stainless steel, ceramic or glass for easy cleaning. Aluminum dishes leach toxins into the food and water while plastic can become covered in microscopic cuts and dings from teeth, resulting in bacteria growth—regardless of cleaning solutions used. Always clean and rinse out the bowl daily, prior to refilling it. Never use a harsh cleaner or bleaches, which not only are detrimental to health but might smell bad or alter the water's taste and discourage your pet from drinking. Water should be kept out of the sun to avoid heating it beyond a comfortable drinking temperature, and all water containers should be made impossible to tip over. Keep outdoor water bowls free of algae, giardia or bird droppings, which could make your pet sick or unwilling to drink from that bowl.

Although water consumption may vary from day to day, and season to season, it is important that you keep an eye on your pet drinking from the water dish. Be sure that they are not changing their normal pattern or experiencing any difficulties which could lead to dehydration. Changes in water consumption can often be the first sign of dis-ease in a pet. Speak to your veterinarian if you suspect that there has been a *decrease* (possible immune reaction, toxicity, etc.) or *increase* (possible fever, diabetes, kidney disease, etc.) in your pet's drinking behavior. On the average, most pets will drink fairly consistently when pure, clean drinking water is available. During crisis, force feed up to one ounce per pound of body weight per day as the more fluids you can get into your animal the better. This also accounts for spillage during oral hydration (force feeding the water).

Average fluid intake

Cats & Small Dogs—minimum 3 to 4 ounces per 10 lbs. of body weight per day.

Medium to Large Dogs—minimum 2 to 3 ounces per 10 lbs. of body weight.

Horses—minimum 5 to 7gallons per day.

Birds—as I know from my own, can consume a lot between their intake needs per day and bathing in it! But, I could not find anything to confirm an actual amount.

Guidelines for Feeding Supplements to Finicky Pets

Dogs & Cats

- Mix supplements well into Azmira® canned food.

- Add warm water, gravy or broth to dry Azmira® nutrition, mix well.

- Add canned food to dry kibble with or without warm water or broth.

- Make "gravy" or a mix-in from a raw egg, yogurt, cottage cheese, apple sauce, baby food, ground cooked turkey, chicken, hamburger. Mix supplements in well *then* mix this into kibble and/or canned food. You can also make a treat out of it.

- Use salt-free chicken or beef broth. Rehydrated Azmira® treats such as **Liver Slivers, Kidney Bits** or **Beef Patties** also make a tasty broth. Cover in hot water for fifteen minutes then add supplements.

- Consider using tuna can water / sardine oil for finicky cats.

- Mix powders with 1/8th tsp. honey, make a ball and place on back of tongue.

- Use a feeding syringe (with oral attachment) to give liquids. Mixed into apple, peach or grape juice. Avoid acidic juices. Vegetable juices such as carrot and parsnip also work well. Use 1/2th tsp. of juice for small pets up to 1 tbsp. for big dogs.

- Use plain bread, or with peanut butter or cream cheese.

- Place drops of herbal extracts on treats or inside open cookies.

- Place liquids or powders in an empty 00 gelatin capsule.

- Hide capsule in cream cheese, hot dog, or peanut butter.

- Wrap capsule in cheese, liverwurst or natural deli meats.

- Sprinkle food with Flavor Shak'R, tuna flakes or treats.

Horses

- Make bran mash, adding liquid and powders with water.

- Roll powders in honey or peanut butter, place on back of tongue.

- Use feeding syringe (with oral attachment) and 1 oz. apple or carrot juice.

- Place extracts on treats or a handful of rolled oats.

Birds

- Use feeding syringe (with oral attachment) and drops (4:1) of apple juice.

- Sprinkle extracts and powders on treats or mix into seed.

- Make a **bird food mixture** of one hard boiled egg ground up with two inches of carrot and one cup or more of whole wheat toast crumbs or oat bran cereal. I use a small food processor and grind this up until I have a crumbly mixture. Add 1/2 Mega Pet Daily and 1/8th teaspoon of Super C 2000 for maintenance, double for illness. You can add a quarter more of these supplements for large parrots. Do not process the egg too much or it will form a paste which is hard to work with. This mixture should be frozen with a bit taken out each day. It defrosts quickly and liquid supplements can be added prior to feeding. Give one teaspoon daily for finches, etc up to two tablespoons for large parrots. They love it in addition to their seed!

CHAPTER SIX

STEP THREE:
SPECIFIC SYMPTOM REVERSAL

Although the basic curative process is the same for all living beings, each one of us has our own unique journey toward symptom reversal and wellness. All symptoms have a history unique to our own experiences. A youthful body can handle a multitude of stresses and maintain some balance, until one day the body gives out, which is why you often see three or four year-old pets *suddenly* show symptoms and develop "conditions." Unfortunately, as the body grows older and becomes more burdened, when its biological processes begin to slow down naturally, it becomes overwhelmed by its past and present environment, diet and medical history (especially vaccinations). Prevention is the best cure, but even in the event that the first third of a pet's life was spent in the worst conditions, or a current injury or infection has slowed a previously well-kept and healthy pet, my three simple steps can help you turn things around.

Having quickly established a good foundation with **Step One's** detoxification and nutritional recommendations, the body is now more receptive to assimilating nutrients and utilizing them for wellness. Providing foundation supplementation through a daily multiple vitamin/ mineral, therapeutic levels of vitamin C and garlic extract promotes this wellness and fuels the body so it can draw strength for the curative process described in **Step Two**. Your animal should be well on its way to reversing its poor health and general symptoms; it is now time to address the specific subtleties *or nuances* within the condition of your individual pet by adding to the basic protocol of detoxification, optimum nutrition and daily foundation supplementation.

Each symptom you still observe, *or which becomes more apparent,* during **Step Three** is now clearly defining the underlying weakness creating it and is providing you with a road map or markers to reverse this condition.

EXAMPLE: A Common Arthritic Protocol

During **Step One**—an arthritic animal should be more comfortable (less inflamed) following homeopathic detoxification, especially with Arsenicum. This remedy is directly noted for both detoxification and joint inflammation, as found with arthritis, since toxins trigger inflammation and inflammation triggers joint pain.

Following **Step Two**—when the LifeStyle™ foundation supplements should provide noticeable relief from stiffness and pain within a few weeks—eighty percent of pets in our clinical studies responded favorably to these two steps alone.

Applying **Step Three**—in an additional fifteen percent of animals whose inflammation was more severe or who suffered numerous other weaknesses, additional herbal and nutritional supplementation or homeopathic care was needed. They did show general improvements initially (ie. less stiffness, improved stamina, appetite, coat condition and attitude) but still suffered some from stiffness and painful bouts, indicating specific weakness to be addressed in **Step Three**. In these cases the addition of Azmira®'s Yucca Intensive *to reduce pain and inflammation,* Joint E'Zer *to grow healthy ligaments and lubricate joints allowing for improved mobility* and an increase in Super C 2000 *to reduce waste that can irritate joints and to help strengthen ligaments to support joint function,* resulted in noticeable *and specific* improvements. Now imagine if this animal also had a digestive/eliminatory problem or organ condition which interfered with the body's ability to detoxify itself— Azmira®'s ImmunoStim'R could then be added to increase the elimination of these toxins which feed inflammation and cause pain. Now you have, in just a few weeks, taken the systematic steps towards addressing your pet's individual needs instead of symptom chasing and shotgun therapies. Once the pet responds, as can be expected, the Yucca Intensive can be stopped and then used only as needed, and the ImmunoStim'R and Joint E'zer reduced.

Each step may happen quickly and, in conjunction, feeding off each other's own curative response or healing crisis. In fact, all three steps can be taken at the same time; the point is that *all* three steps are followed.

When you are faced with a pet in severe discomfort who has not been on the LifeStyle™, then it is appropriate to use all three steps together to address this animal's acute needs. Homeopathic detoxification can be started during the fasting period and continued for the next two weeks as you break the fast with Azmira® nutrition. The foundation supplements and herbs (to address the inflammation and discomfort) can also begin during the fast break.

The process of which remedies to apply and when during **Step Three**, will become evident as you follow the symptom's journey rather than seek to simply suppress it. To help clarify this and to better figure which symptoms need medical attention, it is best to clearly understand the difference between curative responses, such as during detoxification and strengthening, and a healing crisis.

Addressing Common Curative Responses and The Healing Crisis

The curative response and healing crisis is a natural part of the cleansing process and rebalancing an animal goes through during the strengthening of its body's organ systems. Sometimes, the body can get a little worse before it gets better, especially after the application of a remedy. Twenty years ago, we used the term "healing crisis" to describe the complete range of manifestations noted when the body's symptoms got worse after alternative modalities were used. Today I differentiate between more severe healing crises and milder curative responses. It is vital to the ongoing strengthening and healing process in the body to support these symptoms, *and what the body is trying to rebalance,* rather than suppressing them. *But what do you do when the symptoms are not easily minimized?*

How long do you wait until you change remedies? What diet should you feed as symptoms improve or get worse? When is it time to seek medical treatment and how long should it be continued? Is the chosen product and/or protocol failing the body or is the body failing to support the pet's healing?

Questions such as these are common among frustrated veterinarians and owners. They followed natural recommendations taught in seminars and videos, or featured in popular magazines or books, only to chase symptoms and eventually resort to shotgun applications of natural remedies, then drugs out of desperation. By developing Azmira® products I have eliminated the most common aspect which interferes with true healing—unreliability of the natural pet care product to perform as promised. Once you learn the difference between the healing crisis and curative response, as I use them, you will easily answer the rest of these questions as you rule out the product's failure and see instead, how the body is failing to respond. This is why I created the three simple steps to my Holistic Animal Care LifeStyle™. Based on identifying the difference between the processes of the curative response and healing crisis and knowing when to make a remedy change, my systematic approach helps you answer these questions quickly and improves the curative process by steering you in the right direction rather than in circles.

The difference between the Curative Response and a Healing Crisis is in the severity and duration of the symptoms' aggravations, as well as the animal's over-all response to specific protocols and products being used.

When the body is fighting to reverse an acute or chronic condition, and certain symptoms worsen—but the overall condition of the animal is improving (i.e. the skin rash is worse but appetite and energy levels have improved), I see this as a positive thing. It means the body is responding by healing itself. When this happens, it is defined as a *curative response*. A natural approach to continue encouraging detoxification and strengthening suits the pet at this time and warrants the continuation of the chosen products.

The *healing crisis* is differentiated by the fact that overall, symptoms progressively get worse even though there may be some good days (i.e. although a cancerous tumor has reduced in size and the exhausted animal has some better days—the animal is now withdrawing with a fever and the appetite is not returning causing the body to get even weaker). When this is the case, with non-life threatening symptoms such as moderate fever, natural remedy suppression is first attempted for twenty-four to forty-eight hours before veterinarian consultation and further clinical examination is needed.

A healing crisis can be reversed while it is still a curative response (i.e. the use of herbs and homeopathy to reduce the fever and stimulate the appetite) and this progression indicates the body is strengthening overall. The failure of easily reversing a curative response indicates the body is not utilizing its own healing abilities well, thus warranting the continued use of holistic support through more specific remedies. This will also improve the outcome of medical treatment when needed, instead of leaving the body more susceptible to drug side-effects and a further lack of nutrition since drugs cause the body to use up a lot of nutrients simply by the drug's metabolic activity. But if the body continues to decline (i.e. the fever gets higher despite your efforts) then this has become a healing crisis.

This is where knowledge and an understanding of your pet's condition will help you decide which step to take next. Remember, the more you know, the better you will be able to help your pets help themselves. In the symptom-specific chapter you can find a listing of symptoms and proven solutions to try first. In the event of a non-responsive healing crisis, it is imperative that proper veterinary clinical care be sought, but unfortunately many curative responses are treated like a healing crisis and the long-term benefits of symptom reversal are aborted. Your gut instincts are also important in making these judgments, respect them and you'll choose the best way to proceed.

Either way, the safest, most effective way to support all symptom aggravations is through the gentle naturopathic modalities of detoxification, nutritional supplements, homeopathy, flower essences and herbs. In my opinion, chemicals and drugs should only be relied on in life-threatening situations, and only after detoxification, diet changes, my recommended foundation supplements—Mega Pet Daily, Super C 2000 and Garlic Daily Aid—plus additionally needed remedies have been tried first. Please, do not forget the power of love, play, contact, and spending time nurturing your pet (even if only to respect their need to sleep more and be quiet) in helping minimize any stress they may be experiencing during the curative process.

Possible Curative Response Experiences

- **A curative response, such as an acute rash, is quickly improved with homeopathic stimulation and lasts no more than six to twelve hours.** *This is true whether the reaction is the result of a topical or internal allergic reaction. For instance, rashes can be the response of histamine, released when needed to protect the body from the allergen's contact zone. The body is in clear need of quick suppression of the histamine reaction, which can weaken the pet and damage the skin, while stimulating the area which was exposed to allergens to bring in nutrients and healthy cells for repair. As you will read in* **Chapter Ten: Symptoms A to Z,** *the remedy Apis works wonders for these reactions.*

- **Symptoms, such as pimples during detoxification periods or allergy season, last less than a month while the pet noticeably responds quickly to applied herbal and/or homeopathic**

remedies. *Each day the pimples improve, although some symptoms may flare up, needing to be addressed with the additional short-term support of herbs and homeopathy.*

- **Symptoms worsen for a few days, within three to six weeks after beginning the LifeStyle™ protocol, but quickly reverse on their own, or with a short-term remedy.** *Often, after detoxification and the addition of Azmira® diets, foundation supplements and general remedies have begun; the body feels strong enough with enough fuel to take on deep cleansing and reversal of specific weaknesses during the strengthening process. Rapid-onset (acute) symptoms such as fever, irritability and digestive upsets are also commonly seen curative responses, often indicating the body is in a deeper detoxification phase. Curative responses at this time are very normal, although they do not have to be present for the body to be healing.*

- **Symptoms appear or worsen within minutes of receiving a homeopathic remedy and quickly reverse on their own.** *This is a great response, a curative response, often indicating that the chosen remedy was right on target.*

- **The pet maintains energy during a curative response and throughout the healing process.** *Regardless of how severe the symptom may temporarily be, the pet's quality of life and ability to maintain general wellness is a vital indicator that the healing process is proceeding well.*

- **The body shows continued improvement over all,** *strengthening each day, although there may still be some difficult days.*

EXAMPLE: The Curative Response

In the arthritic pet we are using for example, who has followed the protocol as described, it is not uncommon for a curative response to happen within six weeks of beginning these steps, especially following detoxification. Since the body has strengthened, and now has fuel for curative processes, it will take on deeper cleansing to promote the healing of chronic immune weaknesses and organ imbalances that are influencing the arthritic condition. This is what **Step Three** is all about.

It is not uncommon to see a flair-up of chronic symptoms during a curative response and/or the elimination of waste from the body, either through the urine, stool and/or skin. This will create acute symptoms such as diarrhea, or crystals in the urine, even blood and bacteria. Since we know the diarrhea can be a common sign that the body is responding and healing itself, we can "support" the symptom rather than "suppress" it, by using homeopathy, herbs or even oatmeal. This way the body reverses the severity and duration of the episode within its own curative timeline rather than a forced, premature ending. This way the process the diarrhea has begun happens (cleansing the colon of an irritant such as old fecal material), rather than clogging up the intestines with a clay liquid or halting peristalsis with drugs, which leads to further dis-ease.

Each symptom has its *own three steps* to take regardless of how long you have used natural care and followed my LifeStyle™ recommendations. This doesn't change the overall protocol you have been using for the arthritis, but we can follow Step One and fast the pet for twenty-four hours, rather than resort to a constipating OTC (over the counter) drug. Assuming you are utilizing **Step Two's** recommendation and feeding the daily LifeStyle™ supplements, you quickly move on to **Step Three** and apply a homeopathic or herbal remedy. This is certainly not the time for antibiotics or switching the pet's food to a prescription kidney diet if crystals show up in the urine (another common curative response)!

What your pet is experiencing is a temporary condition of the systematic process of achieving wellness. Using suppression will only interfere with the body's attempt to heal itself through detoxification and weaken the pet's health further. Having to deal with the chemical treatment's toxic side-effects may damage the animal's immune system and lead to future conditions such as allergies, even cancer. **Step Three** is where you can fine tune your pet's protocol, if you do not get side-tracked by curative responses (symptom aggravations).

Experiencing a Healing Crisis

- **Severe, difficult to reverse symptom aggravations, are followed by frequent relapses.** *Especially when caring for a chronic condition, symptoms can return as soon as nutritional, homeopathic and/or herbal support has ceased.*

- **Your pet becomes exhausted, despondent and unresponsive to naturopathic care.** *During the healing process, when a pet's energy continues to struggle and cannot be stimulated, a curative response has become a healing crisis.*

- **Your pet's over-all condition continues to worsen.** *The breath or coat smells, eyes and nose discharges increase, fever returns* frequently, appetite falters, sleep or stool patterns change and general energy is depleted.

- **Your pet becomes despondent** regardless of the attention he or she receives.

EXAMPLE: The Healing Crisis

Again, using the arthritic pet as I have, let's explore what constitutes the healing crisis. What if you have applied the logical remedies and your pet still has diarrhea? Here is the beauty of my protocols combined with products that we know should work a certain way in a certain amount of time. If the immune response is not there (symptom support to slow the diarrhea) within a reasonable time (determined by individual remedies), then systematically seek the cause, such as excessive pain, bad food or a bacterial infection that has nothing to do with detoxification or arthritis. Apply additional **short-term** *suppressive* therapy such as herbal antibiotics first, or drugs if warranted, but continue to support the body's process with holistic care.

The history of disease and the applied curative process is determined by the age of the pet, how genetically compromised they are, the quality of their lifestyle, and the severity or duration of the symptoms. I have never seen an animal that was too old, too weak, too young, too sick or hopeless to respond to my Holistic Animal Care LifeStyle™ protocols and Azmira® products. Some respond better than others, but there is always a response. It is a matter of whether or not the process was supported or aborted that counts. More often than not, the process was not followed through.

Your Goal & Reward During Step Three

Unraveling each level of imbalance, to finally address deeper issues which created your pet's symptoms, is the goal and reward of **Step Three**. What is important during this process is providing the proven Azmira® products described since you can rely on these to function optimally so you can clearly understand what the body is responding to, or not. By feeding the correct supplements, herbs and homeopathic remedies, but only as signaled by the body's specific symptoms and conditions, you will quickly help your pet reach full symptom reversal and long-term wellness while saving time, effort and money.

By applying specific remedies in a systematic manner you will be able to decipher what is or is not working for your individual pet's needs. This will eliminate the waste of precious time that your pet may have regarding reversing a weakness which could quickly result in a life-threatening symptom. If the animal fails to respond in a timely manner, then the next approach can quickly be embarked upon instead of wasting time and your pet's energy going around in circles with shotgun approaches.

Is every case a complete one-hundred percent success? That depends on your definition of success and how far you addressed deeper weaknesses. We have clinically proven that each animal's symptoms, when addressed holistically, experienced some positive change. Even death can be seen as a final step in the healing process, the natural course for that individual animal to take, now made peaceful and comfortable through the holistic methods I describe to be used during **Step Three**. Obviously, the further along you follow the LifeStyle™ approach and utilize the appropriate remedies, the more you can help your animals help themselves. Once you are assured that you are on the best route to promote your pet's healing and are working with the right tools and protocol, you will quickly and easily take them through **Step Three** and on to complete symptom reversal.

CHAPTER SEVEN

PUTTING THE HOLISTIC ANIMAL CARE LIFESTYLE™ TO WORK

Knowing that specific symptom reversal and elimination happens in **Three Simple Steps** can give you the peace of mind to truly go after the condition or symptoms your pet is exhibiting. The secret is to work within the LifeStyle™ recommendations, and not deviate, so that you can experience the process for yourself.

I know this information may seem a bit repetitive but it is important to clearly understand how this process works and the consistent results I have gotten by following these steps, so that you can be sure that you are using the process to its potential.

Step One: it has been clinically studied and proven that *fifty percent* of pets do respond to the recommended detoxification and a change to Azmira®'s healthy, wholesome food, often within days. At the very least, the curative process has clearly begun, and markers as to the body's abilities to heal itself begin to show themselves as the overall condition improves.

Step Two: when given the additional nutritional foundation of *Mega Pet Daily, SuperC2000* and *Garlic Daily Aid,* a higher number of animals experience quicker results, with *eighty percent* of pets also achieving long-term symptom reversal. Fueling the body's natural abilities to reverse weakness and dis-ease provides a faster outcome than the application of individual remedies alone.

Step Three: addresses the *fifteen percent* that will still need additional naturopathic care (including exercise, acupuncture or acupressure, chiropractic, energy work and massage), plus specific homeopathic and/or herbal remedies, to complete the curative process begun in **Steps One** and

Two. Remember, this will effectively reverse symptoms by addressing the body's underlying weaknesses. By accomplishing these systematic steps, symptoms and weaknesses will be easier to decipher, allowing you to quickly apply the correct curative support required. Remember, all three steps can be taken initially at the same time in the more debilitated cases. Diet and supplementation, including a **Step Three** remedy, can begin following a twenty-four hour fast or at the same time during a two week homeopathic detoxification.

Unfortunately, if these steps are taken out of order or overlooked, **Step Three** is used without the benefits of the first two steps; the outcome will be less than optimal. For instance, using homeopathic remedies without the support of proper nutrition is a common mistake. Nutritional supplements are needed to fuel complete symptom *reversal* once a curative response is homeopathically stimulated. If not used together, then symptom *suppression* will be your result and relapse with symptom-chasing in the future. In addition, when proper nutrition is provided but detoxification is not encouraged, then overall results may be better, but still not provide optimal healing. At the very least, symptom support will be evident, but slow-coming and short-lived. Therefore, when needed, all three steps should be taken at once with remedies and supplements started at the same time as detoxification. As mentioned, I generally recommend two weeks of homeopathic detoxification when starting the new diet and supplements; additionally if there is a chronic symptom, it should also be addressed at that time. In addition, **Step One's** detoxification can be followed whenever a boost is needed regardless of how long the body has been at **Step Three.**

Five percent of pets will always need medical and chemical support, including drugs and surgeries. Unfortunately, long-term symptom suppression through medication (such as prednisone for life threatening, non-responsive immune dysfunctions) may be needed with acute suppression therapies. When a symptom becomes worse, this may be the most beneficial modality.

Many of these animals will still benefit from *short-term* chemical or drug support until the natural remedies they are receiving take over. Unfortunately, probably half of these animals were given chemicals or drugs because the body's attempts to rebalance during a curative response were misunderstood. Classic symptoms of detoxification were visible, but the owner or veterinarian arrested the process with medical treatment. Some of these owners later returned to symptom support successfully. Others remained in the cycle of symptom suppression for years before they allowed the curative process to be completed. Others simply give up on natural pet care.

Some suffering pets will always have illness or general poor health regardless of what is done. Symptoms can be suppressed holistically and/ or chemically for short-term relief, but as soon as treatment is stopped, the cycle begins anew. These pets are either too genetically compromised or too overwhelmed by their condition to ever successfully reverse their dis-ease on their own. Remember that the more holistic the LifeStyle™, the easier it will be to keep the pet's resistance to toxins high through **Steps One** and **Two** with their biological functions processing to their fullest potential—even if you choose to use medication as well. Each year your pets live a holistic LifeStyle™, their bodies will continue to strengthen, and many symptoms will become easier to handle, or even reverse themselves later on. Detoxification, nutrition and herbs also protect the liver, kidneys and other vital organs from common toxic drug side effects.

Importance of Using All Three Steps Together

Zaezar, my very much missed female Rottweiler, had a genetic predisposition to hip dysplasia and allergies. She was raised on the best natural diets and naturopathic care available at the time and had been healthy, but when my work became all consuming I became lax in her daily foundation supplement regime. Around twelve years old she developed general "aging" symptoms that we addressed with herbal and homeopathic remedies when needed. Overall she continued to look great for her age and was in shape, including having no grey or cataracts, so we didn't take her care as seriously as we should have. Suddenly her mobility was compromised and her allergies so intense at times that we were forced to limit her daily outdoor activity with us.

Zaezar's structural and immune weaknesses were then addressed through **Steps One, Two** and **Three** and within one month she needed fewer doses of her symptom-suppressing herbal anti-inflammatory and antihistamines—she was so much stronger! She again was enjoying wandering the property in comfort. Approximately six months later we decided to manufacture our own Azmira® diets so Zaezar was part of the test subjects on our first batch. It amazed us how much improvement we then saw. Whereas the remedies provided some resistance to her symptoms and reduced pain, the change in diet gave her additional benefits, tightening her "paunch" (without calorie restriction), noticeably improving her mobility and increasing her energy. We didn't realize how healthy *she could be* until we saw the comparison.

We knew we had a winner with this food as part of the LifeStyle™ approach when she began "guarding" the property against coyotes in the wash (she had so much more vim and vigor) and did so until a few months before she died shortly before her fifteenth birthday. Zaezar was in better shape her last two years then she had been the previous two! She is a prime example of the fact that even in older, genetically compromised pets, health can quickly improve adhering to The Holistic Animal Care LifeStyle™ three step process. Having symptoms supported overall by fueling the body, even when temporary suppression is needed, will in time effect some positive change. It may even turn back the signs of aging. Although Zaezar, due to her overall lifestyle had not grayed or developed cataracts, many caregivers have reported that their senior pets on the LifeStyle™ have reversed their own gray and cataracts, often within the first six months!

Getting the Results You Want

Common sense is the most valuable tool you possess for reversing symptoms. Ask yourself if what you are doing is getting you the results you want. If not, re-evaluate, but do continue addressing the problem.

Not doing* something is *NOT* an option. *Nothing comes from nothing.

On countless occasions, people exclaim, "I thought I'd just wait and see if it got any better on its own." They are shocked that the condition gets worse! By the time they get around to doing something, it may be too late, the body too weakened, or the dis-ease too deep, and it is so much harder to regain balance! The only time that it is appropriate to *do nothing* is during detoxification or a curative response, where the health of the animal may temporarily become worse as the body attempts to rebalance itself. To do something (to suppress) during this time only stops the process, and drives the imbalance deeper into the body creating a degenerative effect. This is why we stimulate and support the body's ability to *handle* symptoms such as inflammation rather than let it struggle on its own—to stop any degenerative effect while the overall condition can strengthen.

When It is Appropriate To Address Symptoms Through The Holistic Animal Care LifeStyle™

- Any *non-life-threatening* symptom or *curative response*: remedies are given to support the body in responding through its own immune system's ability to rebalance the body.

- Acute (sudden onset) symptoms from over-exertion or toxins are present: stiffness, digestive upset, discharges, irritations, pustules, irritability or emotional stress, including withdrawal (often the results of exhaustion due to pain or confusion).

- Acute flare-ups of chronic (long-term) symptoms occur, especially during detoxification.

- Known triggers are present, such as during high exertion days or high pollen counts. For instance, many of my symptom reversal suggestions can also be applied as a preventative, such as Azmira®'s *Yucca Intensive* to reduce potential inflammation and minimize the severity of possible symptoms.

- A curative response which has been ongoing for more than forty-eight hours requires that you support the body's attempts to complete it. Homeopathy is very helpful to *stimulate* healing at this stage, while the addition of nutritional and herbal supplementation will *support* the body by providing the fuel required to reach symptom reversal.

When it is Necessary to Address Symptoms through Veterinary Care

As you can learn in the symptom-specific section, there are many homeopathic and herbal remedies that can be used safely in a time of emergency. These will lessen the side-effects of physical and emotional trauma. These can be given on the way to the clinic, during overnight clinical stays or in conjunction with medical treatments given at home.

- Any broken bones, potential internal bleeding from an accident or life-threatening acute (sudden on-set) symptoms are to be addressed medically immediately. Nervous system or spinal injuries, especially paralysis, respiratory difficulties resulting in hyper-panting, an excessive heart rate, uncontrollable seizures and loss of consciousness are other common markers. Excessive dehydration and loss of potassium from repeated vomiting or diarrhea can lead to heart failure so be sure to seek professional care. Uncontrollable shaking, stumbling and disorientation are also acute symptoms which warrant a clinical visit with your veterinarian.

- A high fever present for more than twenty-four hours after applying holistic remedies indicates a deeper infection, warranting allopathic antibiotics.

- Chronic symptom aggravations (curative response) can become a healing crisis, lasting for more than twenty-four hours. This weakness can result in loss of mobility, uncontrollable digestive upsets, urinary dysfunction or other, severe symptoms which become unresponsive to holistic care.

- Unmanageable infectious states, *even if mild,* which have lasted for six weeks or have become chronic and cyclic despite proper holistic care.

- Whenever in doubt, do seek out a trusted professional to support your pet's process and diagnose the situation. Never diagnose and treat a pet's more serious condition on your own.

Be sure that you are first clear on how you want your pet to be treated and always provide information regarding the current diet, supplements and remedies you are feeding. This will allow others to best inform you regarding your individual pet's needs. Also, this will allow you to be able to listen to others' recommendations and determine for yourself, which one will suit your needs best.

On this note: please be wary of what you read on the Internet or in chat rooms. Does it really make sense that yucca is "akin to snake venom?" That a single supplement product can benefit all arthritic pets, regardless of individual needs and symptoms? Or that flax seeds will cure all conditions? They are a fantastic source of fatty acids, but nothing cures all. Think about the consequences of what you choose to believe and the *reality* of what you are told. Especially be wary when there is no data or long-term clinical experiences to back up the "fact."

Think carefully about the recommendation itself: should you really be force-feeding four ounces of vile, strong-flavored herbal immune stimulating tea to a cat who is suffering from cancer—*especially when you can get the same, if not superior, benefits with* Azmira®'s *standardized (reliable concentrations) herbal extract formula* ImmunoS tim'R? *At only four DROPS per day!* Think about the effect force-feeding four ounces of strong tea, almost a day's worth of fluid intake for a ten pound animal, has on the cat. It is different than giving water or diluted fruit juices orally, as is sometimes needed during illness. The taste is difficult to swallow, creating a struggle and strong emotions. The cat can foam at the mouth from the extract's bitter properties.

The stress alone can become very detrimental to the immune system and counteract any benefits. In addition, the cat has to now use its bio-energy (vitality) to assimilate all these compounds, draining itself rather than strengthening its immune response. This energy should be used instead in applying these compounds to fuel healing. When a standardized extract, like Azmira®'s, is given: one drop per five pounds of body weight is mixed with a little apple juice or water and is swallowed with little stress. Standardized alcohol-base extracts are easily assimilated and quickly penetrate the cellular surface to fuel the cell's repair and replacement. All the immune system's energy goes towards healing—as nature intended!—and is significantly less stressful.

Helpful Hints in Applying The Holistic Animal Care LifeStyle™

- *Feed high quality Azmira® diets and supplement with the foundation products at least twice per day*—use Mega Pet Daily, Super C 2000 and Garlic Daily Aid—to improve the body's ability to maintain optimum health. These supplements combined are beneficial to help stabilize blood sugar, fuel the immune system and improve symptom reversal. Wellness is harder to achieve without the proper fuel these vitamins and minerals provide.

- *Supplement with the proper nutrients and compounds, to additionally support specific issues, for your pet's individual needs;* products including glandulars and standardized herbs should be fed as needed, such as for poor digestion or reactive arthritis, as symptoms show themselves. These nutrients are also needed for immune stimulation to support the body's curative response.

  Through the **Three Steps** described in THE HOLISTIC ANIMAL CARE LIFESTYLE™ and following the simple systematical applications of these additional nutrients, your pet will quickly reach optimum wellness. Azmira® manufactures proven formulations I have used for years into herbal, homeopathic and nutritional supplements— now easily and quickly addressing specific symptom reversal for the individual pet's needs.

- *Utilize homeopathy to help stimulate* the body's curative potential, especially the processes of detoxification and specific symptom reversal. Homeopathy is also beneficial to use during a healing crisis to minimize symptoms and to help maximize the curative reaction, maintaining the healing process.

- *Utilize herbs __to help support__* the body's curative potential by providing additional fuel and physical compounds for the reversal of symptoms.

- *Use appropriate synergistic modalities for the condition or present symptoms;* chiropractic care and massage relieves structural problems; touch and energy therapies including giving acupressure therapy at home in between veterinary acupuncture sessions also helps stimulate the curative process. Home therapy will prolong all benefits received in a clinical visit and support daily wellness.

- *Address emotional stress as well as physical discomfort or pain.* Use R&R Essence, Fear and any other of the Azmira®'s Flower Remedies to improve disposition during the curative response or chronic symptoms. Calm & Relax is a proven herbal blend for reducing anxiety and physical pain.

- *Maintain The Holistic Animal Care LifeStyle™,* even in between curative responses or after long-term symptom reversal, to help enhance the body's defenses and further balance the body's weaknesses. Supplements and remedies may need to be adjusted or changed as the process proceeds. With each month the body will continue to gain balance and strength, including joint function, organ support and increased resistance to general sensitivities. Remember, symptom suppression—*even holistically* BUT without the needed ongoing support—only leads to a recurrence of symptoms, not a long-term reversal of dis-ease.

- *Provide a safe environment.* Be sure your pet's home and common yard are free of hazards. Cleaning agents, antifreeze, medications, fertilizers, critter poison, pest control products and other chemicals can potentially toxify the body over time or cause acute crisis, even death.

  Traveling with your pets, boarding with others, transitions through stressful times, and training or competition anxiety can be full of avoidable physical and behavioral hazards.

- *Minimize structural dysfunction* by removing obstacles to free mobility for puppies, kittens, foals, pregnant, older or prone pets. Symptoms are often triggered by a physical stress on the weakened body. This is common to pets who played hard during their early years and now struggle up and down furniture, stairs, and uneven terrain. If the floor is too slippery, causing your pet to go down twisting its legs, use some throw rugs with a rubber backing for better footing. Common injuries lead to chronic structural damage. If the bed or couch is too high, try a cloth-covered stool or carpet-covered box next to it for your pet to get on first. Don't take your pet on difficult hikes. Don't allow them to ride in the back of a pickup or anywhere their footing is unstable. Avoid allowing pets to become overweight, or forcing your older pets to struggle on their footing. This will relieve much of their discomfort and avoid chronic damage to the joints and ligaments resulting in limping and pain. A sound structural alignment supports the body's biological processes such as digestion and elimination. Use Azmira®'s Yucca Intensive to reduce structural inflammation and improve the curative response.

- ***Do not underestimate the power of Mother Nature;*** recognize that Naturopathy can take longer to suppress a symptom then a drug, but often will do the job more completely. Give a product the time to fuel and support healing.

- ***Support the curative power of Nature*** and avoid interfering with it. Use chemicals and medications carefully. Avoid vaccinations whenever possible. Give nature the time to work.

- **Provide the tools needed** by the body to function optimally and it will return to health itself.

- ***Use common sense.*** Address changes in your animal's health or behavior as soon as possible; pay attention to what your pet's symptoms are telling you. For example, if your dog's arthritic stiffness or allergy reaction increases the day after you play in the park with him, don't encourage his tugging on a toy for so long or continue using the same Frisbee routine, avoiding long periods exposing him to the grass triggering the symptoms. Identify such triggers and adjust your pet's LifeStyle™ to address them. Something as simple as keeping nails trimmed off the ground to relieve pressure on arthritic toes or therapeutically shoeing a horse can increase your animal's chances of structural recovery. Stimulating the immune system and using a steroid alternative will minimize, even eliminate, most allergies. Don't be frightened to try something; you can always go back to the old way if the protocol adjustment didn't hit the mark in due time.

- ***Don't sabotage the healing process*** by incorrectly utilizing diets, veterinarian-prescribed medications, or natural supplement products. Read the directions. Ask questions of experts and those around you with similar experiences.

THE MORE YOU KNOW AND UNDERSTAND, THE MORE SUCCESSFUL YOU WILL BE!

Remember, it can take three to six weeks for detoxification and increased assimilation of nutrients, the very fuel needed, to begin establishing the necessary foundation for a successful curative process. During this time old cells are being replaced with newer, healthier cells, which will bring change to the overall condition.

Therefore, it is best to allow the body some time to respond on its own before adding too many other ingredients to the mix. Provide Azmira® foundation supplements with basic herbal or homeopathic support, for the first month or two, until you better understand the specific underlying imbalance. Remember that close to eight out of ten pets successfully reverse their symptoms with this alone. Additional supplements or medications may overwhelm the body with ingredients it doesn't need and interfere with the body's natural curative process. Explore Azmira®'s products to see what they specifically can provide in your situation. Be sure to read ingredient labels carefully, and follow all instructions listed on the products which you choose to use.

Azmira Holistic Animal Care® provides a free help line, six days a week, to educate you regarding your pet's individual needs and the proper products to use. Phone them at 1-520-293-6639, 10_{AM} to 6_{PM} MST, to clarify any doubts you may have or to find the right approach. The more you know the more successful you will be. Azmira®'s professional support staff is available free to you—use them! In any event, if something doesn't seem right or your pet is obviously more distressed than during a common healing crisis then stop the protocol and seek an answer as to the cause.

But always bear in mind: each time the body experiences a curative response or healing crisis, *which has not been suppressed* but rather supported naturopathically, it strengthens. Symptoms return (cycle) less frequently and less aggressively until eventually the symptoms are reversed and eliminated completely.

CHAPTER EIGHT

USING HOMEOPATHIC AND HERBAL REMEDIES

Before applying remedies during **Step Three** to help stimulate (homeopathy) and support (herbology) curative responses, rebalancing and strengthening, it is helpful to understand what they are and how they are best applied for optimum success. Homeopathic and herbal remedies can be used together or separately, although I do not find with most symptoms that the use of a homeopathic remedy alone, without any nutritional or herbal support, is as effective as an herbal supplement is alone. They are best used in conjunction with one another. For instance, using homeopathic *Byronia* for a stiff, arthritic cat alone is not as effective in helping the cat's mobility as combining it with Azmira®'s herbal anti-inflammatory, Yucca Intensive. It's with the application of the herbal anti-inflammatory that the majority of the pain lessens and the mobility improves, whereas the homeopathic remedy will stimulate the body's own ability to reduce inflammation. This is accomplished by a process in which the body seeks substances available to it, such as vitamins, minerals and the saponins (therapeutic compounds) found in yucca, to "fuel" the process of reversing the inflammation.

Therefore, it is in the best interest of your total protocol success that you do not rely on only one modality of symptom reversal, rather work each symptom with a combination of nutrients, herbs and homeopathy. For instance, an acute ear infection is not an appropriate symptom to address homeopathically without the support of Azmira®'s Garlic Daily Aid and Yeast & Fungal D'Tox (both potent natural antibiotic herbs). Without herbal support there would be nothing *physical* (i.e. saponins) to fight off the infection. Homeopathic remedies can lessen the pain in the ear and encourage healing by fighting the infection but it is the herbs which kill off the organism.

This is why my three step LifeStyle™ approach works so well. You build the body's nutritional resources to fuel the curative process of detoxification, rebalancing, strengthening and maintaining while utilizing homeopathy to stimulate certain physical and/or emotional curative responses, flower remedies for emotional stability and utilizing herbs to support the complete process to its optimum outcome.

WORKING WITH A HOMEOPATHIC REMEDY

Homeopathy is safe to use in addition to herbs or medications, although drugs may interfere with a remedy's potential to stimulate a curative process. Do not give remedies within thirty minutes of feeding or giving strong medicinal herbs. This will protect the remedy's potency. Utilize homeopathy to its fullest potential by following these few simple suggestions. It is very helpful in reducing acute flare-ups, such as curative responses during detoxification or allergic reactions and during the process of rebalancing and maintaining.

Homeopathic remedies support symptom reversal on a deeper level than herbs or supplements alone. I recommend you use these remedies to stimulate the body's participation in its own healing process. The body will respond by utilizing support, or fuel, being provided by other supplements and herbs. This can often be the key to reversing a deeper acute or chronic weakness. Although a lot of emphasis is placed on potencies, I have found many to be successful in a wide range of potencies, so today I'm more inclined to support getting what is available to you regardless of whether it is a 6X and not a 30C. For the majority of acute reactions, even if due to chronic conditions, utilizing the lower potencies will affect change. These potencies range anywhere from 3X to 30C. For long-term reversal of a specific disorder, utilizing the higher 200C potency will be effective, once lower potencies have brought the acute reaction under control. High potencies, such as M's which create the deepest constitutional changes, should be used under professional guidance. By giving the body a boost with homeopathic remedies, other supplements act more quickly and effectively.

I recommend building up a homeopathic remedy's action in the body through frequent dosing. You cannot overdose your pet homeopathically; each repeated dose simply strengthens the involvement the remedy might have in regard to the ongoing process.

Acute symptoms of dis-eased or allergic-reactions can be successfully "suppressed" with a few doses of *homeopathy,* given five to fifteen minutes apart in lower potencies (3X to 30C). Sometimes this type of symptom suppression is necessary to reduce the acute stress experienced by the body until the foundation supplements and therapeutic herbs can fuel and support reversal of the symptom. This protocol will prevent a process of cellular deterioration from occurring; reversing any possible long-term damage and future health concerns.

Give one dose orally, according to the manufacturer's recommendations, every fifteen minutes for the first hour, then every hour until there is relief. To maintain relief, dose a minimum of twice daily for an additional week or two. More frequent dosing, every five minutes, can occur as needed and at any other time you feel that your pet might need a little extra boost detoxifying or reversing a symptom. Resume this or any other appropriate remedy whenever the symptom presents itself and follow this schedule until there is complete reversal. Long-term maintenance is also possible through a weekly dose of the most beneficial remedy. For instance, with a cat who suffers from an irritable bowel disorder, one dose of Phosphorous 30C given weekly will help maintain a stress-free bowel and lessen the reoccurrence of bloody diarrhea. A monthly dose can follow in six to eight weeks, until the symptom remains stable for three more months. Once your pet is symptom-free for six months it's a safe bet you have completely reversed the condition, given that you remained on the LifeStyle™ program.

I prefer liquid remedies because they are easier to give. If the dropper touches your hands or your pet, rinse it off before returning to the bottle. Most remedies come in sugar pellets (use as is applied to the inside of the lips) or tablets (crush inside a piece of paper first to pour into the mouth for best application). To avoid contamination and a reduction in efficacy, do not handle remedies with your bare hands. Rather, use the cap or a clean piece of paper to administer the dose and remember to always allow at least fifteen, preferably thirty, minutes apart from food or strong extracts when giving homeopathic remedies.

UNDERSTANDING HOW FLOWER REMEDIES HEAL EMOTIONAL DYNAMICS

Helping the body heal physically and emotionally can often be very frustrating, especially when certain tools known to work in most other cases, seem useless. One physician and botanist, Edward Bach, pondered years ago why this was. He often saw that a patient who seemed not as ill or weakened as another did not respond as well to standard treatment. *It was as if the patient lacked the will to improve.* Dr. Bach successfully identified several emotional and psychological traits which influenced the patient's emotional "filter" through which he viewed and reasoned his illness and various plants that helped to alleviate these filters. I modified this for use in animals over twenty years ago.

The use of flower remedies as a gentle, chemical-free method to provide natural emotional pet care is especially exciting. Unlike many humans, animals never, ever doubt the true power of something simply because they do not understand it or how it works. They simply respond to the highly successful support they are provided with, to alter their mental filters, so that the emotional healing needed to reverse their negative behaviors may occur. If one remedy chosen is not successful, at least it will do no harm, and you will know rather quickly what is or is not working by your pet's behavior.

Owners who choose to use flower remedies to help alleviate a pet's emotional stress, aid in rehabilitation or to be used in preventing behaviors or disease triggered by stressful situations, do appreciate the subtlety of these wonderfully healing remedies. The result is often remarkable, overnight in fact. Generally, slowly eliminating the behavior in question, over a period of a few days to a few weeks, is more the norm. Some pets, who have suffered over extended periods of time, may take six months to a year for total reversal. At times, for the very few, negative reactions are happening on such a deep level that reducing the behavior over time and then periodic dosing of remedies as needed for flair ups, may be the best you achieve. Many pets and families have coexisted like this and appreciate how much of an improvement it is over what they have experienced before, knowing also that they may be preventing far worse from developing.

Physical and emotional stress can also severely cripple the immune system and the body's ability to support itself. As I have stated before, it is not uncommon to have a pet with a history of emotional stress develop health problems. Pets respond to stress much as humans do, developing heart disease, kidney or liver dysfunction and cancer, I believe, primarily in response to stress. When this stress is reduced, the body often responds much more quickly to whatever modality is being used to reverse the disease in addition to the fact that training will become easier for the pet.

I have worked with flower remedies since 1983, in both humans and pets. Since 1996, Azmira®'s flower remedies have been clinically proven faster-acting than Bach® flower remedies and used successfully with the protocols described for the use of homeopathic remedies. This is because we homeopathically potentized each flower remedy to 30C (acute behavior) and 200C (chronic issues) and combine these potencies together in each product for a faster and more long-term healing response. Since you can never know exactly what came first, is this simply a reactive symptom or reflective of an underlying long-term behavioral condition? Your pet may fear riding in the car TODAY but that stems from a bad experience YEARS AGO. Address both issues. Bach® Flower Remedies are not homeopathically potentized therefore they are simply less effective.

Azmira®'s flower remedies are a very important tool in eliminating the emotional "filter" from which a pet "perceives" the actions around them. If a pet associates hands with pain from a previous beating (even years earlier by another owner) then it will automatically react negatively to your hands on or near its body. Given a remedy such as **R&R Essence** or **Fear**, this filter may begin to change and the pet will not react as strongly to hands the next time—providing a more positive learning experience. Each time this is repeated, the pet will continue to positively respond with this new behavior because the remedy has changed its reaction.

To successfully use flower remedies to reverse more specific emotional issues, first identify what personality trait or "filter" you associate more closely with your pet's problems and utilize one or more remedies to reverse this trait. By reversing the emotional issues that may be interfering in your pet's ability to learn (due to warped perceptions) and improve on positive behaviors, you will realize the benefits of your training program more quickly. Often, removing this trait by altering the pet's emotional filter can be enough to fully realize a difference in your pet's most difficult behavior.

WORKING WITH AN HERBAL REMEDY

Herbs are powerful agents of change when given correctly and in the right form. They come in many forms (liquid, powdered, etc.) and various potencies (tinctures vs. standardized extracts). Understanding which form of herb is best suited for which job will increase its availability to further the curative process. When I explain this in my seminars, especially to the veterinarians, I most often hear participants exclaim that they have finally realized why it was taking so long for some previously-used herbal products to work and why minimal results and secondary symptoms (such as nausea) were often the case.

I recommend very few dry herb remedies as they are the least potent. The pet has to ingest too large a quantity for any therapeutic support—

adding stress to the digestive system and often causing refusal to eat on the part of the patient. Dry herbs generally provide good adaptogenic doses, those used for daily maintenance. Many of Azmira®'s dry herb supplements have been treated with a standardized extract to improve their performance.

Liquid extracts come in various extraction levels. Tinctures are teas made by steeping the herb in water and represent the lowest potency available—I don't even bother recommending these as you can not guarantee consistent results. The volume of fluid (approximately four ounces per ten pounds of pet per day) needed to be consumed can also lead to gastric upsets, not to mention the stress of force-feeding it. Standardized extracts, the process of which brings out the highest concentration of therapeutic compounds, is the process Azmira® uses. It is this method which renders the best herbal remedies while standardizing the extract that <u>guarantees</u> reliable and repeatable results. Not all *extracts* are *standardized* due to the expense involved.

The alcohol used not only extracts the largest quantity of compounds available in the herb, it also provides a carrier for the compound into the cellular structure it is meant to support. The alcohol allows it to be easily assimilated into the blood stream through mucous membranes in the intestines and again through the wall of the cell to directly feed it (or kill it as in the case of antibiotic and antiparasitic remedies).

Glycerol-based remedies are now popular for those fearful of the alcohol (the amount of which in herbal extraction actually represents in a daily dose the equivalent of alcohol naturally found in one banana). But consider this: glycerin forms a protective barrier on tissue (including inside the digestive tract and cellular bodies). Have you ever used a glycerin-based hand cream in the winter? It repels water off your hands! Glycerol inside the body, when used as a carrier for an herbal compound, interferes with absorption into the blood stream and then into the cell's structure. Children, cats, alcoholics, weak puppies, old mares: I've exposed them all to alcohol-based extracts for over twenty years and I have never had a negative reaction to the alcohol in an herbal extract. Would you not feed them a banana?

The most important reason that I recommend and manufacture standardized herbal remedies is the fact that they are so easy to digest. The amount required of an Azmira® herbal remedy is generally one drop per five pounds of body weight per day. This is very easy on the digestive system and even easier to hide in the pet's diet. A few drops in a teaspoon of water, broth or diluted apple juice in between meals gives you the most bang for the buck. For finicky pets or those with very sensitive tummies, just add the drops to your daily menu or Azmira®'s canned food and mix in well. They rarely even notice it's there and if they do, they do not mind the taste. It can't get any easier than that.

To avoid having your animal develop a resistance to the beneficial herbal compounds being fed over an extended period of time; give herbal supplements for six weeks on and one week off. The only exceptions are animals who are severely debilitated by a symptom (i.e. cancer, inflammation or pain). For these cases, taking one day off from the remedy every couple of weeks will also encourage optimum results and benefits to continue.

Now that you understand The Holistic Animal Care LifeStyle™ three step approach and the use of flower remedies, herbs and homeopathy it is time to embark on addressing the specific needs of your companions.

CHAPTER NINE

Addressing a Specific Symptom or Condition

Do not allow yourself to become consumed by a diagnosis: The word "CANCER?!!!" for instance, can scare you into stupidity. Address the obvious weaknesses (symptoms) your pet is suffering such as a depressed immune system, inflammation, pain and anxiety. In this chapter are the most common symptoms associated with acute and chronic dis-ease. Your pet may be experiencing multiple symptoms or a slightly different version of the symptom than what I have described. Please try to match your pet's particular needs *as closely as possible* to the symptoms listed in the next chapter. Work from the most apparent symptom on. For instance most skin infections will respond to the recommended "infection" protocol, in addition to the standard "skin" support, such as topical applications and nutritional supplements. I have added many more nuances of various symptoms then I was able to in my previous books due to volume restrictions, so I think you will be better able to create a protocol which is specifically geared towards your own pets' individual needs.

What you will also come to recognize is the fact that many symptoms respond to the same remedies; for instance, the homeopathic remedy *Arsenicum* (to stimulate symptom reversal) with Azmira®'s herbal ImmunoStim'R (for therapeutic, physical support of that reversal). Their general benefits are detoxification which encourages improved nutrient utilization which fuels good health. As I have explained, the over-all weakness of the immune system, the digestive system, the urinary tract, the respiratory system, the nervous system, skeletal system and such is fundamentally caused by a toxic reaction (system overload) that interferes with nutrient utilization, including therapeutic compounds in herbal remedies. The body runs low on fuel, biological processes malfunction and dis-ease sets in. This can be from dietary, environmental and even emotional triggers which create a negative reaction (symptom) or a negative behavior (emotional stress, often resulting in an organ imbalance and physical symptom). Azmira®'s homeopathic D'Toxifier (containing Arsenicum) and herbal ImmunoStim'R could work for all these organ systems when they are in weakness and symptomatic. But there's so much more!

You will come to find that working the "symptom" is even easier when you break it down to its most common denominator. Remember to look beyond the diagnosis: address and support *how* the body is reacting, *and to what.* Feline Leukemia—this is a viral condition—use Azmira®'s herbal Viral D'Tox. Support detoxification for two weeks with homeopathic D'Toxifier *and see some improvement, but* is the immune system still *severely* dysfunctional? Add ImmunoStim'R and increase vitamin C. It's as simple as that.

Each body will develop and move through various markers within its own dis-ease.

You will see a multitude of suggestions listed for each symptom or condition-specific subject in the next chapter. **I am not recommending you use all of the listed remedies at once, but rather see which ones most accurately fit your animal's condition.** In some cases, you may start off with one remedy and switch to or add another, days or weeks later, as the symptoms progress towards reversal. Some pets may require two remedies at the same time for two different symptoms. This is why the LifeStyle™ approach quickly *and permanently* reverses the cause of dis-ease when so many other methods give temporary suppression at best, conflicting symptoms at worst. You are addressing what really needs to be reversed. Most other products are too broad. The animal must deal with a lot of ingredients it doesn't need. This takes energy, needed to utilize the appropriate ingredients and strengthen the body, away from its task. This energy is diverted towards digestion and elimination of the unnecessary ingredients instead.

These recommendations include the most relied upon Azmira® products for general symptoms and specific remedies to address the individual nuances of dis-eases and behavioral problems such as seizures, digestive conditions, allergies and aggression. Your animal will tell you, through these various markers (symptoms and behaviors) where its curative process is. Animals are very clear about feeling well or not, although some pets can be stoic; there is no "pretending" with them. This is why I choose to dedicate my life's work to animals after working with humans for several years. They simply get better or they don't. You know with animals that what they are experiencing is witness to their weakness. Certainly I would have preferred at times that an animal could give me greater detail about cramps or a pain pattern, but for the most part I reaped more accurate feed-back about dis-ease and reversal from my animal clients than from my human ones.

When you use Azmira Holistic Animal Care® Products you know what to expect from the supplement and remedies so if the animal is still struggling you can easily work with what the symptom present is telling you. You are assured that it was not the product that failed but the body's ability to respond due to other underlying weaknesses. It's up to you to watch these markers *and their nuances,* adjusting your protocol to support what it is the body is trying to accomplish. If you have taken **Steps One** and **Two** this will be even easier to follow.

Use Nuances of the Animal's Condition to Guide You

For instance: viral infection, suppressed immune function and compromised vital organs are markers within the diagnosis of Feline Leukemia and all cases would need to address this illness with the herbal formula Viral D'Tox But the facts that your cat may also tremble, with acute skin lesions and swollen glands are dis-ease nuances that respond to the use of a homeopathic remedy called *Mercurius* and the addition of the herbal formula Yucca Intensive for inflammation and pain. Yet, another cat may have bladder irritation and pain urinating due to a build up of catabolic waste in conjunction with his Feline Leukemia. This individual's case would respond instead to the individual homeopathic remedy *Cantharis.*

Homeopathic remedies help stimulate the body's curative action towards a particular area of imbalance (i.e. bladder irritation) while the herbal formulas support the body's effort to reverse the symptom by providing therapeutic agents that physically address the problem (i.e. reducing the inflammation). This process is fueled by the daily nutritional supplements recommended in **Step Two.** As you can see, there is not, nor will there ever be, one product that can cure all but rather, there is a symbiotic relationship between remedies that provide various functions and results.

Remember Before Proceeding: Detoxify the body and change your pet's diet as recommended in **Step One**, adding the foundation supplements listed in **Step Two.**

Without following **Steps One** and **Two;** the body remains toxic without the ability to assimilate nutrients well, and is lacking the reserves of optimum fuel needed to complete all biological functions and necessary curative responses needed for symptom reversal. Before adding too many different products together allow these fuel reserves to build over a few weeks to provide the strength needed to heal. If not, you can stimulate and support an animal in addressing the symptom through homeopathy and herbs, but the body will only temporarily *suppress* the symptom. Without a systematic approach, the pet fails to reach total symptom *reversal* and this can lead to chronic conditions.

The same holds true when using one modality singularly. As I have mentioned, nutritional changes without detoxification minimize proper assimilation. Homeopathy alone can stimulate symptom reversal, but without a high quality daily vitamin and mineral program, the body has no fuel to complete the process. This is evident when herbal products are used by themselves. This is also true for all protocols used without the **Three Steps** recommended in the Holistic Animal Care LifeStyle™; symptom reversal will be short term, difficult to obtain quickly and less beneficial to the animal's over all wellness. Be sure to give your pets the best chance they have to reverse their poor conditions by following these proven protocols and using the right tools.

If you wanted to build a pool you could use a spoon, a shovel or a backhoe to dig the hole; all move dirt and can get the job done… but which one would you rather stake your time and back on?

HOW TO USE PROTOCOL RECOMMENDATIONS

I have listed the most promising protocol, with products *listed in order of their potential benefit,* for each symptom or condition described. What I am hopefully setting in motion for you is a systematic approach to reversing each symptom as you discover it, address it and reverse it. Regardless of whether it is an isolated problem or chronic condition; the body heals in layers. As an onion sheds its skins so does the body shed its weaknesses and imbalances (symptoms) to return to wellness. These layers must be removed in the reverse order they were created to truly reach the core disease. It is not important that you know the order, such as the case where you may have adopted a pet with an unknown history. As you apply one remedy and reverse a symptom associated with the condition, then the next symptom to be addressed will become more apparent, and so on, until you reach core symptom or condition reversal, and long-term wellness. The greater the reliability of the remedies you use, the quicker you can recognize the true underlying weaknesses and be able to address those, fully reversing symptoms and re-establishing your pet's optimum health.

My Azmira Holistic Animal Care® Products are listed in <u>this font style</u> to help you identify them from other general remedies I recommend, if you choose to follow the complete Holistic Animal Care LifeStyle™ approach for optimum results. Azmira® diets, supplements, herbal formulas and homeopathic remedies are guaranteed to work as promised when used as directed. If notable results fail to show within a reasonable time or additional symptoms surface, *then you know the animal's system (immune, digestive, nervous, eliminatory, cardio, etc.) is still deficient* and needs additional stimulation and/or support for a proper curative response.

Unfortunately I may have missed the specific symptom or condition you are seeking, so simply consider what the symptom is telling you and address it accordingly. Is the animal's severe diarrhea a digestive problem, such as colitis, or an acute ingested poisoning? Track down the potential cause by analyzing the symptoms most clearly presented and deal with them from there, a layer at a time. For instance:

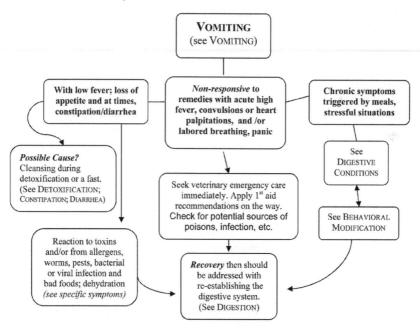

If you have not yet read the prior chapters, please do so before embarking on symptom care: These previous chapters explain The Holistic Animal Care LifeStyle™ **Three Step Process** I have used for over twenty years. Proven in clinical studies to be safe and effective, we have followed thousands of animals through long-term reversal of their dis-eases and generations of healthy, illness-free animals living on my prevention protocols. Understanding and applying this systematic approach properly will increase your ability to reverse your individual pet's symptoms and chronic conditions with the recommendations listed in this chapter.

Dr. Newman's Holistic Animal Care LifeStyle™

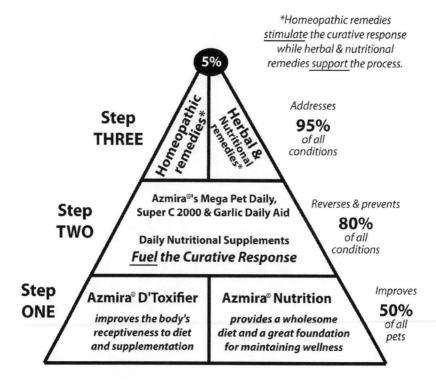

Homeopathic remedies stimulate the curative response while herbal & nutritional remedies support the process.

5%

Step THREE

Homeopathic remedies*

Herbal & Nutritional remedies*

Addresses **95%** *of all conditions*

Step TWO

Azmira®'s Mega Pet Daily, Super C 2000 & Garlic Daily Aid

Daily Nutritional Supplements
Fuel the Curative Response

Reverses & prevents **80%** *of all conditions*

Step ONE

Azmira® D'Toxifier
improves the body's receptiveness to diet and supplementation

Azmira® Nutrition
provides a wholesome diet and a great foundation for maintaining wellness

Improves **50%** *of all pets*

This systematic approach was created to eliminate the guesswork associated with natural pet care. As you take each step, you reach a greater depth of wellness and symptom reversal. The use of Dr. Newman's naturopathic protocols with specific Azmira Holistic Animal Care® products has been proven to promote rapid, reliable and long-term results. If an animal fails to improve on the next Step, taken with a proven product, then it is likely the body failed to respond rather than the product failed to work. This allows you to uncover the true weakness, based on the symptoms you witness, and adjust the protocol as needed, rather than simply supplementing blindly.

5% of chronically ill pets will still need medication. The LifeStyle™ approach will help prevent toxic build-up and provide support to maintain health while lessening the need for higher doses and possibly, the drug itself. It is not uncommon, for instance with diabetic pets, that insulin need is cut in half from previous use, and within months possibly eliminated.

CHAPTER TEN

Symptoms A to Z

Abandonment

The feral cat is a great example of the abandoned pet dynamic for which this specific flower combination works well. They fear our confinement yet desperately need our shelter and are torn between many feelings. Dogs and cats that become very vocal or destructive when left alone are indicative of this dynamic. Being isolated longer, or in other ways punished for their behavior, only makes this pet more desperate to act out.

This emotional dynamic is also associated with difficulties with homesickness; where changes in the family or home, isolation for extended periods such as during hospitalization or kenneling and the loss of routine may be a trigger for depression and anxiety. Nervousness, fear, obsessive behavior and even aggression can be secondary behavioral symptoms to being abandoned. But the primary effect abandonment has on any living being is generalized stress which can lead to illness as well as behavior problems such as barking. This pet may try to hide its distress, seem friendly and easy-going, yet experience fur pulling, minor obsessive behavior and other stress-related symptoms triggered by being left alone. Frustration will also quickly lead the abandoned pet to act out aggressively; therefore, their emotions need to be stabilized. Abandonment can be based upon deep-seated feelings that may have originally stemmed from an experience long ago, but are fresh in the pet's mind and filter.

Pets suffering from chronic abandonment issues are often later stricken with kidney, bladder and/or digestive ailments as well. This makes daily

LifeStyle™ supplementation, especially for the B-Complex in Mega Pet Daily, even more important. Behavior modification and environmental changes (self-access to outdoors, increased playtime) can also benefit in creating a safe home, with little stress, and one the pet can appreciate, improving the pet's emotional wellbeing.

- Flower combination—Abandonment or R&R Essence

Homeopathic remedies

Give two doses of remedy, spaced fifteen minutes apart, prior to when you leave and also put in your pet's water dish.

- *Arsenicum* is for the pet who reacts to their perceived abandonment with destruction or aggression. There is great vocalization. Arsenicum is included in D'Toxifier.

- *Aconite* or Fear helps those who suffer fear or anxiety when left alone.

- *Gelsemium* for when being left alone creates lethargy or withdrawal, possible "housetraining accidents" or destructive chewing is the result of abandonment.

- *Ignatia* is for the pet who becomes hysterical when you leave.

Behavioral Guidance

- These pets need reassurance that you are returning or that they will not be "ignored" too long and/or that things will remain the same. They respond best to a set routine, such as being fed in the same place at the same time each day, until they feel more secure. You should first try desensitizing your pet to being left alone in addition to working with my homeopathic flower remedy.

Herbal Support

- For very stressed pets, the addition of Calm & Relax will physically relax your pet to help minimize its reaction to being left alone. Often four to six weeks of this herbal remedy is all that is needed to help change your pet's focus.

(see Behavioral Modification for additional information and exercises)

Abrasions

ABRASIONS can occur for a number of reasons, and are best addressed topically, so I recommended you use Rejuva Spray for its antibacterial properties to protect against infection. This product also contains herbs to soothe the tissue and reduce pain/itching on contact, while improving healing time. If needed when scabbing has occurred or deep scarring is a concern, Rejuva Gel can then be applied to reduce scarring.

Homeopathic *Arsenicum*, as found in D'Toxifier, stimulates the process of skin repair quickly while reducing irritation and inflammation.

Abscesses

Boils can erupt topically especially around the chest and back. This occurs most often during a curative response and especially during the detoxification process where the body is attempting to release waste products through the largest eliminatory organ, the skin. The body, as one of its defenses against toxins, will pocket this irritating substance, even an allergen (sometimes for years) to keep it from establishing a deeper hold on the body. Detoxification releases these toxins from the fatty tissue they are stored in and moves them back into the blood stream for elimination, resulting in skin eruptions such as hot spots and pimples, which can become infected and cause pain.

A puncture or bite wound will introduce bacteria and viruses which can become toxic and create an abscess. *R&R Essence* will help reduce the initial emotional and physical trauma associated with the bite. The best cure for these wounds is prevention through daily supplementation recommended in **Step Two**. Garlic Daily Aid and Super C 2000 help kill off any organisms before they can infect the body. But if the body is too overwhelmed, even when supplemented, then it will allow the abscess to occur.

Topical Remedies

- Treat topically at least once a day, twice a day or more if the abscess is large and angry. Apply a warm, damp cloth to the area for fifteen minutes at a time to encourage eruption of the abscess. It will also soothe your pet.

- Once there is drainage, be sure to keep the area clean and dry.

- It is helpful to trim away a little fur around the site to expose it to more air. This encourages healing, and makes it easier to address the abscess topically.

- Rejuva Spray prevents the spread of infection and helps eliminate it while soothing and repairing tissue. Reduces pain and inflammation on contact. Clean the area with a solution of *fifty percent hydrogen peroxide and fifty percent water*, rinse well and then saturate the area with Rejuva Spray, allowing it to air dry. This encourages healing, prevents the infection from spreading and kills off bacteria. Rejuva Spray alone can be used in between cleanings to reduce scratching or biting/licking of the area.

- Goldenseal Extract can be added by *four full droppers*-worth to the Rejuva Spray bottle to increase its antibiotic properties for serious, severely angry infections or those who have been non-responsive to topical treatment for twenty four hours.

- Rejuva Gel can later be used, once healing and scabbing have begun, to reduce the likelihood of scarring as the result of a serious abscess.

Homeopathic Remedies

- D'Toxifier contains *Arsenicum* with complementary remedies which help reverse the abscess and secondary symptoms (i.e. fever) through improved nutrient utilization and waste elimination. Promotes tissue repair and a reduction in inflammation and pain. D'Toxifier is good in reducing the physical and emotional trauma of a bite or deep scratch. Helps prevent the development of abscesses when given as a weekly maintenance dose.

- *Belladonna* and/or *Sulphur* may discourage the full formation of an abscess when given at the first sign of swelling and accompanying heat.

- *Calcarea Carb.* is beneficial for abscesses deep inside the muscle; surrounding organs.

- *Silicea* encourages eruption and drainage, whether or not you suspect a foreign object has caused the abscess. Actually, since the abscess itself is a foreign object, Silicea has generally worked well in expelling it. Can be used with *Calcarea Carb.* for stubborn internal pockets of bacterial or septic tissue.

- *Mercurius* is used especially if thick pus has formed and the skin surrounding it has become angrier or is painful to touch. This pus can be a runny, greenish, putrefied discharge streaked with blood.

- *Hepar Sulph.* is the best remedy for abscesses too painful to touch. It can be used in conjunction with other remedies.

- *Phosphorous 30C* with doubled the herbal remedies of Garlic Daily Aid and *Yucca Intensive* combined are exceptionally helpful in eliminating internal abscesses including old bacterial pockets, surrounding or in organs often filled with cancerous tumors, which are commonly the root of pain and fever. Phosphorous is also indicated for rotten teeth in abscessed, bleeding gums. All these symptoms are generally treated with antibiotics and steroids, yet respond quickly to naturopathic care with this protocol.

Herbal Remedies

- Yucca Intensive reduces the inflammation, tissue deterioration and pain associated with abscesses.

- Garlic Daily Aid, in double the recommended daily foundation dose, will provide natural antibiotic support and tissue repairing nutrients.

- Blood & Lymph D'Tox added during the acute phase of severe abscesses will help the body fight this infection and invasion. This is also a good remedy to use twice a year (one bottle at a time to detox and strengthen the immune response) for the chronic tendency to develop abscesses such as when fighting cancer.

- ImmunoStim'R, either started with the Blood & Lymph D'Tox (for severe infected tissue especially internal abscesses), or used alone for a few months can help clear out diseased, infected and cancerous tissues and the resulting catabolic wastes. Should be used for maintenance in the cases of debilitated pets or those who suffered many years of a toxic lifestyle and which led to the chronic development of abscesses.

(See Infections, Cancer)

Abused Pets

ABUSED PETS can live a lifetime of dysfunction and illness, long after the abuse has stopped. Addressing the physical symptoms of acute abuse should be done, followed by the emotional outcome, notably fear, anxiety, and aggression.

The homeopathically potentized flower remedies—Fear, Neediness, Aggression and R&R Essence (to Rescue and give Relief)—should be used as required.

Herbal Calm & Relax can help physically lower the pet's anxiety and lessen their behavioral issues. It should be used for six weeks on and one week off until the pet becomes less reactive around you.

Desensitizing the pet to those situations which remind them of the abuse is vital, especially if facing these situations triggers negative behavior (ie. your pet sees a rolled-up newspaper and fears it or becomes highly anxious when you leave). The sooner these after-effects can be dealt with, the less likely long-term damage, both physically and behaviorally, will be done. Since emotional stress is often at the root of physical dis-ease, it is also important that previously abused pets be given emotional/ behavioral support when they manifest symptoms later in life such as allergies, cancer or specific organ weakness, especially when they still exhibit or lapse back into negative emotions.

(see Behavioral Problems)

Addison's Disease

ADDISON'S DISEASE (hypoadrenocorticism) is a condition of inadequate corticosteroid production. Mineralocorticoids, in addition to the glucocorticosteroids produced by the adrenal glands, are deficient— causing fluid and electrolyte imbalance (dis-ease) throughout the body. This can be a life-threatening situation in addition to the causes of this dis-ease; includes tumors, infections, catabolic waste, chemical reactions and autoimmune dysfunction. Chronic use of corticosteroids can also trigger an onset of Addison's disease.

The best way to reverse Addison's is through symptom-specific remedies and support. This is a dis-ease which may trigger a host of symptoms, from heart conditions to vomiting and diarrhea, based on the individual animal's constitution. Your veterinarian must give you a clear picture of how this condition is manifesting itself in your pet so you can support symptom reversal while strengthening the adrenal gland.

(see Adrenal Malfunction and Symptom-specific subjects)

Adrenal Malfunction

ADRENAL MALFUNCTION is common in animals who are also exhibiting chronic symptoms, especially infected skin conditions and liver dysfunction. Often, it can actually be caused by previous cycles of steroid and antibiotic treatments which are commonly used to suppress reactive symptoms associated with previous conditions such as allergies.

Clinical testing for hormonal or cortisol levels many benefit you, no matter what you decide to do. If nothing the LifeStyle™ has to offer has seemed to work, utilize any medication that is appropriate for you and your animal. But this is generally in a very few, severely dis-eased cases. Pets who have not responded well to natural modalities are often diagnosed with deeper glandular malfunctions including thyroid dysfunction, which, when addressed, help stimulate the curative process for the adrenal disorder.

There are many wonderful, natural glandular products available. I prefer *glandulars in powder or tablet form* to homeopathic ones. But do not disregard a homeopathic remedy combined with a potentized glandular *in addition to* a tableted form. Homeopathic glandulars work on a deeper level and are beneficial to overall support, whereas tableted glandulars actually feed the gland directly, providing more substantial support in reversing glandular weakness. *Multi-glandulars*, a combination of several glands, are beneficial in supporting the weaker gland, but be certain the combination contains sufficient amounts of the particular gland you do need to stimulate and support. Add another single adrenal glandular product to the multiple, if needed.

Herbal Remedies

- Stress & A'drenal Plex is a therapeutic formula geared towards reestablishing proper adrenal and thyroid functions (thyroid imbalance is often in conjunction with adrenal disorders) in all cases of adrenal imbalance. Helps replenish vitality, repair tissue and balance hormones. Benefits the pet in either case of hypo- (Addison's) or hyper- (Cushing's) activity of the gland.

- Yucca Intensive helps control inflammation of the adrenal gland and the body, reduces edema and supports detoxification. This product does provide natural steroidal compounds that are beneficial in the reversal of Addison's disease—and supports the body to balance the gland when it is dealing with Cushing's disease. Although Cushing's is a condition of too many corticosteroids circulating within the body, Yucca seems to benefit rather than harm when reversing the symptoms of Cushing's (namely skin conditions). Certainly, if you have any concerns, then work with the Immuno Stim'R and homeopathic remedies for an anti-inflammatory protocol.

- Immuno Stim'R can reduce the stress that catabolic waste can place on the glands, improving cellular respiration and nutrient assimilation, which will restore vitality to the adrenals.

- Calm & Relax is indicated for the pet who has severe nervous energy and weight loss with their imbalance. The hallmark of this formula is the restoration of brain chemistry and hormonal balance and wellness.

Homeopathic Remedies

- D'Toxifier contains several remedies including *Arsenicum* and *Iris* which are excellent at rebalancing and maintaining glandular function. In addition, *Phytolacca* has marked effect on adrenal imbalance associated with aggression. D'Toxifier also addresses numerous secondary symptoms such as weight loss and skin changes.

- *Adrenalin* in the lower potentizes has a stimulating and balancing action on the glands; benefiting adrenal function in Addison's Disease and condition-related symptoms when used daily. To benefit Cushing's by regulating function, a weekly 200C dose can help.

(see Addison's Disease, Cushing's Disease and Symptom-specific subjects)

Aggravations

AGGRAVATIONS occur at various times, generally as the body is balancing itself, and especially in response to a homeopathic remedy which was on target for the individual pet's condition. During this process, symptoms will temporarily worsen or return. Generally this lasts for less than forty-eight hours. An aggravation is a curative response. It is vital the aggravations be supported and not suppressed for complete symptom reversal to occur.

A variety of products can be used to suppress symptoms although it is best to allow the aggravation to run its course without interference, unless the symptom is life-threatening. Then it is considered a "healing crisis" and warrants intervention. Homeopathy is a wonderful tool to use during an aggravation. It allows the body the ability to continue with the curative response while minimizing noted symptoms and their outcomes.

Homeopathic support for a curative response

- D'Toxifier contains several homeopathic remedies including *Arsenicum* which is excellent at rebalancing and maintaining proper bodily functions such as digestion and assimilation, cellular waste elimination and immune response. It also improves the body's use of products needed for symptom reversal. In addition, several remedies have marked effect on thyroid/adrenal imbalance associated with severe curative responses. D'Toxifier also addresses numerous general symptoms such as appetite loss and skin irritations.

Aging

AGING comes gracefully when The Holistic Animal Care LifeStyle™ is followed. Unfortunately, that is not often the case with other types of lifestyles. Today we are told that dogs and cats should be considered seniors at six and seven years old. Watch the pet food advertisements that convince you that you need a special formula for that aging pet.

This dismays me. When I first started in pet care during the 1970's "senior" was applied to dogs when they reached nine to eleven years of age depending on the breed. We considered a cat to be older only when it was around sixteen years old! Why has the veterinary community changed the guidelines on "age" rather then question why most animals are prematurely aging today?!

As both a naturopathic doctor and pet product manufacturer, it is easy to answer this question. Dogs and cats raised on the LifeStyle™ today do not "age" that quickly. All the chemicals in other pet foods and products, lack of proper nutrients or ones which can even be assimilated and excessive vaccinations are destroying healthy, youthful tissue and have rendered pets' immune function too weak to fight off aging.

Also as a manufacturer I can share with you that all the trade magazines I receive are full of encouragement to market a variety of life-stage diets (growth, adult, senior), in addition to "specialty" ones (kidney, allergy, weight issues), so that the average consumer who has more than one of each breed and age of pet will have to buy more than one type of food in the brand's line at the same time! Dry food purchases take longer to feed, often going rancid in the opened bag or plastic tub. Even refrigerated kibble loses its flavor and nutrients within a few weeks. Pets do not like to consume old, tasteless food and become finicky. Old food has also lost it nutritional value due to oxidation and become harder to digest. This increases toxicity in the body which leads to premature aging, and so on. Certainly, a variety of protein sources such as ostrich, lamb or fish and palatability changes are warranted to appeal to a variety of individual animals, all with their own taste buds (to provide a healthy menu variety as Azmira®'s diets do—buy beef one month, lamb the next). But let's market it like it is and not under false promises that can actually harm the pet in the long run. This is done for increased sales and profits. Period. It is simply to encourage your purchases of several bags at a time.

This is not necessary. It is certainly cheaper in the long run, to use a good basic canine or feline diet and supplement according to your individual animal's needs and life-stage, and you will get more results from your dietary investment. In addition, when you can buy a larger bag for all your dogs or cats that can be finished within a month, your pet's food will be fresher and also cheaper.

For your information: Zaezar, one of my Rottweilers, lived to be fifteen years-old and Gucci to sixteen years-old (and I rescued him at the age of twelve in very poor health and near death!). Another one of my Rotties, Golda, is nine years-old and in perfect health despite having rescued her at three months-old malnourished with a bad case of cystitis and Valley Fever, an often fatal fungal infestation. People are always mistaking her for a three or four year-old dog. Sometimes, I do wish she had a little less energy like the other "seniors" I see at the dog park, but the life just shines from her today, and she has no trace of the fungal infestation in her blood—unheard of in traditional veterinary circles when treated with antifungal drugs.

Preventing Premature Aging Homeopathically

Azmira®'s D'Toxifier was formulated to encourage optimum nutrient utilization and waste elimination through organ stimulation and balancing. This is the key to a successful wellness protocol. Without the body's cooperation in digesting and utilizing the improved diet and supplements in **Steps One** and **Two** you are feeding while eliminating immune suppressing wastes, you may be wasting your money.

(see Symptom-specific subjects)

Aggression

AGGRESSION can be a problem in pets suffering from acute and chronic conditions, pain and/or emotional stress. Most common feed ingredients—especially sugars and chemical preservatives—contribute to the sensitivities which result in the symptom reaction and trigger the aggression as well.

Be sure to also follow my desensitizing exercises and seek professional training when needed for biting, barking, stalking and fighting. Aggression is often related to the liver, so be sure to detoxify on a weekly basis, after the recommended two week process during **Step One**. Many aggressive pets have noticeable improvements in their dispositions shortly after a detoxification process; therefore, proper diet is especially important to prevent a build-up of toxins. In addition, some animals cannot tolerate the constant itching and irritation caused by allergies, the stiffness and pain of arthritis, the confusion of old age or seizures, often becoming exhausted from the symptoms and lashing out when approached.

Although aggressive behavior is most often associated with biting, destroying personal property and malicious vocalization, the overly concerned and possessive pet who demands constant attention in a bullying fashion is also being aggressive. Difficult to handle often describes these pets. Azmira®'s flower combination helps to minimize general negative feelings that cause a pet to be quick to act out, before thinking about the consequences. Anxiety or fear can also trigger aggression. Fear-aggression is a dynamic that commonly results in biting accidents—when a nervous pet is cornered. These pets may also be troubled and easy to panic, often suffering physically from poor digestion, liver problems or arthritis.

- Homeopathically-potentized Flower Remedies—Aggression, Fear and/or R&R Essence

Nutritional and Herbal Recommendations

- B-Complex 50 provides additional B-vitamins necessary in reducing the aggressive tendency by helping to bring brain chemistry back in balance—use until the aggression is under control, *for at least three months,* then wean off over a two week period. Use 100 mg. per day for cats and small pets; 200 mg. a day for large dogs. This is *in addition to* the available B-vitamins in Mega Pet Daily.

- **L-TryptoPet** is a pharmaceutically pure amino acid that is a precursor to seratonin and essential for regulating brain activity. Excellent supplement for hyperactive, irritable pets, or those with aggression and other mood disorders. Helps with pain relief, promotes sound sleep, and alleviates depression and nervous conditions.

- **Grape Seed Extract** is a powerful antioxidant which reduces free radicals known to irritate the brain, resulting in aggression. A toxin, drug and ammonia-free environment for the brain promotes proper balance of the hormones and chemicals responsible for a stable mood.

- **Herbal Calm** can be given to a pet at least one half-hour prior to exposure to a stimulus which creates an aggressive response; lasts approximately four hours.

- **Calm & Relax** is a stronger relaxant which also has herbal properties to help balance and stabilize brain chemistry. Better suited for long-term, daily use to reverse aggressive tendencies and the anxiety often associated with fear-aggressive pets.

Homeopathic Remedies

*part of D'Toxifier

- **Arsenicum* for liver involvement and/or chronic illness with mean disposition.

- *Apis* reduces aggression with anxiety from scratching and biting at bodily irritations.

- *Gelsemium* is good for aggression from fatigue, especially chronic scratching or fighting pain. Benefits the pet whose aggression seems to have come on suddenly for no reason.

- *Ignatia* helps the fear-aggressive pet, or one who turns suddenly when seemingly happy.

- **Iris* benefits glandular function, primarily thyroid imbalance associated with aggression.

- *Phosphorus* supports the overly-sensitive pet or one who has become weak from illness.

- **Phytolacca* has marked effect on adrenal imbalance associated with aggression.

Behavioral Guidance

- These pets need reassurance that you are in control and/or that things will remain the same. They respond best to a set training routine; additional play/exercise time will help to reduce tension and reinforce good communication skills between you and this pet. Also avoid stress, sudden movements, and the abrupt awakening of an aggressive-type pet. These situations tend to trigger an outburst.

(see Behavioral Problems for desensitizing exercises)

Allergies

ALLERGIES in general are the result of a depressed immune system and a toxic lifestyle. Be sure to follow **Steps One** and **Two** first when addressing any allergic condition or homeopathic and herbal remedies will simply suppress the symptom temporarily and make the condition worse over time. The LifeStyle™ approach is very important when dealing with an allergic condition as these conditions are often the precursor to more serious conditions such as cancer (especially when suppressed with a lifetime of steroids, antihistamines and antibiotics). In addition, the LifeStyle™ will provide the daily fuel to help prevent a recurrence of symptoms when exposed to allergens since you can limit exposure but you can not eliminate the culprits in our environment totally—strengthening the immune response and minimizing waste in the body is a far easier task.

Remember, it can take a while to reverse the underlying weaknesses which are at the root of allergies. It is not uncommon to have an animal strengthen the first season and successfully overcome their reactions only to begin again the next year. The good news is that if you didn't use chemicals during the year, vaccinate heavily, or rely on shotgun medications then the symptoms should be much tamer, easier to address and reverse more quickly. Continuing with the allergy protocol and LifeStyle™ process will probably eliminate the allergies totally by the following season. The older the pet is, the longer it may take to reverse their weakness. Allergies are the most common thing I hear about *and a protocol with which we have a very high rate of success.* But it can be a frustrating condition.

Acute allergic-reactions can be successfully "suppressed" with a few doses of *homeopathy*, given five to fifteen minutes apart for up to one hour, in lower potencies (3X to 30C).

This does not affect the body like chemical suppression does but rather allows the body to stop fighting the allergens and focus on improving the immune response. Give one dose orally, according to the manufacturer's recommendations, every five to fifteen minutes for the first hour, then every hour until there is relief. Generally, there is relief within the first two doses, give one dose in an hour to help the curative process. Repeat as needed. When in doubt, treat the most obvious symptom first (i.e. stress, watery eyes), then focus on any specific ones that manifest later, such as their sensitivity to grass and fear.

Do not overlook the emotional stress your pet is exhibiting around the allergic reaction itself or to life in general. During our clinical studies we confirmed that pets with the worse allergies were more likely to be of the nervous or fearful types. They did not respond as well to the allergy protocol until their behavioral issues were also addressed in addition to their physical needs.

One client's Siamese cat in particular, who tore out her fur each spring, was in the first stages of cancer at the age of nine years-old and had a diagnoses of allergies (from the age of four years-old) and a history of veterinary prescription diets, steroids and antibiotic use for three years. She had been seeing a holistic vet for two years prior to when I first met her. She did not respond well to a prior regime of natural care including acupuncture, glandulars, nutritional supplements and herbs (she was being force-fed twelve pills and three ounces of teas per day; all symptom-suppressors, *not stimulators or supporters working together as with the LifeStyle™ approach!*) and now was prescribed steroids again however, she could not tolerate them well despite the holistic remedy for liver dysfunction, Milk Thistle herb, the vet had also prescribed.

The first thing I recommended was to fast her, with no medication or supplements, for two days. Then we switched to a home-cooked diet and added **Mega Pet Daily** (1/2 capsule mixed right into her meal), **Super C 2000** (1/8th teaspoon), two drops of **Yucca Intensive** (for inflammation & liver), and four drops of **Blood & Lymph Detox** (for the cancer and blood toxicity/allergics/liver). We repeated this twice a day. Two weeks later, when she got stronger with a better appetite, we added (½ of a pearl) **Garlic Daily Aid**.

Within a month her fur was growing back, her energy was stronger and her blood tests (eosinophils, RBC, WBC and liver enzymes) had improved, but she was still pulling her fur out despite the addition of **Aller'G Free** (antihistamine). I suspected that she did not have true allergies (as we can rely on the **Aller'G Free** and **Yucca Intensive** to suppress whatever true allergy there is and it wasn't working!).

I spoke more with the owners and found out that she was also a very vocal and high strung cat so I recommended we try Azmira®'s homeopathic flower remedies. We stopped the Aller'g Free and switched to Neediness. Well, that did the trick! Within two weeks she had noticeably reduced the amount of fur she was pulling out (not to mention spitting up). They also built an outdoor enclosure for her to be in during the cooler parts of the day. She had not seen the outdoors since her move into this current home at the age of three years-old (nine months prior to her first "allergy" episode that first spring, which now was obviously due to spring fever rather than spring allergies).

The following spring, not only had her cancer gone into remission, but there was no fur pulling and none of the emotional fits that used to overcome her, as long as she got some time in her outdoor enclosure. Unfortunately, a few years later, the family got lax on her maintenance protocol (common when the animal has been doing so well) and then went through a divorce. The fur pulling started again and was not responding to the Nervousness remedy so I recommended they go back on the LifeStyle™ and this time add Calm & Relax. The fur pulling stopped and four months after she was moved into a new home. They stopped the symptom-specific remedies, switch to a maintenance protocol and life went on as usual until she passed at the age of seventeen years-young from the cancer (yes, we never "cured" the cancer but she got eight more *healthy, symptom-free* years! Certainly many chemically-raised animals live on with cancer, but often full of dis-ease and pain).

Another consideration, in a pet who is not responding to my allergy protocol, is to rule out structural misalignment. A pinched nerve can create numbness in the extremities causing the pet to lick and bite at their feet, tail base or sides, mimicking an allergic reaction. Once the allergy protocol has been followed but with minimal success, it behooves you to seek an animal chiropractor to rule out spinal misalignment. One of my own dogs suffered a pinched nerve and we first addressed it as an allergy after he chewed off fur behind his hind legs. It wasn't until he was structurally adjusted by a chiropractor that he finally stopped his tiny bites back there and grew the fur back. Twice he has started chewing again and immediately gets relief after an adjustment.

Most Common Homeopathic Remedies for Allergic Reactions

- D'Toxifier contains *Arsenicum* and other remedies used for general irritations, pimples, hot spots, digestive imbalances or toxicity-related allergy symptoms such as reactive arthritis. The animal may also be a bit ill tempered or suffer from aggression, snapping at anyone who touches their itchy areas. They may suffer exhaustion due to their allergy condition. Weekly maintenance dose helps minimize or prevent the onset of symptoms.

- *R&R Essence* is used for generalized stress-related reactions, when emotional stress can trigger sensitivities, or excessive scratching, etc. has made the pet anxious. Can be used in addition to booster other homeopathic and herbal remedies.

- *Obsessive* benefits the pet whose chewing and scratching has become obsessive in nature, rather than a necessity. This remedy is good for a pet whose allergy "symptoms" persist despite the lack of allergens; use when the season is over, but the behavior is not.

- *Apis* is good for intensely itchy skin that is aggravated by warmth, including the warmth the body may give off when covered in angry rashes. Use when the skin, eyes and/or ears are noticeably red and warm to touch.

- *Euphrasia* is another excellent remedy for allergy-related eye and tear duct irritations. Use with cases of excessive tearing.

- *Nux Vomica* addresses the majority of digestive imbalances, including gas, vomiting, diarrhea, or lack of appetite often associated with allergy conditions. Do not use while dosing with D'Toxifier as Nux and Arsenicum antidote each other.

- *Rhus Tox* is helpful when the animal is rubbing or scratching its skin; when the animal gets wet, or cold weather seems to aggravate itchy skin. It is especially good for irritations about the head and reactive arthritis. For swollen, red eyes. Pet becomes listless fighting allergies.

- *Sabadilla* is a popular hay-fever remedy, addressing common upper-respiratory symptoms such as asthma, dry cough, spasmodic sneezing, watery nasal discharge, facial itching, irritated ears and red, runny eyes. Animal may lack appetite or thirst and be of a nervous or timid nature.

- *Sulphur* is used for a wide variety of skin conditions, especially dry and scaly, associated with intense itching or symptoms which are worse at night and in warm surroundings. Scratching may seem to satisfy the pet temporarily, but often will result in increased itching and burning. Sulphur is also good for greasy skin conditions and digestive upsets. Helps sooth an ill-tempered pet.

- *Urtica Urens* addresses extensive eruptions, hives or welts that are very itchy. Usually the skin is dry and aggravated by warmth or bathing. (These conditions are non-responsive to Apis or Sulphur.) It is also good for profuse discharges from mucous membranes. Symptoms may be localized to the right side of the body.

Herbal Remedies for Allergic Reactions

Herbal antihistamines and anti-inflammatory products are very effective and a good alternative to over-the-counter antihistamine drugs or veterinary prescriptions, such as steroids. I highly recommend that you use a combination of homeopathy for acute reactions and herbs to lessen sensitivity and repair irritated lungs, eyes, ears and skin, which may reduce a more severe reaction and lessen the damage to sensitive tissues. Herbs also promote the long-term reversal of chronic allergies and should be used in conjunction with daily supplementation. It is best to keep up the maintenance protocol in-between allergy seasons (minus acute symptom-specific remedies) to build a better immune response and ultimately resistance to the upcoming seasonal allergens.

You can also begin an allergy-specific product six weeks prior to the start of the upcoming season to build up a resistance before the body becomes burdened by allergens and is then asked to fight back. For instance, your pet responded well to Aller'G Free and Yucca Intensive during the thick of it last year and you noticed that grass seemed to be a culprit. So you begin with Aller'G: Grass & Pollen six weeks before the arrival of spring to prepare the immune response. This will reduce the need for other symptom-specific remedies and keep the animal from getting so bad, eventually eliminating future allergic reactions.

General Herbal Remedy

- *Daily Boost* helps reduces sensitivity to allergens and fights infection, stimulates resistance against food or reactive allergies. This is an excellent daily tonic for the blood, skin, colon and liver. Prevents the onset of an allergy condition. Chinese Mushrooms, included in Daily Boost's formula, have been used by the Chinese for centuries to prevent and treat allergies associated with the digestive system. A dramatic reduction in food sensitivities is often the result of long-term supplementation.

For Acute, General Symptoms *these products can be used as needed:*

Yucca Intensive is made from a desert root which has been used for centuries by native cultures to reduce general inflammation. It is an herbal steroid alternative.

- Recent studies conducted by Azmira® have confirmed that bio-available steroidal saponins perform as effectively as their chemical steroid counterparts without the serious drug side effects. Up to 87% steroidal saponins are found in the mostly pure extract form Azmira® uses, rather than the low single digit percentages available in the fibrous powder (that is a waste by-product of extraction) used in capsule or powdered products.

- Yucca enhances the action of other, more specific-use herbs and nutrients, in working more effectively by supporting liver function and detoxification.

Aller'G Free, our OTC antihistamine alternative, is a formulation of dry herbs and powdered extracts which noticeably reduce symptoms within the first hour of use.

- Reduces inflammation in general, is helpful with detoxification of histamine and in reducing respiratory stress. A powerful combination when used with **Yucca Intensive**.

- Helps address most allergy symptoms affecting the eyes, ears, respiratory system and skin. Is useful in minimizing skin eruptions such as pimples, hot spots, rashes and pustules, as well as reducing wheezing, coughs and bronchitis. Supports general immune function.

- Reduces redness and irritation of the skin, eyes and ears. It can also help reduce irritation of the anal glands and inflamed intestinal tracts or joints from reactive arthritis.

For Chronic Allergy Symptoms

These remedies help with reversing the actual weakness itself and should be used for no less than six weeks at a time for optimum benefit. A bottle six weeks prior to *and during* the season can do wonders, especially with the severely affected animals, in reducing the likelihood of a reaction or its severity. These can be used in addition to any acute symptom-specific remedies which may also be needed from time to time.

Aller'G: Grass & Pollen:

- Builds resistance to air-borne allergens.

- *C*ontracts swollen mucous membranes associated with respiratory ailments such as asthma and air-borne allergies (hay fever).

- The antibacterial properties of this formulation help prevent and reverse chronic infections of the eyes, ears and respiratory system.

Aller'G: Skin & Digestive:

- Protects the liver from circulating antigens and allergens, thereby reducing infections and skin or intestinal irritations associated with air-borne, urea and food-related allergies.

- This combination of standardized extracts supports the adrenal glands when epinephrine is needed by the body during inflammatory responses generated by allergens.

- It also is indicated for all disorders of hypersensitivity, including allergies, asthma, dermatitis, irritable bowel syndrome, reactive arthritis and food-related digestive disorders.

Aller'G: Skin & Pimple D'Tox:

- Purifies the blood and drains excess lymphatic fluids. This formula improves metabolism by carrying more blood and nutrients to the cells and thereby promoting greater assimilation at the cellular level. It is useful for eczema, psoriasis, tumors, cysts, pustules, acne, chronic hot spots and other skin disorders such as mange. Helpful for lymphatic edema and toxemia (common side-effects of fighting toxins and allergens), including reactive joint inflammation.

Stress & A'Drenal Plex:

- Promotes vitality, restoring integrity to the adrenal and thyroid glands when allergies have exhausted the animal. As an adaptogenic formula, these herbs reduce the stress on a body that is constantly exposed to excessive physical or emotional conditions preventing or reversing a severe loss of energy, with anemia, low blood pressure and anxiety. Helps the "borderline" thyroid cases often diagnosed with allergies, and vice versa.

Anal Glands

ANAL GLANDS can become impacted in dogs who have been fed poor quality diets and whose digestive and eliminatory systems do not function properly. The glands become impacted with waste (the odiferous secretion) that the body is attempting to rid itself of (and these dogs may be using to mark their territories with) but "pockets" instead; another of the body's defense mechanisms. This creates inflammation, irritation and itching around the anus. The dog will scoot their rear ends across the floor, lick the glands and even chew at them, eventually infecting the area.

If the pet caregiver squeezes or drains these glands incorrectly, it will only damage them further, making them even more susceptible to refilling and impacting, often worse with each time. The skin will toughen and scar. Please have these glands professionally expressed by an experienced groomer or veterinarian. In order to avoid damaging these sensitive tissues do this no more than every six weeks at first, and then tapering off until you can go yearly, if needed at all.

Topical Recommendations

- You can encourage drainage of these glands naturally by holding a compress, soaked in a warm solution of *6 ounces pure water, 2 ounces witch hazel, with 20 drops of* Calendula (for tissue scarring), *10 drops of* Goldenseal (eliminates infection) *and 10 drops of* Yucca Intensive (reduces inflammation, pain and itching). Rinse area well with fresh solution.

- Followed by a topical application of Rejuva Spray (soak a cotton pad and hold it gently against the area for a few minutes, or spray it on as needed) to soothe and heal sensitive tissue while reducing infection and inflammation. Refrigerate for added anti-inflammatory benefits.

- Apply homeopathic Rejuva Gel afterwards, as needed with more severe conditions. This keeps anal tissues from toughing up and creating further discomfort. Keep some in the refrigerator; it will feel especially soothing on irritated and inflamed tissues. Repeat twice to three times a day until swelling and redness is gone. Great to use directly after having the gland sacs drained.

- Apply Vita E 200 directly to severely toughened or scared tissue to soften it. Tough anal gland tissue creates its own discomfort and problems with future eliminations. Avoid petroleum-based products (check product labels!) which will further irritate the area, encouraging bacterial infection. Besides, such products can become poisonous if ingested frequently by your pet.

Nutritional & Herbal Remedies

- Azmira® has a wonderful product call NaturFiber that includes these ingredients: Dried *Chinese mushrooms,* such as *Shiitake* and *Reishi* which are very healing to anal gland tissues, together with other *fiber producing ingredients (apple pectin, guar gum, psyllium)* can help stimulate a complete evacuation of stool from the colon, which will reduce toxic waste from backing up the anal glands. This should be a staple for the chronically gland-impacted or constipated pet. Psyllium used by itself can be too harsh and create additional problems so I highly recommend this product instead.

- Skin & Liv-A-Plex (history of poor diets or digestion) or Blood & Lymph D'Tox (additional immune-related dis-eases such as arthritis) should be used to detoxify the digestive system, strengthen liver function and improve elimination in the case of severe anal gland impaction. Choose the one which most closely matches your pet's total health picture.

- Goldenseal Extract benefits the antibiotic protocol for severely infected glands or a severely debilitated, chronically dis-eased pet.

- Immuno Stim'R reduces catabolic waste in the blood which interferes with proper digestion and elimination. Can be used in maintenance supplement protocol to prevent recurrence.

- MSM is concentrated nutritional sulfur which helps to repair and strengthen the sensitive tissues of the anus and its glands. This is a proven remedy for scarred tissue, returning elasticity to toughened skin. Should be used in severe cases for a total of three months, following the last crisis, and definitely after surgery.

- Increased use of **Garlic Daily Aid** which provides nutritional sulfur to feed healthy tissue and antibacterial support to prevent infection. Double the recommended level during crisis as it is beneficial to proper anal gland function; excellent maintenance supplement.

Homeopathic Care

*part of D'Toxifier

- *Arsenicum* is used for detoxification and can greatly reduce discomfort, especially with chronic inflammation. This is a very important remedy to help prevent or reverse an episode. D'Toxifier benefits the body through improved nutrient utilization and waste elimination.

- *Apis* will reduce the itching and irritation of impacted or sensitive anal gland tissues.

- *Berberis Vulg.* stimulates regulation of the anal gland.

- *Hepar Sulph* can help reverse infected glands and *is more effective when combined* with an herbal antibiotic supplement such as **Goldenseal Extract** and/or **Blood & Lymph D'Tox.**

- *Hypericum* is for pain and tissue damage when used <u>before and after</u> expressing or surgically removing the glands. This is the definitive anal gland remedy.

- Don't forget flower remedies, such as **R&R Essence** or **Fear** if your pet refuses to allow you near the rear without a fight. Give two to three doses, five minutes apart, prior to approaching your pet and dose again during expressing the gland or topical treatment.

(See Abscesses, Infections.)

Anemia

ANEMIA is a common symptom in dis-ease suffering pets. I believe that many cases of anemia associated with various conditions are the result of complications from liver toxicity due to the body's inability to process toxins. Common side effects of anemia include lack of stamina, a depressed appetite, poor coat condition with slow tissue repair, poor immune function, muscle weakness, increased respiratory and heart rates, pale colored gums, and dull eyes. Sometimes the faint odor of metal is present on the breath. More serious anemia needs proper diagnosis and specific remedies during **Step Three**, but borderline anemia is commonly reversed during **Step One** and **Two** with detoxification and proper nutrition.

Anemia is the body's inability to produce more red blood cells to counteract the liver discarding its cells when this valuable organ becomes burdened, and begins malfunctioning. Iron supplementation is a well-known treatment for anemia, and will quickly reverse symptoms. Always use a good quality source such as an *iron proteinate*, iron chelated with an amino acid, for superior absorption. Be careful not to overdo iron supplementation, as it can easily become toxic; the first symptom of toxicity is constipation.

- Limit daily iron supplement levels to around 10 mg. for cats and small dogs, and 20 mg. for medium to large dogs as found in a recommended dose of Mega Pet Daily. In addition, Mega Pet Daily also provides *Chromium* to aid in iron assimilation, which reduces the body's need for higher levels of iron. The next step is to improve iron metabolism.

- I also recommend *Alfalfa*, both in herbal (nutrient rich) or lower potency homeopathic form. This improves iron metabolism to build up the blood.

- Daily Boost also contains herbs that help boost red blood cell production.

- *Taraxacum,* found in D'Toxifier, is also a good homeopathic choice as is its herbal twin, Dandelion, an ingredient in Herbal Boost. Both products are beneficial for red blood cell production through improved nutrient utilization and waste elimination. One product stimulates the process while the other supports it with therapeutic herbal compounds. *Iris* is another homeopathic remedy found in D'Toxifier which also regulates metabolism to improve blood health.

Although feeding cow's liver is a popular remedy for anemia, avoid feeding it to your pet on a regular basis. Liver is a primary detoxifying organ and stores excess toxins it has filtered from the blood. When you feed this organ to your pet, you are also feeding these concentrated toxins, including growth hormones (steroids) and antibiotics! I am not discussing liver treats (unless you feed a lot each day) or when liver is added to our canned diets as flavoring, but rather the feeding of ounces of it daily as a main ingredient in the diet. One or two meals of liver weekly is appropriate in a home cooked menu—more than that and you are leaving your pet prone to toxic build-up. This seems especially true when you combine yeast with the liver as is often the case in pet foods and treats.

Anxiety

ANXIETY is a condition that affects many pets for many different reasons but especially those who have been physically or emotionally abandoned or mistreated in some way. In addition many breeds have anxiety bred into them as an unfortunate negative by-product of genetic manipulation. Cats such as Siamese and small dogs in particular seem to be susceptible to these conditions. The use of human antipsychotic or antidepressant medications has grown in popularity to treat a variety of behavioral issues in pets. Unfortunately these drugs are very hard on the animals' systems and often leave pets living like zombies. Addressing your pet's anxiety should not be causing you more concerns and leaving your animal toxic, encouraging premature aging.

Anxiety most often comes from a lack of communication or understanding of what is expected between the animal and caregiver—more importantly, what can be trusted. Therefore, the use of daily training exercises which improve understanding between the owner and the pet and increases the pet's confidence, as well as regular (reliable) outdoor playtime together, will help to reduce the pet's anxiety.

Homeopathically-potentized Flower Remedies

According to a clinical study conducted in 1997, Azmira® flower remedies are faster and deeper acting than traditional Bach® remedies, which are only effused in water rather than homeopathically potentized like Azmira®'s. They can also be used *as a preventative,* given prior to and during exposure to the source of stress which results in anxiety, for instance, when company visits or for a trip in the car. This will greatly help minimize their reaction to the stimulus and allow them the clarity to learn from you that there is nothing to fear. Each time you repeat this successfully your pet will learn there is no reason to react. Give a few doses orally *five minutes apart* shortly prior to leaving (and during desensitizing exercise) plus place a few drops in their clean water dish.

- **R&R Essence** is an excellent choice for generalized stress, regardless of the source, resulting in anxious behavior (i.e. shaking, whimpering).

- **Neediness** (anxious to please) is more specifically intended for the animal who has a tendency towards these behaviors

- **Fear** (phobia-based anxiety) will help improve the animal's ability to settle down quickly and minimize their reactions. Works on fear of known or unknown things.

- **Abandonment** if the anxiety is from being "abandoned" or staying at home alone, placed in a kennel or left at the vet clinic or groomer's for the day.

- **Obsessive** remedy is for anxiety due to obsessive thoughts or desires; the pet stays glued to the window all day watching for the car to drive up and Dad to return home.

Homeopathic Remedies

- **D'Toxifier** contains *Arsenicum* with complementary remedies which help lessen anxiety through improved nutrient utilization and waste elimination. Anxiety is greatly reduced and remains minimal when given as a weekly maintenance remedy.

Herbal Remedies

- **Herbal Calm** can reduce acute anxiety in thirty minutes and maintain a sense of relaxation for three to four hours, on an as needed basis. Can be double dosed.

- For animals with severe anxieties, the use of **Calm & Relax** on a daily basis will help to physically relax and soothe the pet's nervous system until it can live peacefully amidst the situation which previously caused its anxiety (unless it is an over-stimulating/abusive environment. Remember, you have to change the stimulus as well as minimize the reaction to it). It can be given in a one-time triple dose for an emergency situation to immediately calm the over-anxious animal, when **Herbal Calm** has proven itself not strong enough for your pet in past situations. Safe to use with other calming remedies, but give regular dose if you have already given **Herbal Calm**. This herbal formula's similarity in properties acts as a natural form of valium. It is very important to minimize your pet's daily, chronic anxiety. Anxiety can be the root cause of many behavioral problems and physical conditions such as premature aging, allergies, kidney problems and cancer.

(see Behavioral Problems: Training without Trauma)

Appetite

APPETITE is the best gauge you have to decide when there is an imbalance present and further detective work is warranted. Certainly, as with any symptom you do not understand or are uncomfortable with, it is best to seek a veterinarian diagnosis to rule out any more serious of an underlying condition such as an inflamed organ, viral infection or parasitic infestation. Whenever there has been an increase or decrease in appetite it is best to first ask yourself: "Is this related to changes in environment?" Simple things like hiking for the weekend (increases appetite) to warmer weather (decreases it) can have an effect. Early summer is a notorious time for pets to stop eating, or to reduce their intake, in response to the heat. Some animals are simply being fed too much food and are not hungry until every other meal or so, therefore, controlled portions are a primary tool in maintaining a good appetite. Watch for patterns in their eating to help you understand their problem. One of my own dogs refused dog food in the mornings until we figured out that he was a dairy lover. We tried everything at first, dry then canned food and he held out until dinner when he would eat it. Then we tried cottage cheese and he loved it. Now breakfast is an egg with oatmeal or cottage cheese and dinner is dry and canned food. You have to find what works because two meals a day is optimum for stable blood sugar.

Some animals will gorge themselves when palatable food is available to them in unlimited quantities. This can distend the stomach and cause serious complications, even death. Others, especially dogs, have the urge to eat whatever they can get in their mouth, be it rocks, paper or rotten meat. Some refuse even the highest priced kibbles for days on end in response to stress, or rancid pet food ingredients. Understanding and monitoring your pet's appetite will help you create the perfect nutritional plan and succeed in your overall LifeStyle™ protocol.

Excessive Hunger

If the animal has not regulated its own appetite shortly after **Steps One** and **Two**, then additional homeopathic and/or herbal remedies are needed. Always consider this question—Is the urge to eat emotional or physical?

Insatiable appetites: Some pets will continue to eat regardless of detoxification and nutritional supplementation. If the animal is not gaining any weight (and worms have been ruled out) then a deeper physiological issue is at hand. First step would be to give an acute homeopathic dosing of *Phosphorus* which is a great general appetite remedy. Add DigestZymez to the diet (in case the body is not fully digesting and assimilating the improved nutrition) and if the appetite still does not regulate within two more weeks, or there is appetite with weight loss, then tests should be ordered.

If the animal is recently gaining weight from their insatiable appetite then regulation is in order to rebalance their metabolism. Feed four to six small meals per day for two days never exceeding their daily recommended intake for their preferred weight level. For instance: if the daily recommended amount is two cups per day for a fifty-pound dog—you would feed one-half cup, four times a day. On the third, fourth and fifth days feed three meals per day and then two meals a day from then on. Work with herbal Calm & Relax during this time to aid in the brain's regulation of its appetite "department." Generally six weeks to three months is sufficient. If the animal is already chronically overweight, please refer to WEIGHT LOSS recommendations in this chapter.

Obsessive eating: One of my dogs was obsessed about little rocks approximately one-half inch in size. When stressed (or when Zaezar sensed I was) she would gobble them down as quickly as she could. Due to her fine digestive system and NaturFiber (a bulk-producing vegetable and fruit fiber product) they always found a way out. Some dogs are not so lucky and all need to be monitored for distress. Rocks and other foreign objects can become lodged in the digestive tract requiring surgery.

The use of R&R Essence would diminish Zaezar's need to hunt and swallow rocks. I would feed her well prior to leaving for our walks and administer the remedy, then check my own stress levels (sometimes do a few drops of R&R myself) and have a journey free of rock eating. When she got older and began eating small rocks everywhere in her yard and the R&R did nothing, I put her on a six-week protocol of Obsessive remedy and cleaned up as many rocks on the surface as I could find. In two weeks it had improved *but not substantially* so I added Calm & Relax, a hormone and brain chemistry balancing herbal formula. After the initial six weeks she was no longer obsessively hunting them down. I never did find out what triggered that episode but the systematic approach allowed me to quickly bring balance back into her life and reverse the symptom.

Loss of Appetite

Loss of appetite can occur during curative responses to dis-ease or drug toxicity. First, however, be sure there is no fever, vomiting, diarrhea, constipation or distended stomach present and that your pet is not dehydrated. These are more serious problems; by addressing these symptoms the appetite will likely return on its own. Same advice holds true if any viral diseases such as Feline Leukemia, Parvo or Corona may have infected your pet. (See symptom-specific headings for additional protocol recommendations to these listed below.) Also determine the level of stress your pet may be experiencing and address that with R&R Essence and/or Calm & Relax, as stress can also interfere with appetite (see Behavioral Problems.)

For nutritional support, be sure you are feeding up to 100 mg. of B - Complex vitamins per day for cats and small dogs and 200 mg. for large dogs and horses, adding B-Complex 50 to the Mega Pet Daily you are already using since **Step Two**. This should be doubled if appetite has not improved in forty eight-hours. You should only need the additional vitamin B supplementation for six weeks until the appetite is well regulated (ie. remains stable for at least two to four weeks prior to lowering the dose.) Vitamin B supplementation, in addition to a short twenty-four hour fast with homeopathic support (if it has been more than a month since you began the LifeStyle™ or last fasted), can quickly stimulate the appetite. This is because a lack of appetite is often the result of a toxic overload and common during a curative response to dis-ease.

Herbal Remedy for Appetite Stability

- Daily Boost contains herbs which help cleanse the digestive tract and regulate function which helps regulate the appetite regardless of disorder.

Homeopathic Remedies for Appetite Disorders

- D'Toxifier contains *Arsenicum* which reverses general appetite loss due to its action upon the liver and digestive system. Benefits the pet who also suffers allergic sensitivities which are suppressing appetite. Helps reverse need to eat "whatever." Additional remedies included, such as *Taraxacum* and *Iris,* help regulate metabolism.

- *Alumina* is used for abnormal cravings; to stimulate passing of small hard knotty stool, or when difficulty is present in passing stool of any shape or consistency.

- *Belladonna* benefits the pets with mostly nausea, empty retching and vomiting as well as an aversion to drinking. A dose or two daily of Belladonna, *especially 15 minutes prior to feeding,* can also help to stimulate appetite.

- *China* benefits the anorexic pet who suffers from great prostration, debilitating dis-ease and irritability. May suffer symptoms secondary to chronic fevers.

- *Nux Vomica* is appropriate when appetite loss is accompanied by one or more symptoms including nausea, vomiting, stool problems and/or flatulence. Also stimulates appetite. Dose apart from D'Toxifier.

(see Symptom-specific subjects)

Arthritis

ARTHRITIS can flair up in conjunction with, or as a direct reaction to a prior accident or injury to the vertebrae or joint, a genetic predisposition (hip dysplasia), an infection (feline leukemia, tick fever) and even from certain "reactive" (allergies) or autoimmune conditions where the body attacks its own joint and tendon tissue cells (lupus). Weakened organ systems, especially involving congested or malfunctioning liver, kidneys, adrenal, and thyroid glands, seem to go hand-in-hand with chronic arthritis. Symptoms can best be suppressed and possibly eventually reversed homeopathically and/or herbal while the structure (joints, bone, ligaments, tendons and muscles) is strengthened through nutritional supplementation. Remember that homeopathy stimulates the body into symptom-suppression while the herbs and nutrients support (symptom-suppress temporarily) and fuel the body repairs (plus strengthening) for long-term symptom reversal. Acute arthritic-reactions can be successfully "suppressed" with a few doses of *homeopathy*, given five to fifteen minutes apart in lower potencies (3X to 30C).

Environmental Considerations

- **Slick floors (tile, wood, linoleum; wood shavings or torn newsprint on hard surfaces, etc.)** do more damage resulting in or worsening arthritic conditions than all the car accidents and broken bones combined—plus *it is so preventable.* Keep birds, foals, puppies and kittens on non-slick surfaces for the first six months of their lives to allow the full strengthening of their ligaments and the proper growth of their bones, reducing the instances of slipping "spread-eagle." This position can tear the vital tissues stabilizing the knees, elbows, shoulders and especially the hips. For elderly pets, slick floors can twist ligaments, tear tissue, break bones and create anxiety resulting in pain, a loss of mobility and life enjoyment. Please consider carpet or carpet runners for your home. Keep nails trimmed as these can cause poor footing and arthritic toes.

- **Exercise** is vital to strengthening the bones, muscles and ligaments when preventing or reversing an arthritic condition. Daily play, running and rolling on the ground helps maintain the flexibility needed for optimum structural ability. Jumping high off the ground to catch a flying disc or ball is not recommended, as it puts too much pressure on the joints, back and neck each time the pet lands, including cats. Asking a small dog to jump up into and down out of a car and up and off a high bed or couch will soon lead to arthritic pain. Always provide another means of access. As a rule of thumb—do not ask any aged dog or cat to jump higher than twice their height or comfort level.

Herbal Remedies for Arthritis

- Yucca Intensive is a very effective anti-inflammatory. The roots contain steroidal saponins, which react in the body as chemical steroids do, without the side effects; they also reduce tissue inflammation and pain. Be sure to use a cold-pressed extract found in Azmira®'s rather than the low potency by-product powder or even weaker, teas or tincture. Standardized extract contains up to eighty-five percent more bio-available saponins and is easier on the digestive tract then any other forms.

- Garlic Daily Aid, *doubled the daily dose,* is a wonderful supplement for joints affected by inflammation. Regular foundation dose is excellent maintenance to prevent inflammatory reactions. Provides sulfur for connective tissue repair and strengthening.

- **Daily Boost** contains six excellent dietary herbs for liver and blood detoxification, reducing free radicals that can irritate joints, and improving nutrient utilization for structural support.

- **Calm & Relax** promotes arthritic pain control through restful sleep, relaxed muscles and a greater sense of wellbeing. Especially effective when combined with **Yucca Intensive**.

- **Blood & Lymph Detox** helps detoxify the body of impurities which, when left circulating in the blood, feed the inflammatory response by settling in the joints and surrounding tissues. This formula works more towards a reversal of the weakness which leads to chronic inflammation and joint deterioration. Helps repair damaged tissues and regulates the body's immune system. It is excellent to use when a pet suffers arthritis due to autoimmune disease, or a multitude of other ailments in addition to the arthritic condition.

- **Viral D'Tox** protects the joints from further deterioration while reducing inflammatory reactions in infectious arthritis from both viral *and bacterial* sources. Joint inflammation is *secondary to an infectious state* as seen with cases of tick fever (ehrlichiosis), feline leukemia, FIP, parvo and even periodontal disease.

- **Yeast & Fungal D'Tox** was formulated to fight infectious arthritic conditions associated with Northwest and Valley Fevers and other fungal infection/infestations.

- **Skin & Liv-A-Plex** is beneficial for cases of skin, liver and joint inflammation.

- **Immuno Stim'R** also removes the catabolic waste which feeds the inflammatory response and makes the joints stiffer and hotter. This formula is well suited for maintenance of an arthritic pet, especially one who suffers reactive symptoms associated with allergens or toxins. Can be used to give the other herbal remedies a boost when needed for severely debilitated pets.

- **Stress & A'drenal Plex** promotes vitality, restoring integrity to the adrenal glands when arthritic pain has exhausted the animal. As an adaptogenic formula, these herbs reduce the stress on a body that is constantly exposed to excessive physical or emotional conditions preventing or reversing a severe loss of energy, with anemia, low blood pressure and anxiety.

Nutritional Supplements for Arthritic Pets

in order of benefit

- Increase Super C 2000 (up to 1000 mg. per twenty-five pounds of body weight per day) helps strengthen ligaments and tendons, reduce inflammation, and allergy sensitivities.

- MSM is a sulfur-based product, which not only helps reduce inflammation, repair connective tissue and strengthen the joints but is also wonderful for the poor skin and coat conditions which often affect arthritic animals. This is a great supplement for the whole body, especially the hips. For general arthritic conditions; MSM used with herbal Yucca Intensive is a powerful combination.

- Joint E'zer, pharmaceutically pure Glucosamine and Chondroitin Sulfate, helps repair connective tissue and lubricate the joint for stability and improved movement. These ingredients, contrary to popular belief, do not reduce inflammation well so Yucca Intensive is also recommended in severe cases.

- Glucosamine aids in the repair and strengthening of connective tissues to stabilize joints. "Tighter" joints, which do not slip in and out of the joint capsule, reduce pain and bone destruction which can lead to more severe arthritis. Glucosamine is especially beneficial for arthritic conditions of the neck, back, knee, elbow and hips.

- Shark'Rah is supportive to Glucosamine or MSM by providing *Chondroitin sulfate.* Acts as an additional pain reliever by replenishing synovial fluid, a shortage of which can create the rubbing of bone upon bone (causing pain and encouraging calcium build up) which can result in more severe arthritis.

- GlucoMChondro is formulated with Glucosamine, MSM and Chondroitin sulfate. For those pets with more advanced cases— who would benefit from all three supplements combined.

- Calcium with Boron-3 aids in proper calcium absorption and strengthens bone density. It helps the body avoid calcium build-up or over-calcification, common in arthritic conditions, especially for joints which are breaking down from excessive grinding through hard work or old age. Three months on Calcium with

Boron-3 is a must for any pet who has broken a bone or cracked a vertebra—to help prevent severe arthritis from developing.

- L-Pheny Pet is a powerful, non-addictive analgesic found in clinical research to be as effective in relieving pain as morphine or opiates. It seems to be responsible for increasing the brains endorphins and is beneficial to add when Yucca Intensive and Calm & Relax are not enough to reduce and manage pain.

- Coenzyme Q10 may be used to aid in the prevention or reduction of fibromyalgia (a debilitating disease in pets who suffer severe, chronic arthritis). This supplement is an excellent over-all nutrient for older, arthritic animals.

- Mega Omega-3 fatty acids have been found to help prevent the development of arthritic conditions when added to the daily diet. A reduction in inflammation and stiffness is often reported with omega-3 oils as well as a reduction in muscular tension.

Homeopathic Remedies for Arthritis

- D'Toxifier contains *Arsenicum* which is an excellent general homeopathic arthritic remedy, especially in an animal with a history of poor nutrition and a toxic lifestyle. Many arthritic animals respond well just to **Step One's** homeopathic detoxification for this reason. Additional remedies are found in D'Toxifier which improves nutrient utilization and waste elimination, vital to the management of an arthritic condition. It aids in slowing or reversing premature aging.

- *Arnica* reduces swelling, general muscular pain, and discomfort. Excellent after trauma occurs or after a hard day running the trails.

- *Bryonia* helps when the pet is stiff upon standing and *cannot* walk out of it.

- *Rhus Tox* is for the pet that is stiff upon standing but *can* walk out of it.

- *Hypericum* reduces nerve irritation and pain. Found in animals who are constantly licking their legs and feet, sometimes even their backs, with no evidence of an allergy present. They are licking at the numbness they feel from impinged nerves in their inflamed arthritic joints.

- *Ruta* is best for severe tendon or ligament strains, common in nutritionally-depleted pets. Combine with *Hypericum* for degenerative intervertebral disc disease.

Asthma

ASTHMA is common in animals raised with a toxic lifestyle where the lung tissues are not well nourished and there are many immune-suppressive wastes and chemicals floating in the body. Lack of nutritional sulfur is a prime trigger of weakened lung function. Since the respiratory system is prone to irritation due to its direct contact with allergens and environmental chemicals, it is often overwhelmed and develops irritation and inflammation, even infection. Animals with a history of respiratory allergies are most often diagnosed with asthma and I believe that it has become an all too common diagnosis for upper respiratory stress in general.

An obvious tip to reducing asthma is through the environment. Absolutely do provide a smoke-free environment clear of the scent of perfume, chemical-based cleaning products' fumes or dust. This allows nutritional augmentation and herbal detoxification to go a longer way in reversing the physiological weakness which leads to bronchial stress and asthma. Homeopathic remedies are wonderful in stimulating the reversal of acute asthma-related symptoms.

Herbal Remedies for Asthma

- Aller'G Free is Azmira®'s incredible anti-histamine, proven to open up the airways and reduce acute attacks of wheezing and constriction. Works as well as over the counter antihistamine drugs with no side-effects.

- Yucca Intensive is an outstanding anti-inflammatory remedy, as effective as steroids without the side-effects. Reduces bronchial spasms.

- Aller'G: Grass and Pollen promotes the strengthening of the respiratory system, building resistance to triggers, including dust or mold, which may constrict the bronchial tubes and create chronic wheezing. This is a remedy which supports long-term reversal of asthmatic symptoms.

- Yeast and Fungal D'Tox is specifically for fungal mycosis, such as Valley Fever, which can settle in the respiratory tract creating the asthmatic symptoms.

- Blood & Lymph D'Tox is for the severely debilitated pet who suffers chronic bronchial infections in addition to their asthma. This animal is debilitated from a toxic lifestyle and needs a great deal of support to reverse their respiratory ailments.

Homeopathic Remedies for Asthma

- D'Toxifier contains *Arsenicum* with complementary remedies which help lessen all symptoms of asthma through improved nutrient utilization and waste elimination. D'Toxifier relieves wheezing and the occasional cough in an animal who suffers from a toxic lifestyle but has no clear signs of upper respiratory infection or allergies; borderline asthma. Just the wheeze and occasional cough. Comes and goes.

- *Aconite* is for oppressed breath in the animal who is also debilitated with chronic, severe asthma. Spells can come on suddenly, especially after moments of stress.

- *Carbo Veg.* is for the animal who suffers wheezing and rattling of mucous in the chest. A spasmodic cough with gagging and vomiting of mucous. Worse in the evening and in the open air. Can bring up bloody mucous from chronic cough and bronchial irritation.

- *China* benefits the animal whose periodic episodes of asthma are marked by great prostration.

Nutritional Supplements

- MSM is a wonder sulfur supplement to aid in the repair and strengthening of lung tissue and bronchial tubes. Helps reverse sensitivities and reduce deterioration of the lungs. Builds resistance to pollution, dust and allergens.

- Super C 2000 builds resistance to asthmatic attacks and slows the deterioration of the lung's tissues; increase daily dose to 1000 mg. for cats and small dogs, 4000 mg. for large breeds.

- Grape Seed Extract promotes a reduction of free radicals which are known to trigger asthma-related symptoms.

Bacterial Infection

BACTERIAL INFECTION is often marked by fever and damaged tissue of some type, be it a topical wound (now reddish and probably oozing) or internal pocket of irritation/pus created from a parasite, cancerous tissue, chemical organ damage or stone which allowed anyone of the millions of bacteria floating in the body to take hold and develop into an infection. Bacterial infections, when left untreated, can cause permanent damage and sometimes death. The standard treatment is a course of antibiotics which can be very disruptive to the digestive tract and need to be exactly the *right* ones to treat that *specific* organism. Herbs are much safer and easier to use; they kill off *any* bacterial infection and then stimulate and support the body's immune response to reduce inflammation, repair damaged tissue and avoid recurrence of infection.

(see Infections, Inflammation)

Behavioral Problems

BEHAVIORAL PROBLEMS can be frustrating to reverse because they often result from subtle physical symptoms. Be sure to check for underlying conditions or environmental problems first. Common environmental problems include inconsistent meals or not enough to eat or drink (hunger and dehydration cause nervousness and aggression), lack of a peaceful corner with a bed to sleep in (increases fear-based behavior), extreme weather conditions (creates stress) for an outdoor-only pet, difficult training schedule, etc. Discomfort and illness can also trigger aggression, though some animals respond with nervousness, shyness or complete withdrawal.

Unfortunately, nervousness, fear or any intense emotion, regardless of its cause, will reduce immune function and leave a pet very susceptible to physical weaknesses. Be sure to address the emotional needs of any physically ill pet or a vicious cycle will occur. Their illness leads to emotional suffering which leads to further physical stress/illness. As we know from human health care research (often first done on animals!), this produces stress hormones such as adrenaline, which damage the sensitive tissues of the heart, muscles and digestive tract. They also create thyroid and sugar imbalances and will flood the brain with ammonia which leads to learning and memory difficulties. Therefore, it is not uncommon to find behavioral issues due to physical symptoms and physical symptoms arising form negative behaviors. Physically caring for the pet's needs, in addition to behavioral modification, will help best in these cases.

Alternative medicine acknowledges that organ system malfunction can create specific behavioral problems and vice versa; therefore it is wise to seek a medical diagnosis and address *that* condition with non-responsive chronic behavioral problems. You might have a cat with chronic kidney dis-ease who is not responding to protocol and the animal has been exhibiting fearful behavior. Address the emotional stressor (fear) before changing the kidney protocol again when the stress is relieved or reduced, the body should respond better. Once the body's dis-ease is in balance, the fearful behavior should not return or return infrequently.

Organ Relationships to Negative Behaviors (in general):

Kidneys *are related to* fear
Liver *is related to* aggression
Lungs *are related to* grief and shock
Low back *is related to* guilt
Colon *is related to* repressed emotions, anxiety and jealousy
Brain (seizures) *is related to* nervousness and hyperactivity
Heart *is related to* obsessive behavior and abandonment

Naturopathic remedies work really well at addressing both the underlying emotional and physical aspect of most behavioral problems.

Herbal Remedies *create physical changes and help rehabilitate the nervous system*

- Calm & Relax helps relax the pet and controls pain, allowing them to rest more comfortably and sleep more deeply—all necessary for supporting the curative process. In addition, this herbal remedy can help rebalance the brain's chemistry.

Homeopathic Remedies *also help to change perceptions and resulting behaviors*

- R&R Essence is an excellent first line of defense to prevent negative behavior from developing when there is an emotionally charged situation. It can also be used as needed to reduce the reaction a pet may be having to a situation or stress in general.

- *Aconite* addresses behavior that is the result of situations that produced sudden shock or fear. Can be used with R&R Essence. Excellent for fearful or nervous conditions in general.

- D'Toxifier contains *Arsenicum* with complementary remedies which help lessen negative behavior through improved nutrient utilization and waste elimination. D'Toxifier relieves anger and aggression. Helps stabilize other emotions. In addition to traumatic encounters with humans, toxic lifestyles and diets create toxic behaviors. The liver is a primary organ of anger and this is a wonderful detoxifying remedy.

- *Ignatia* helps to reduce symptoms related to grief or loss. Can be given at the time of the loss to prevent issues or years later when the grief and depressive behavior just won't pass.

- *Thuja*, another remedy in D'Toxifier, helps balance functions of the brain responsible for anger and aggression.

Nutritional Remedies *fuel physical changes and help rehabilitate the nervous system*

- B-Complex 50 provides the additional B vitamins needed to augment Mega Pet Daily, for serious nervous/behavioral cases. Rehabilitates the nervous system and calms nerves. Daily maximum total: 100 mg. for cats and small dogs, 150 mg. for medium sized dogs and 200 mg. for large dogs and horses.

- L-TryptoPet is a pharmaceutically pure amino acid that is a precursor to seratonin and essential for regulating brain activity. Excellent supplement for hyperactive, irritable pets or those with aggression and other mood disorders. Helps with pain relief, promotes sound sleep, and alleviates depression and nervous conditions. Calms aggressive pets.

Prevention of a behavioral problem is still the best cure. Many of the suggestions made in this section can also be applied preventatively. For instance, a pet given a calming remedy prior to a new, potentially difficult situation will be less likely to have a negative reaction due to the stress experienced or perceived. The easier the situation is for the pet, the more likely that this pet will look forward to repeating the experience. From negative experiences an animal learns to react in an emotionally unhealthy manner creating a behavior problem.

The Eight Emotional Dynamics of Behavioral Problems

During my years as a consultant, while working closely with both the pets, veterinarians and owners addressing various emotional issues and behavioral problems that were common to many households, I found that certain emotional dynamics followed suit with certain chronic behavioral problems. Specific flower essence combinations, homeopathic remedies, nutrients and herbs worked the majority of times—better than any others I used, within a specific emotional dynamic and predictable period of time with predictable results.

I set out to prove the eight dynamics existed and later, based on data collected the first time, how good Azmira® remedies performed as compared to Bach® Flowers and in which protocol. Each pet had first been evaluated individually, ruling out any veterinary issues. Behaviors would carefully be identified and described. Each pet was then muscle tested for the most beneficial modalities noted (within the study guidelines) and given an individual remedy or combination until the need no longer existed and the behavior was modified. Remedies were reevaluated every other week, if needed, and changed to continue addressing any emotional traits that surfaced. Other nutritional changes or supplementation would be followed as needed. No physical training happened, only daily bonding/play exercises, massage and another ten minutes of personalized attention directed towards each pet's needs—with remarkable results.

First, I was amazed by how easily so many pets fit into one of eight specific emotional dynamics categories that seemed prevalent to the specific behavioral symptoms which resulted. In addition, each dynamic required both multiple remedies and varying potencies (30C to 200C mostly). Having been classically trained in homeopathy (one remedy, one potency at a time) I needed to have my own attitude adjustment to accept this fact. We simply found that a higher majority of pets documented responded quicker to combinations than single remedies and the remedies far out-performed all other modalities—even when used alone. This is why I later developed Azmira®'s flower combination remedies.

Second, I began to see a pattern of the same remedies coming in clusters, following a specific pattern of behaviors (ie. spraying or biting). After three years I had hundreds of documented successes to validate this truth and continue to follow these recommendations. Especially, I recommend the use of flower combinations as a great starting place. It benefits the process of reversing the emotional dynamic which may be at the root of your pet's behavior.

The Eight Emotional Dynamics

- Abandonment issues
- Aggressive behavior

- Fearful, anxious pets
- Jealousy and resentment
- Needy behavior
- Obsessive behavior
- Shock and grief
- Spraying and marking territory

A good example of using emotional dynamics to understand a pet's behavior and adjust their perception (or emotional filter) to encourage and maintain the appropriate behaviors is expressed in how I have taught hundreds of owners to guide their pet's actions around food and eating. In order to get a dog or cat to respect the fact that when food is being prepared or can be seen it does not mean that they are going to get any and it is not tolerable to the family for them to misbehave, steal food or beg, you must understand what motivates them to act out.

Are they restless because their emotional filter perceives during food preparation that they may starve if they fail to "get any food" due to past experiences of not being properly fed or having to fight for their share? This would be the <u>fearful, anxious dynamic.</u> The second most common, <u>the aggressive dynamic</u> behind food issues such as begging or stealing food, is because they are stimulated by a natural urge to dominate the family—common to their wild cousins whose stronger pack members prove themselves by dominating feedings and getting their share first. If you push this pet away or hit it, it will only reinforce their urge to fight harder to get to the food.

The urge to dominate must be addressed—so the message that (or new urge), "it is okay to sit quietly and even ignore the food unless you are invited by the pack leader" develops—in order to be followed by the appropriate behavior. Reinforcing this new behavior must also occur through the use of a specific treat given after mealtime is complete and the pet behaved properly during that time. It is one of the few times I incorporate treats in my teaching of new behaviors because it's like dessert.

Once you identify and understand their dynamic, you can use the appropriate remedies to help modify your pet's bad behavior. On occasion, a pet can exhibit several dynamics at once. I recommend addressing the most overt symptoms initially and then moving on to whichever emotional issues become more prevalent. For instance with fear-aggression the trigger is fear so I recommend you address the fear first. If the aggressive behavior does not subside then you can add the aggression formula.

Desensitizing Exercises: *Exposing Pets to Their Emotional Triggers to Modify Behavior*

Focus on desensitizing the pet to whatever triggers you suspect (ie. food on the table causes begging or being left alone results in vocalizations) by using small periods of time to expose them to their trigger, over and over, while giving them the appropriate remedies. This is a good weekend project. Use the flower combination and/or appropriate individual remedies before each desensitizing experience and all throughout the day. Desensitizing will continue as often as needed, during the remainder of the time required to reverse the emotional dynamic. It can take a few days or a few weeks, and may return during stressful periods but should continue to improve with time and each positive resolution experienced.

Simply expose the pet to their trigger (i.e. food on the table) for no longer than one to five minutes. Praise them when they relax and remove the trigger or remove them away from it. If the trigger can not be moved, ask the pet to sit in a specific spot in the kitchen away from food but still involved with the family, reinforcing the correct behavior with focused positive attention on them, including play time for five minutes (after the food is put away). Then return to regular routine for a while and repeat cycle each hour or so. I have done this technique up to ten times a day, and by the end of the weekend, the animal was more relaxed and less concerned by the trigger. This has worked on pets who have engaged in certain behaviors for years—even jumping up on guests and demanding attention, which is a very powerful position for a pet and a difficult habit to break. It breaks their preconceived notions and alters their reactions to the trigger by altering their filter, helped along by the repetitiveness and flower remedies. Simply put, they stop *reacting* to stressful situations negatively and start *acting* (behaving) properly as guided.

Desensitizing Exercise (example):

I found Maverick (the cutest mixed breed dog in the world, thank you very much) when he was only approximately ten to twelve weeks old, abandoned on the street. He has had a safe and loving home with me for four years, I have never given him cause not to trust I will be there for him. I recently left him with someone he knows well and loves *but since Mav was away from our home* he reacted with whimpering, pacing, and yelping in protest and rejection. Apparently he only stopped long enough to eat a cookie or two from Artie. His anxiety was palpable and my time in the in-laws' pool was short (no dogs allowed so we hoped he would stay inside with Grandpop Dorfman who doesn't enjoy the pool). Because I want to swim more often, and he does so like to visit their house, I taught him that it's fun to stay with Artie while I'm outside at the pool with the rest of the family.

During the next few visits I gave him a dose of **Abandonment** remedy on the way to their house and continued dosing every few minutes when I got there, before I left him inside to go to the pool. Coming back inside to dose him again every few minutes (and to reassure him) I then left him each time with longer intervals—upon returning inside a few *longer* minutes later—I lavished Mav and Grandpop with love and treats each time "they" behaved and played inside without whining. There's no sense in punishing Maverick to shut him up because he'd rather be outside swimming with my grandchildren. This will only serve to alarm him more. Instead I encouraged him to enjoy playing inside and we taught Maverick the phrase "hush" because he is a whiner when anxious, and at least then I can get him to be quieter about it. The command helps focus him and he becomes less fearful, instead of being allowed to escalate his anxiety. If he is quieted down and not allowed to participate in this behavior he is more likely to learn what it is I am trying to share with him. There is no sense moving on until this is accomplished.

After he got praised and another treat I stepped outside again. If he stayed quiet for a few minutes I stepped back inside and praised him again. If not, I hushed him (with no treat). Then I again repeated the process; leaving him for longer periods of time. I may not have gotten to swim the first few times, I was so busy running in and out but I have helped him learn this way—that staying inside with Artie and several other situations he has encountered since are not so scary.

This negative behavior (the whining and pacing) is stressful for him, limits his being taken along (it is more stressful being left behind all the time) and is embarrassing for me to have a vocal chicken for a dog. So I help him learn to be strong by simply exposing him gently *and consistently* to his fearful triggers. It doesn't take him long at all now to accept new situations or things since he has learned the general routine of "hush, it's okay." He understands now that if he trusts me and experiences what he fears he will be more comfortable with it—so he readily joins in these exercises.

In describing the eight emotional dynamics, in this chapter under their specific headings, I have included Azmira®'s flower combinations and additional homeopathic remedies and handling considerations known to work best in these situations. Although each pet is an individual and each situation is unique, you will find that your pet is very likely to fit into one or more of these categories and that by following the recommendations you will see a decline in negative reactions within a few days. Some pets may need weeks or months of ongoing support for full modification or reversal of certain behaviors, but you should clearly see positive changes to their perceptions, reactions and behavior during this time. Each episode that the pet acts out should be less severe as time goes on and happen less frequently. The pet should become more responsive to you, or you will need to examine other issues at hand and possibly try a different approach. Although changes can happen more subtly or slowly than might be desired, you should be able to identify and rely upon those changes—or you are not working within the correct dynamic.

Behavioral issues are also on the rise, as more pets exhibit aggressive or fearful attitudes and have trouble learning to get along with their human families. Although many breeds are predisposed toward these behaviors, they are more likely to be triggered by chemicals and sugar in their diet, as well as early experiences of abandonment or mistreatment; therefore—these behaviors are preventable, regardless of "poor" genetics. This is what The Holistic Animal Care LifeStyle™ is all about—stimulating the most positive genetic potential your pet has to prevent or reverse problems.

Understanding Your Pet's Behavior

Dogs and cats are pack animals who crave the familiar and need close family contact. Love is as vital to them as the air they breathe. If they cannot be near you and are not allowed to live within the family unit, they will seek contact any way they can—including drawing negative attention to themselves.

Dogs who are left outside or kenneled for the majority of the day live shorter lives and suffer a higher incidence of behavioral or physical problems. Even if you are away at work, if they have access to both the house and yard, they will feel more like they are contributing by protecting the "cave". If left isolated to one area or outside, they feel "banished" from the house (your cave) and will stress from feeling abandoned.

A feline companion can be quite difficult to understand at times. If left isolated, they demand to be noticed. Given attention, some seem to prefer to ignore us. Unlike dogs who have a strong urge to "cave" with their human pack, cats can be quite happy *seemingly* spending their time alone, yet will also feel stressed and "abandoned." Whether you do or do not notice the distress in your pet, this may eventually manifest itself as a symptom. Your dog or cat may then develop a behavioral problem and/or a physical condition.

Horses and birds identify themselves as prey. Your actions are often regarded as suspect until a great level of trust has developed. This can cause a great deal of stress and behavioral issues. They too need to be bonded and can suffer a sense of abandonment, especially boredom, resulting in physical ills. It is not uncommon for a bird to engage in feather picking when alone without daily companionship from their human. Horses are well known to also develop bad habits, such as cribbing, when left isolated in a stall for long periods of time.

The majority of behavioral problems are created by miscommunication between the caregiver and the companion—because you are speaking two different languages. Consider for a moment if you were in a foreign land and trying to understand your tour guide who did not speak anything familiar to your own language. What a relief it is when you both develop some familiar signals. Dogs and cats, along with our other companions such as horses, ferrets and birds, are looking at us constantly for signals and trying to decipher what we are saying, since they desperately want to please us. Begin understanding your animal by putting yourself in his or her point of view. Ask yourself if your companion can rely on:

- **Your love**—consistent, fair and gentle; focused and sincere

- **Your attention**—daily regard for their emotional and physical well-being

- **Your care**—responsive to disorder, accident or illness; acute or long-term

- **Your home**—to be a safe and loving shelter; free of fear or stress

- **Your devotion**—during the easy, fun times *and* the difficult ones

Providing your animals' well-being and raising them well, exploring and changing certain things to fit their needs—rather than only your own—can prevent a lot of struggle on both your parts.

Training Without Trauma

You should never raise your hand to any animal, large or small. Many people think large breeds and animals such as Rottweilers and horses require more brute force when in fact they are often gentle and more responsive than the toy breeds and cats. When you raise your hand to animals, they will only think that you are attacking them—you are being an aggressive threat. This is especially true for animals such as horses and birds who identify themselves as prey, and respond as such. Most people hit their pets out of frustration due to poor communication. Animals learn by repetition. It requires numerous repetitions for an animal to hear the command and correctly associate it with the desired behavior. Then you can rely on the fact that your companion *understands* and is not simply reacting to your cues.

Be absolutely clear and consistent in the signals you are giving:

- Do not say "shoo" one time and "no" the next—use No! only as NO! Mean it.

- Do not use "no" indiscriminately—your pet will simply become deaf to it.

- Give a warning **"NO!"**, if behavior continues—say it deeper, with more growl-tones. A shot of water from a spray bottle or water pistol, *at the moment of sin,* does help.

- If a second warning is needed: *for dogs* grab at their collar or loose jowl skin and *for cats,* grab the loose skin at the back of the neck, applying slight jerk. This method of discipline should be used immediately if biting or scratching is involved. Also, keeping your fingers, hand or arm in the animal's mouth—until they try to get away—will quickly take the fun out of their "attacking" you. Besides there is no leverage for them to actually get a good "bite" with something already filling their mouth. Remember to keep anger and emotions out of the interaction. *Do not hurt them, just frustrate them!*

- Third & *final warning*—only if needed for discipline—is to hold cats or ferrets back by the collar or loose skin, keep horses standing still or backing up with repetitive cues and hold birds into submission for 10 seconds (count it off)—don't let them move. Animals hate being "held back" and they will quickly do what is needed to regain their freedom. They will behave.

- Third & *final warning for dogs*—only if needed for discipline—is to roll them onto their back by the collar or jowl skin and pin them into submission for 10 seconds (count it off).

- If behavior escalates—isolate the animal in a quiet place, no longer than 15 minutes, or they will forget they were "banished." Allow them back into the fold without fanfare, yet quickly praising the next positive behavior they exhibit.

This method of discipline helps focus a bird's or horse's attention. It also more closely resembles how a bitch or queen will discipline her own babies—which is how the puppy or kitten (and adult) is "wired" to be disciplined (it's their language). Therefore, they will quickly respond and understand that this is not acceptable behavior—without the need to chase them about, screaming and hitting them or ignoring them until the problem gets worse, possibly to the point of no return.

Sometimes, you do have to get creative as did a client of mine because her African Grey was very naughty, at times putting himself in danger. Easy to have these birds get in trouble as they are the most intelligent of all. Ollie was full of pranks and one day he went too far. After three warnings his human companion told him how disappointed she was in him and covered his cage for a timeout. This was the second time this had happened. But this time, Ollie cried out to watch his favorite television show and was told he had to wait his fifteen minutes to be up. That did it. It was enough consequences for Ollie. When he came out of time-out he kept his back to his companion for another fifteen minutes while enjoying his show, ruffling his feathers every now and then, but he never did pull her teaspoon out of her hot teacup again.

To avoid any additional behavioral problems during your training, always use the same room, such as a bathroom, for your "banishment." Horses can be put back in their stall while you take a break elsewhere; the separation for them is perceived differently and is effective. Birds need to be covered and lose treats, as did Ollie, if they keep acting up. Select a room where your pet would not normally choose to be. Do not banish them to their bed or if you are crate training, then do not use your crate for banishment; your pet will think of the crate as a bad thing. Same goes for the backyard. This will cause a lot of stress when you use the crate or yard for keeping your pet in when you leave the house. These are methods I do not advocate. Instead, close off the kitchen or utility room to give them room to play during the day with their potty area in a far corner away from the sleeping area, favorite bed and toys. This is even better with access to a yard for dogs to potty and run in or an outdoor enclosure for cats. Excessive retention of urine and stools are also a primary cause for chronic kidney and bowel conditions as well as an unhappy, restless animal.

This is how the LifeStyle™ works: everything you do helps (or hurts) all aspects of your pet's life, emotional, physical and behavioral, while prevention is the best cure. Avoid major behavioral and health conditions from even starting by taking a few moments to see life from your animal's point of view and creating, with just a few changes, a life in which your pet will thrive… not just survive.

To help your pet understand and develop a fondness of learning from you:

- Do not work with your animals when they are hungry or you are in a bad mood or short-tempered. Concentration and clear emotions are fundamental to a positive learning environment.

- Begin each session with play/exercise—this will focus the animal and let off nervous energy for both you and your charge.

- Always use the same signals and commands and follow the same routine.

- Set aside time each day to practice communicating together, by working together.

- FIRST understand what you will teach, go over it in your head— THEN teach it.

- Be very clear in your praise-phrase and use the same words/tone each time.

- Go over new commands until perfect—BEFORE learning another new one—this builds confidence in you and your pet. Confusion will erode effective communication quickly.

- Always end training sessions with a few minutes of exercise/play/ fun.

- End the session with your animal eager to continue learning—not freaked out.

I do not advocate that you only rely on clicker or treat-based training. I have seen too many pets become unruly when these training aids are missing. Such as when you are bringing in the groceries and your hands are full. It is best, in my opinion, to train through communication and emotional reward for daily, long-term benefits. During my years as a professional animal behaviorist, I had the opportunity to work with clients who had previously trained their dogs through clicker and/or treat methods, and then had to seek my services after repeated incidents.

Regardless of the behavior issues such as biting, pulling at the lead, and unwillingness to behave in general, they all turned out to be triggered by poor communication. The dogs simply did not know how to respond to everyday commands when the training gear was not out. Once the owners and dogs went through the exercises described in my *Training without Trauma* book (Crossing Press, 1997), they learned to communicate and appreciate daily demands of family living versus tricks. The remedies used to help reverse behavioral tendencies such as aggression, fear, neediness, obsessive behaviors, etc. are all described in Chapter Ten, <u>Symptoms A to Z</u>. These issues can severely interfere with an animal's ability to behave properly and respond quickly to herbal and homeopathic support, in addition to behavioral guidance.

Seek professional help when needed, especially with aggressive pets, but be sure that you feel comfortable with your trainer and do not trust someone your pet does not trust. The best training is more than training; it is behavior modification through teaching, best started from day one. Any pet at any age can learn to behave, once you clearly explain the rules and follow them yourself. Just be sure to teach at their level. For instance, do not try to teach a kitten a complicated trick until they are at least nine months old and can mentally comprehend what is being asked and have the concentration to follow it. Kittens, puppies, foals and other young animals can only function at rudimentary levels, just like human infants. Teach the simple stuff well (come, sit, stay, etc.) to build confidence; the harder exercises and tricks will easily follow later.

Taking the time to properly educate your pet will provide you with a better, more reliable companion. An educated animal is less likely to be destructive, to run off and get hit by a car, to hurt another pet or human, or to develop bad habits—because you are correcting this before it becomes a problem. More importantly, educated pets are less likely to get sick because you are spending more time with them—due to the fact that they are pleasant and fun to be around! Interestingly, many people do not consider a cat to be "trainable", but anyone who has opened a can of cat food and had their cat come running from another part of the house knows how "trainable" a cat is. One of my clients once shared with me that her cats even knew the difference between an electric can opener used for their food and the one used for opening the family's fruit-filled cans. They never showed up if the other one was turned on...yet the owner herself could not hear any difference between the two. Possibly, it was the difference in the cans themselves?! This is repetitive action and reward at its best.

Teach Your Pet To Stand For Examination and To Be Transported

The most important thing to teach an animal is how to be handled properly without fuss. Animals such as dogs, cats, ferrets, birds or horses should stand still for all examinations and treatments. They do not mind being handled by you or any other person. An educated pet should allow him or herself to be picked up and held or kenneled indefinitely without stress, if ever needed for an emergency trip to the vet or a neighbor's house. They do not mind being put in a carrier for transportation or riding in a moving vehicle. (These are the only two reasons you should crate train.) Even if your pet allows you to hold them, you must be able to touch all over their body and paws, look inside their ears or mouth and do anything else that might need to be done if ever they are hurt or ill. The additional stress of *fearing* being held and examined can do more harm than the injury or illness itself. This is easy to teach; **pet your pet everyday.** Rub your hands all over their body at least once a day, it will make them very happy (especially if you throw in a massaging action once in a while), give you the opportunity to examine them for bumps, scraps or stickers to be dealt with, and give you a moment of peace, love and wellness (it is a scientifically proven stress reliever). Remember that many animals, horses and birds in particular, perceive themselves to be prey; approach with care and do not startle.

Choosing The Right Animal, Especially Your Dog or Cat, Prevents Many Problems

If you have not already brought home a puppy or kitten and are considering a new addition to your family, then consider what kind of pet will suit you best—to avoid clashing with your pet's needs. Many behavioral problems are really genetic markers at work. For example: a Terrier is bred to dig—if you are a gardener and don't like another digging up your flowers—then think again. A Sheltie might be small, but they require a lot of running around or they can become destructive. A Great Dane does not require a lot of exercise, but can be a handful to train for a senior citizen. Poodles do not shed, but they require a lot of grooming. So do Persian Cats... and they shed! Siamese cats are extremely vocal and needy—not for those who cherish their peace and quiet. Even if you have owned your pet for years, research the many breed books available. Talk to a veterinarian and trainer to learn about the feeding, exercise and care required of any particular breeds that interest you before bringing home a lifelong partner or to improve the care of those you already love. The more prepared you are, the less problems you will encounter.

Noah's Theory

I have long advocated that dogs, cats, birds, horses and others be raised in two's of the same species since most are such pack animals and we (as pack leader and primary friend) are often not available to them. An animal pal can keep another from going crazy and acting out or becoming ill from turning the loneliness inward. That's not to say that having only one pet at home is detrimental, especially when you spend a lot of time with them and socialize them often. Since cats play differently than dogs, and birds or horses have their own ways, you can see why two horses would be better companions than a horse and a cat. Certainly a horse and a cat can have a wonderful, loving and playful relationship together as I have witnessed with my own; it's just that they can't meet as many needs as another of the same type so I have two horses and two cats. Although there may be a lot of fur static and hissing initially, most cats take to each other rather quickly if not forced together. Birds' feathers will ruffle while horses may nip and kick a bit but soon find their place. Never force any issues with a bird, horse or feline or they will make an emotional beeline as far away from the situation as possible. They are also not as forgiving at times as a dog might be, so plan new changes carefully. Regardless of breed, never force the issue. Use remedies when needed as listed under the specific headings of FEAR, AGGRESSION, etc.

More than two of a kind and too many kinds around the house, and you run the risk of not having enough of yourself to go around. I believe you should never have more pets than you can pet at the same time! Those who keep all the animals they rescue, which end up numbering in the double digits, are the most generous souls but can often have many animals lacking in basic care and health. Of course, financially, if you cannot afford to give good food and care for two, four or six then have only one of each. Spread too thin, in any direction and you will hurt both yourself and your animals. It is best to care for one really, really well—than two poorly.

The more attention and quality time a pet spends with their human, the healthier and more well-adjusted they will be. Another pet to play with is not to be a substitute for your love and attention, but can make a difference in your relationship, considering that you will better enjoy the company of two well-behaved dogs or cats, than one neurotic one. Some pets do prefer to have you all to themselves but if you do not have a lot of time during the week for your animal, please consider another so they can have each other's company.

The more time and attention that you take in understanding your pet and his or her needs, the easier it will be to prevent behavioral issues from ruining your relationship. A happy, well-adjusted animal is one who is less likely to suffer from disease as well. Emotional stress can have as much to do with immune dysfunction and the manifestation of symptoms as diet can. A pet who is fed the very best diet and is supplemented but lives stressed out or fearful all the time will have trouble assimilating nutrients and maintaining good health. Providing a loving, stable home will help support your animal's well-being as much as anything else you can do.

(see Abandonment; Aggression; Fear; Jealousy; Needy; Obsessive; Shock; Spraying & Marking Territory)

Bites

(See Abscesses, Infection)

Biting

(see Aggression)

Bladder or Kidney Disorders

BLADDER OR KIDNEY DISORDERS sometimes occur in conjunction with other conditions, especially during the elimination of waste products during fasts or curative responses. The deeper stages of detoxification can also produce *the very* symptoms more commonly related to bladder or kidney problems such as difficulty when urinating or incontinence, discharges and infectious states (WBC's and bacteria seen in urine sample), and metallic or sweet-smelling urine. Once detoxification is complete, these symptoms suddenly clear up on their own. Avoid drug-based antibiotics to treat any minor infections during this time.

Following several studies, Azmira® proved in clinical studies that acute symptoms of kidney, urinary tract or bladder infections from detoxification cleared up within a couple days with the continued LifeStyle™ protocol. With the more serious symptoms, in pets with chronic blockages the addition of Kidni Flow (with a lot of dis-eased tissue and crystals to eliminate) or Kidni Biotic (to reverse or prevent infection) gave over eighty-percent symptom relief within seventy-two hours. Once symptoms have abated, give the body at least four to six weeks of holistic support to completely reverse infections or blockages and strengthen new, healthy urinary tract tissue on its own.

The urinary tract is a vital component to the body's eliminatory system; the removal of toxins, metabolic or catabolic wastes, and parasitic organisms from the blood is paramount to maintaining wellness. It is helpful to be familiar with your pet's urinary habits, including water intake, and output. Stool and urine are the best indicators of health, or imbalance, and can help you determine quickly the next change in protocol.

Healthy urine does not have a strong smell

For instance, strong ammonia-smelling urine indicates a diet heavy in animal by-products or difficult-to-digest proteins; an infection present will often produce a putrid metallic urine smell while a sugar imbalance can shed a sickly sweet odor through the urine. Be sure to seek a veterinarian's diagnosis if your animal's elimination and urine changes dramatically and/or is non-responsive to remedies within a few days.

Healthy urine is sunny yellow

While on Mega Pet Daily, in recommended therapeutic levels, your pet's urine should be a deep sunny yellow and have no offensive odor. Once you know what your animal's normal output and drinking behavior is, you can easily see these various markers show themselves and make necessary protocol adjustments to continue on path. I've listed the most obvious triggers first for you to rule out. Try adjusting supplements first— the B vitamins color the urine and can be misleading. Consider if the body is detoxifying; when an animal's thirst demands more fluid to help cleanse cellular tissue and remove catabolic waste from the body, which then presents itself in increased urine output.

Clear urine to light yellow color may indicate that the animal is:

- not receiving adequate amounts of Mega Pet Daily , especially B vitamins, for their individual needs. *(check recommendations on label and add 50 mg. of* B-Complex 50 *if you are already feeding the highest therapeutic level of* Mega Pet Daily.*)*

- drinking excessive water *(check for salty foods and treats, seek diabetes screen).*

Dark yellow color may indicate that the animal is:

- not drinking enough fluids or is suffering from slight dehydration (first: *be sure the pet can physically drink,* second: *check fresh water source and provide a drink of diluted fruit juice in water. Fruit-flavored ice cubes make great treats).*

- detoxifying from a rancid meat diet/liver cleansing/vaccinosis (*follow detoxifying recommendations and provide remedies for specific symptoms/weaknesses).*

- too alkaline, with potential crystallization/gravel/bacteria (*double* Super C 2000 *and consider a six-week round of* Kidni Flow *to support a deeper detoxification of the urinary tract)*

Dark yellow-orange urine may indicate:

- too high of a dose of Mega Pet Daily (*lower daily intake by 25% until urine is sunny yellow again).*

- dehydration (*loss of fluids through stress, illness, diarrhea and/or vomiting requires oral syringe feedings of fluids; give up to one ounce of water per one pound of body weight per day).*

Chronic dark yellow-orange urine <u>with smell</u> may indicate:

- advanced dehydration and/or potential kidney tissue damage, including loss of blood cells *(use* Kidni Kare, *Phospherous30C and seek medical advice regarding subcutaneous fluids).*

- advanced stage infection (Kidni Biotic).

- crystallization, potential blockage (Kidni Flow).

Nutritional and Herbal Recommendations for Bladder and Kidney Problems

- *Provide plenty of fresh pure drinking water* and monitor daily water intake. Add water to food to increase fluid intake if needed.

- *Increase* Super C 2000 to therapeutic levels—at least 1000 mg. for cats and per 25 lbs. of dog's body weight per day—to acidify the urine, kill off bacteria and support tissue repair.

- *Decrease therapeutic levels* of MSM as this <u>alkalizes</u> the urine which discourages the elimination of debris, crystallizations or stones.

- Calcium with Boron-3 provides calcium to prevent the body *from storing calcium.* Boron improves assimilation and tissue repair. When the body is lacking in minerals (or leeching them from bone tissue due to dis-ease) it attempts to store this mineral to ward off *starvation,* or total loss. Unfortunately, where the body chooses to store minerals (resulting in bladder stones, bone spurs and calcified joints) can be detrimental in the long run.

Although traditional veterinary logic is to reduce minerals when this occurs—I saw another connection over twenty years ago and began working with therapeutic levels of calcium and magnesium to reverse arthritis and bladder stones with great success.

In 2004, Harvard Medical School published reports that backed up my theories and recommended mineral supplementation for bladder stones. One-half dose per day for cats and small pets to one dose per day for larger dogs and horses provides ample additional supplementation to the current recommended levels in Mega Pet Daily.

- Kidni Flow was formulated for increased urine output and to dissolve blockages. It is an excellent stone emulsifier, urinary tract detoxifier and disinfectant (antiseptic) which help eliminate recurrence of F.U.S. and infections. This compound also works as a restorative and is beneficial during cleansing periods as it stimulates the removal of catabolic waste (waste from the blood and tissues) and encourages elimination via the kidneys—minimizing the recurrence of troublesome symptoms during periods of detoxification. This is safe and effective renal support in even the worse cases, regardless of history. Remember: the evidence of traces of blood, infection or debris in the animal's urine during times of detoxification is a good sign—the pet is *eliminating* this waste—and it is a perfectly normal part of rebalancing and strengthening the urinary tract system. Continued support through the LifeStyle™ protocols and Azmira products will quickly and effectively reverse most urinary tract blockages, when followed as directed.

- Kidni Kare is a combination of herbs that work well together controlling incontinence by restoring, regulating and strengthening the musculature, toning membranes and helping to balance hormones associated with the urinary system. Can be used with Calm & Relax for severe cases of hormonal dysfunction due to spaying, neutering, old age, etc. Relieves minor irritation and general weakness. Can be used as a restorative tonic to strengthen the musculature of the general pelvic organs after surgery, injury or atrophy. Excellent support for senior pets becoming weak in their urinary function.

- Kidni Biotic contains herbs which are very fast acting, powerful antibiotics for urinary tract infections, including cystitis (inflammation of the bladder) and nephritis (inflammation of the kidneys). Can be safely used with Yucca Intensive for severe cases of inflammation and pain. Kidni Biotic contains certain therapeutic agents known to target the very bacteria which create the irritation and inflammation. These herbs are safer for long-term treatment and crisis care in older or more debilitated pets, and can be used safely with prescribed antibiotics if needed (for life-threatening infections). While drugs only attack the acute infection, these herbs also increase the pet's natural resistance and repair eliminatory system organs. When the pet is weaned from the chronic drug use, the herbal properties will take over the task of protecting the urinary tract and reduce the likelihood of infection recurrence.

- Yucca Intensive can relieve inflammation and pain in the urinary tract. Use instead of steroids to control symptoms. Proven in clinical studies to be as effective as drugs yet without the side-effects. Has added detoxifying and liver supportive benefits.

- Stress & A'Drenal Plex promotes vitality, restoring integrity to the adrenal glands when the bladder or kidney dis-ease has exhausted the animal. As an adaptogenic formula, these herbs reduce the stress on a body that is constantly exposed to excessive physical or emotional conditions preventing or reversing a severe loss of energy, with anemia, low blood pressure and anxiety.

Herbal Kidni-*Maintenance:* One bottle (approx. four to six weeks) of either standardized herbal Kidni-formula, every four months, works wonders in eliminating the recurrence of that group of urinary tract symptoms. It's an inexpensive insurance policy—keeping your pet symptom-free. When used at the first sign of symptoms it can quickly reverse the onset of these symptoms before a problem can occur. Continue to use for six weeks after symptoms are reversed to prevent reoccurrence.

Homeopathic Remedies for Bladder and Kidney problems

- ***Thlaspi Bursa* for the most urgent, emergency need without urine presenting; frequent F.U.S. with blockages.** Use every five to fifteen minutes until urine passes, then every hour for four hours until pet is resting well. Use twice a day for four days to promote full reversal of the blockage.

- D'Toxifier contains *Arsenicum* in addition to other remedies* which improve kidney function, bladder tone, nutrient utilization and elimination including improved urine flow. Relieves scant, burning, involuntary urine which may contain epithelial cells; clots of old tissue and globules of pus and blood. This way, D'Toxifier prevents the blockage of waste in the urinary tract during detoxification by stimulating the organs of elimination. It is a recommended part, used as described in **Step One**, of the F.U.S. prevention protocol. If the kidneys are cleansing (and flowing) they can't be blocking up with the additional waste the body is sending their way during everyday detoxification. This is always a good remedy to try first if it is not an emergency situation. If the situation is an emergancy, begin D'Toxifier and follow with whichever other remedy or medical treatment is appropriate for your pet.

- *Cantharis,* the most popular remedy for bladder and kidney problems, is used for pets with a frequent, strong urge to urinate, possibly with pain—but not passing gravel or blood. When painful elimination is interfering with output, it can help stimulate flow of urine. It is also beneficial in reversing incontinence due to bladder irritation. Pet is often irritable.

- *Apis* provides great relief to those who experience kidney and bladder inflammation. There is much discomfort straining to pass only a few drops of urine. The abdomen is sensitive to touch, and the pet's attitude is bleak.

- *Belladonna* is an excellent remedy for incontinence due to acute urinary infections, or when high levels of phosphates are present in urine. Urine is almost continually being released by the body; can be dark and cloudy.

- **Berberis* is helpful with obvious back pain from urination or motion afterwards.

- *Gelsemium* supports control of urine flow, especially when incontinence is due to partial paralysis of the bladder. Urine is often profuse, clear and watery.

- **Juniperus* promotes the healthy flow of urine while addressing kidney inflammation, congestion and cystitis.

145

- *Lycopodium* is best used when there seems to be red sand in the urine. This pet may also suffer fatty growths or poor coat conditions.

- *Mercurius* is indicated for a small volume of dark urine, often present with infection. Often painful at beginning of flow, with uncontrollable urges. Pet may become aggressive.

- *Sarsaparilla* addresses even the most severe pain, especially when accompanied by dribbles of urine. *Best to be used in addition to* Yucca Intensive *and/or* Calm & Relax.

- *Urtica Urens* is another good general remedy for kidney and bladder symptoms. Promotes the flow of urine, reduces pain and discharges. Reduces crystals, stones, gravel and blockages. This pet often suffers an arthritic or allergic condition as well.

- *Uva Uris* also addresses chronic blockage and can be used as *Thlaspi Bursa* when that is not available. For cystitis; bloody urine and calculi (gravel) inflammation. Urine has grit in it, pus or slime, and causes much pain in passing.

WARNING: Serious problems during urinating, such as excessive straining with little or no urine output for twelve hours or more, should be evaluated immediately by a veterinarian.

(see Detoxification and Infections)

Bleeding

BLEEDING problems can be quickly quelled:

- Internal bleeding, gums, and other general bleeding problems respond to acute dosing of homeopathic *Phosphorous*. Use this in addition to these listed suggestions.

- For cuts to the quik of the nail, apply pressure with a dab of baking soda, corn meal or sugar till the bleeding stops.

- For cuts and bleeding scraps, apply pressure with a clean cloth saturated with Rejuva Spray. This will stop acute bleeding plus help the skin heal quickly.

- With severe, deep cuts requiring veterinary attention, spray with Rejuva Spray then wrap the area well and apply pressure on the way to the clinic. Apply a tourniquet above a badly bleeding limb. Dose with homeopathic *Phosphorous* and R&R Essence.

Blind Animals

BLIND ANIMALS can lead very normal lives given a little understanding and support. They are very adaptable to their surroundings, becoming perfectly at ease with each step as they move around their quickly memorized locations. Obviously, if the route has been memorized and the chair is suddenly left out away from the dining room table, then there's going to be a collision. Learn from your animal how it is that they are dealing with their predicament and support that. Teach them some cues for when they are approaching a potentially dangerous situation and commands for "left," "right," "back up" and "forward." Common sense and a little awareness on your part can make the life of a blind animal easy and fulfilling.

Reversing blindness has been accomplished but it is a process which depends on the condition of the eyes and brain connection themselves. Some animals, having suffered a viral dis-ease or genetic mishap, are missing actual tissue behind their eyes from which to see. Seek out the advice of a top rated veterinary eye specialist for a proper diagnosis and explanation of the condition, then approach each weakness to see if there is any possibility for recovery. For example: Has there been a history of vaccinosis, a common cause of blindness? Apply recommendations to reverse the effects of vaccinosis and feed additional nutrients for eye health. Is this related to trauma to the head? Use the anti-inflammatory protocol. Cataract growth? Follow the cataract protocol.

Spontaneous blindness can occur from a severe reaction to a vaccination or allergic reaction and can be very responsive to detoxification and curative stimulation as listed in those respective symptom-specific subjects. When there is pressure on the eyes or brain from injury or in response to a substance resulting in blindness, then herbal support is often beneficial and successful in reversing these conditions.

(see Cataracts, Eye Problems and Symptom-specific subjects such as Infection, Inflammation)

Bloat

BLOAT *or gastric dilation* is a condition common to large, deep-chested dogs, especially Great Danes, Irish Setters, English Sheepdogs, Standard Poodles, German Shepherds, Dobermans, Boxers, Labs and Rottweilers. Some long-bellied dogs, such as Dachshunds, may also be more prone, particularly when fed only one meal per day or poor quality diets. Cats are also susceptible to bloat while horses have a particularly fatal form of bloat called colic. Both would also benefit from these suggestions.

Bloat is a gastric backup of gases resulting in a distended, *bloated* belly with excessive salivation and rapid breathing. At the onset, pets will be very restless due to pain, possible seeking to eat grass. As the disease progress, vomiting (except in horses) with severe constipation, weakness and eventually shock will set in. It is possible that without treatment the stomach may actual twist itself over—requiring surgical intervention.

Improper diet and infrequent or unscheduled feeding (only once a day or at different times each meal) are more to blame than any breed predisposition. Digestive difficulties due to soybean and other poor quality or inappropriate ingredients—commonly used in commercial dog food— can lead to a build-up of waste product in the form of gases. Flatulence is the first symptom, often ignored until the situation becomes a more serious and chronic, life-threatening condition.

Prevention is the best cure! But in the event that bloating still occurs in your pet, homeopathic remedies can be life saving. Given individually or together, every five to fifteen minutes until there is some relief and then hourly until total reversal of the attack, these remedies can address the majority of indications. But get to the vet immediately if within a half-hour of dosing there has been no relief.

Homeopathic Remedies

- D'Toxifier contains *Arsenicum* with complementary remedies which help lessen bloating through improved nutrient utilization and waste elimination; benefits chronic conditions of a toxic lifestyle; general restorative to prevent reoccurrence. Targets all the organs of elimination, helps relieve gas and reduces shock.

- *Carbo Veg.* reduces stomach distention with gas; possibly bluish tint to the tongue and gums; reverses shock. This is a well known and trusted bloat remedy.

- *Nux Moschata* has been successful for severe gastric stress with a painfully tight belly; dry mouth with unsuccessful attempts to vomit; final stages of bloat with shock or disorientation.

- *Nux Vomica* is for the initial symptoms and anxiety; to prevent or reverse twisting of the stomach; excellent first-aid remedy to have on hand for digestive disorders and bloat symptoms, but do not use with D'Toxifier, antidotes each other.

- *Raphanus* is for extreme and sudden bloating—without the ability to pass gas.

Preventing Bloat Recurrence

- D'Toxifier, when given as one weekly dose, helps maintain a bloat-free pet

- *Homeopathic Sepia*, especially if hard, dark stools are common or *Belladonna* which addresses chronic, colic-like symptoms can also help prevent a reoccurrence. Use these remedies two to four times per day for two weeks while **Step One** detoxification and diet changes are implemented, then taper off to one weekly dose for another month.

- Daily Boost is an herbal blend which helps prevent bloating and colic when used as a daily supplement.

(see Digestive Disorders)

Body Odor

BODY ODOR is a common complaint among pet owners, especially dog lovers. The skin is the largest eliminatory organ on the body and what waste is not exuded through the kidneys and liver is cleansed through this organ. This creates odor and feeds bacteria, which creates more odor. The next most likely culprit is scent glands and anal glands, both of which are affected by a toxic body and lifestyle.

Permanently Eliminate Pet Odor

- Follow **Step One** recommendations in Chapter 4.

- D'Toxifier contains homeopathic *Arsenicum* with complementary remedies which help lessen body odor through improved nutrient utilization and waste elimination; minimizes odoriferous glands and skin secretion (sebaceous cysts). Benefits chronic conditions of a toxic lifestyle; general restorative.

- Homeopathic *Mercurius* is an excellent choice when the body's odor smells foul.

- Immuno Stim'R, which is an herbal catabolic detoxifier that helps eliminate body odor-causing wastes. Works wonders during a maintenance protocol to permanently eliminate and prevents stubborn body odor.

- Skin & Liv-A-Plex is an excellent herbal product for more severe cases of body odor from the skin.

- Blood & Lymph D'Tox, another herbal formula, should be considered for severe cases of glandular dysfunction.

Boils

(see Abscesses)

Breath, with a bad odor

BREATH, WITH A BAD ODOR is always the sign of toxicity, including teeth and gum problems, infection associated with oral abscesses, a recently ingested or mouthed "yucky thing." If these are ruled out; *think compost heap.* When you turn over a well-decayed compost pile, the trapped gases are released. Same thing occurs in the digestive tract, releasing these gases either down towards the flatulence factory or up through the mouth. Bad breath means garbage (old, undigested food) is built up inside the digestive tract due to poor quality ingredients and/or improper digestion and slow elimination.

(see Chapter 4: **Step One**, Digestive Issues, Infections, Teeth and Gums)

Breathing Difficulties

(see Upper Respiratory Illness)

Bronchitis

BRONCHITIS is a dis-ease of the bronchi (branches) of the respiratory tree inside the lungs and is the leading cause of coughs in animals. More appropriate is the term tracheobronchitis due to the fact the inflammation often occurs in both the trachea and bronchi. Incessant coughing is the marker for this dis-ease. Generally we see a dry, hacking cough whereas in other cases of chemical irritation or bacterial infection we are faced with a wet cough, productive with mucous.

(see Asthma, Cough)

Burns

BURNS can be very painful and difficult to heal in animals. Obviously for severe burns you will need veterinary support but these recommendations can help with all types of burns.

Nutrition is paramount to growing healthy skin quickly:

- MSM, in addition to double the daily recommendation for Garlic Daily Aid provides sulfur for tissue repair while garlic is also a natural antibiotic.

Herbal Remedies

- Yucca Intensive can reduce pain and swelling. It has been proven as effective as steroid medications without any of the side-effects. Promotes circulation, important for bringing nutrient-rich blood to the injured area. Helps reduce scarring.

- Calm & Relax worked wonders for a cat—burned over sixty percent of her body—to stay calm and better tolerate the pain without the drugs she couldn't stomach. Reducing the stress that the pain caused improved her healing time so she could go home early.

- Topically, use Rejuva Spray for its antibacterial properties to protect against or fight infection. This product also contains herbs to soothe the tissue and reduce pain/itching on contact, while also improving healing time. I personally treated a severe burn on my own hand with this product alone and not only did not need additional treatment, the doctor could not believe how rapidly (and with little pain) I healed.

- Rejuva Gel protects healing tissue from scarring. Use after Rejuva Spray, once the pain is gone and the burn is not angry (first twelve to twenty-four-hours). This will prevent scarring while decreasing the healing time needed. Good for sun burns on snouts.

Homeopathic Remedies

- D'Toxifier promotes tissue repair and a reduction in pain through improved nutrient utilization and elimination of damaged cells. Addresses inflammation and pain.

- *Arnica* and/or *Hypericum* are remedies which can help reduce the pain associated with burns.

(see Skin Conditions)

Cancer

CANCER can often be the end result of a long-term bout with other poor health conditions, such as allergies or thyroid imbalance. Vaccinosis is also often a trigger while additional vaccines or exposure to toxic substances will only worsen a cancerous condition. Cancerous cells take so much energy from the body that it becomes very susceptible to allergens and toxins, in addition to infections and infestations, it becomes a vicious cycle. Unfortunately, I have seen many immune system problems, including Feline Leukemia, FIP, Tick Fever, Valley Fever and chronic anemia (a possible pre-cancerous state), in pets originally diagnosed and treated chemically for "allergies" or other chronic conditions. In addition, pets who are vaccinated yearly or suffered from other chronic diseases, behavior problems and glandular disorders seem most susceptible.

I believe that the constant stress upon the body, due to symptoms such as allergic or inflammatory reactions—as well as the chemicals and drugs used to treat them—weakens the animal's constitution and their curative potential. This encourages damaged cells to mutate into cancerous cells. Some animals are born prone to cancer and may develop it early in their lives depending on how poorly the weakness has been addressed in the mother. Passing a strong immune system on through the supplementation and health of the mother provides the best opportunity with cancer prevention for the baby's whole life!

A recent discovery of Azmira®'s product support staff, headed by Lisa Marie Davis, validating my belief that the primary cause of cancer is a toxic lifestyle, has been through the random sampling of approximately thirty new customers who contacted us because their dogs have lymphoma. We found out that one hundred percent of these lymph node cancer cases had ingested a monthly dose of heartworm preventative medication for a minimum of three months prior to their initial symptoms! Believe me; the lymphoma will kill them before they ever could have been infected with heartworm. Think about the odds of mosquitoes infecting your pet versus your animal getting cancer because it was poisoned monthly in the chance it could be bitten by an infected insect?

Many of the symptom relief recommendations in this book are applicable to the treatment and prevention of cancerous conditions. In both cases, the underlying imbalance to be addressed is the immune system. Other markers, even the cancer itself (i.e. blood, lymph, bone), are simply symptoms to be addressed and reversed. Don't fear the diagnosis: step back and evaluate the whole animal. The goal is still to strengthen your pet's ability to heal while minimizing a degenerative process. Detoxification with improved nutrient utilization, foundation supplementation and specific remedy use based on weaknesses presented (i.e. liver dysfunction or anemic blood) are the same *Three Simple Steps* to take regardless of the name of the cancer.

The only added consideration is when using a nosode. This is a homeopathic remedy made from the actual dis-eased tissue of other cancerous growths or blood cells. This can include a remedy made from a cancerous piece of bone tumor or swollen lymph node. They are listed by the cancer's name (i.e. Osteosarcoma) so it is best to have a proper diagnose and choose a nosode that fits as closely as possible. I highly recommend Newton's® Homeopathic Laboratories. Their information is listed in the back section of this book under "Resources." You may also order through Azmira®, who is also listed in the back.

(see Symptom-specific subjects such as Feline Leukemia, including Immune Dysfunction, Vaccinosis, etc.)

Cataracts

CATARACTS occur in a large number of pets who suffer toxic lifestyles, often with season after season of allergy problems (not necessarily only in the eyes) and the chemical treatments of these problems, infections, diabetes or genetic predispositions. A lack of nutrients such as *vitamin A, E and Zinc* (often depleted during prior illnesses and a toxic lifestyle) is often a primary cause in the formation of cataracts. Some sources suggest that vaccines have contributed to the rise of cataract cases. What I do know from the case histories I have documented is that cataracts most often share a common background: histories of a toxic lifestyle resulting in irritants and toxins, from environmental and dietary sources, damaging sensitive eye lens tissues and causing them to cloud over.

This is also the case in lens opacity caused by the normal aging process (lenticular sclerosis). A holistically-raised animal simply does not develop a cataract. My fifteen year-old Rottweiler, Zaezar, never did develop any cataracts. As a matter of fact, on the morning she passed away she could still see joggers along the wash behind our home—which is over three hundred feet away! Her eyes sparkled with vitality until the end.

Reversing Cataracts

Along with the LifeStyle™ recommended detoxification protocol with homeopathic D'Toxifier, daily foundation supplements and nutrition, I have successfully reversed cataracts with homeopathic *Silicea 200C daily* for four weeks, then a course of *Silicea 1M weekly* for four weeks, with *Silicea 10M weekly* for four more weeks. A single dose of *Silicea 200C,* given once a month as a maintenance protocol, can retard the progression of cataract formation.

During this time I also applied, for at least six months, herbal Blood & Lymph D'Tox, to help stimulate the breakdown of tissues which form the cataracts. It eliminates them through the eliminatory system and brings nutrients to the eye for repair and strengthening. I also maintained weekly homeopathic detoxification and the Holistic Animal Care LifeStyle™ recommendations for the life of the animal. We did have relapses, but *only* in those pets whose caregivers were not following the prevention protocol to its fullest potential, especially when they stopped regular periods of detoxification and feeding the foundation supplements or used numerous medications.

(see Eye Problems)

Cherry Eye

CHERRY EYE can not only be unsightly but very irritating to the afflicted pet. When a prolapse occurs of the gland of the third eyelid occurs, a "cherry eye" appears. This is very common occurrence for certain dog breeds, notably the cocker spaniel, Pekingese, Lhasa apso and Beagle.

- D'Toxifier contains homeopathic *Arsenicum* which is an outstanding remedy for Cherry Eye. Give daily for one month, then weekly for maintenance. At this time add Arsenicum 200C weekly for one month then give a monthly dose for maintenance.

- Vitamin E, 100 IU's per day for cats and small dogs, up to 200 IU's for larger dogs as found in Mega Pet Daily, protects eye tissue from the degenerative nature of Cherry Eye. Vita E 200 can be added in severely prolapsed cases.

- Supplement with herbs such as Eyebright (nourishes eye tissue) and Yucca Intensive (anti-inflammatory).

- Use Azmira®'s Goldenseal Extract (for infection) and Calendula Extract (reduces irritation and inflammation), which can be used separately or in combination to make a natural eye cleanser. Add six drops each to two ounces of distilled water in a clean dropper bottle available at most drugstores, apply a few drops directly to the eyes two to four times a day.

Although surgery was often performed to remove the gland, today veterinarians are recognizing its function in tear production and opting for less radical means of therapy. I have had great success in reducing the inflammation (and size of the prolapse) naturopathically, allowing the dog to live comfortably and without infection.

(see Eye Problems)

Chewing

CHEWING can drive both the pet and the owner nuts. There are three types of chewing; the results of tissue damage ("reactions" to allergens, chiropractic needs, toxins, wounds or punctures, i.e. splinters), parasites (flea, ticks and fungal pests), and emotional triggers (obsessive or nervous behavior). One or all three triggers may be happening at the same time. Sometimes it seems as if it will never end. Excessive chewing is potentially very harmful to your pet. The constant stress of chewing and licking the body quickly leads to emotional and physical exhaustion, further weakening the immune system.

Chewing can also become a nervous habit—rather than just a symptom. Obviously, you need to first rule out any rashes, abrasions, cuts, flea or tick bites, etc. that may be triggering the chewing and address them topically. Follow recommendations in Chapter 4: **Step One** and Chapter 5: **Step Two.** If this fails to address the chewing, or it has become a habit, utilize herbal and/or homeopathic remedies for irritability and nervousness. You will be amazed how effective these are; even if you do not believe that your pet has any emotional issues. Flower essences, such as my Obsession formula, work well also.

Homeopathic Remedy Reduces Chewing

- D'Toxifier contains *Arsenicum* with complementary remedies which help lessen chewing through improved nutrient utilization and waste elimination; reduces skin irritations. Benefits chronic conditions of a toxic lifestyle; general restorative.

Herbal Remedies

- Calm & Relax is an excellent nerve tonic and helps rebalance the nervous system which helps balance hormones and brain chemistry to provide a sense of well being and calmness. It also acts as a sedative and improves pain relief. Supports the nervous system and helps control seizures and pain. Is an effective calmer and works well, especially for chewing possibly triggered by anxiety.

- **Skin & Liv-A-Plex** is beneficial with the animal who is toxic and may be producing a gout-like condition in the paws, has allergies (hot spots) or other triggers. It will cleanse the body and liver, reducing the eliminatory effect creating the need to chew on skin irritations.

- **Stress & A'Drenal Plex** promotes vitality, restoring integrity to the adrenal glands when chewing has exhausted the animal. As an adaptogenic formula, these herbs reduce the stress on a body that is constantly exposed to excessive physical or emotional conditions preventing or reversing a severe loss of energy, with anemia, low blood pressure and anxiety.

(see Obsessive Behavior, Allergies, Skin & Coat Problems, Parasites)

Circulation

CIRCULATION is often prohibited by inflammatory responses, fluid retention and heart conditions. Good circulation is vital to wellness and the curative process. It is the circulatory system which carries nutrients to each cell and removes metabolic or catabolic waste to prevent it from harming the cell and disrupting normal biological functions—the heart of dis-ease. Other than **Step One's** nutrition recommendations and detoxification, the herbal formulas **Blood & Lymph D'Tox** (for circulatory support) and **Yucca Intensive** (for venous tissue and heart inflammation) are excellent tools.

Homeopathic Remedies *can stimulate specific changes in the circulatory system*

- **D'Toxifier** contains *Arsenicum* with complementary remedies which help the heart and circulatory system through improved nutrient utilization and waste elimination; reduces chronic conditions of a toxic lifestyle; general restorative. This is a good remedy to start with for most cases.

- *Belladonna* has marked action on the vascular system, especially with pets who are often frightful or aggressive. These pets might lack appetite and stamina. Seem sluggish.

- *Calcarea Phos.* is an important tissue cell salt for poor circulation. These pets are often overweight—their mouths and feet may feel cold to touch.

- *Phosphorous* is indicated for any internal bleeding problems.

Colic

COLIC, especially in horses, is often the result of a sandy pasture, poor water utilization and/or coarse (not much nutrient-rich leaf) and/or moldy hay (which causes gassy build-up). This is another digestive disorder which responds well to The Holistic Animal Care LifeStyle™. I have lived with quarter horses most of my life and worked with hundreds more. Here in the Southern Arizona Desert. I know colic. The worst kind: sand colic. To prevent colic I feed soaked burmuda/alfalfa pellets once a day as a 25% feed replacement to their grass/hay mixture. That's two to three pounds of pellets per horse. I soak these in a gallon of water to promote intestinal hydration and I add the LifeStyle™ foundation supplements **Mega Pet Daily and Super C 2000** plus **NaturFiber, Yucca Intensive** and 1/8th cup of corn oil with one cup of bran. In case of colic: I did once have to call the veterinarian to oil a serious case but the rest of the times my horses moved through their episodes within a few hours of repeated homeopathic dosing, belly massage and a few walks. Colic has only happened during periods that I became lazy and stopped supplementing with the soaked pellets, especially when the weather got hotter and the horses had not increased their fluid intake to keep up. This is true for coarse and moldy hay colic.

Acute reactions of colic can be successfully "suppressed" with a few doses of *homeopathy*, given five to fifteen minutes apart in lower potencies (3X to 30C).

Homeopathy is very effective in reversing acute stomach aches, liver inflammation (especially due to vaccines, moldy hay or pesticides), constipation, intestinal spasms and underlying stress that often accompanies colic.

Homeopathic Remedies for Colic

*part of Azmira®'s D'Toxifier

- D'Toxifier contains *Arsenicum* with complementary remedies which help the digestive and eliminatory system through improved nutrient utilization and waste elimination; given every five

157

minutes apart for one hour will stimulate symptom suppression and promote a release of trapped gas and manure. Reduces chronic conditions of a toxic lifestyle to prevent colic; general restorative to help regulate the bowels.

- **Arsenicum* is used for digestive imbalances from poor quality diets or general toxicity and will alleviate most digestive disorders, especially if there is liver or spleen involvement. This remedy is especially effective when the disorder has been triggered by a bad batch of moldy hay, vaccines, chemical wormers or other drugs. Alternate weekly doses of Arsenicum 200C with daily doses of D'Toxifier for severe cases of toxic reactions.

- *Belladonna* is for the sudden onset of gastrointestinal symptoms. After initial use, should be tapered off slowly and then followed by a more specific remedy. **Acute colic** is a marker for this remedy.

- **Berberis Vulg.* stimulates liver function, reduces uric acid and regulates anal glands.

- *Bryonia* addresses those horses that are also severely cramping or whose stomach rumble, but they avoid laying down or respond in pain when their stomachs are rubbed.

- *Carbo Veg* is helpful when the horse is also overweight, has chronic colic, seems to have trouble digesting well, and feels discomfort soon after eating. This is a good senior pet tonic.

- *Colocynthis* is indicated for horses who are cramping or whose stomachs are rumbling. There may be other symptoms. They want to lie on a hard surface or they will respond to positively when you rub their belly. Movement, drinking or eating will aggravate symptoms. Another excellent colic remedy.

- **Iris* benefits glandular function, primarily the thyroid, pancreas, and liver. Also improves digestion.

- *Nux Vomica* also addresses the majority of digestive imbalances, including gas, lack of appetite or stool problems (especially alternating between constipation and diarrhea). Use this when D'Toxifier is not available.

- **Taraxacum* stimulates liver function and proper bowel evacuation. Promotes general rest and recovery of the digestive system. Helps prevent chronic colic conditions.

Herbal remedies can support reversal of many symptoms associated with colic. Simply mix one half teaspoon of standardized extract in one ounce of apple juice and give with a feeding syringe.

- Yucca Intensive extract provides natural steroidal saponins, which effectively reduce inflammation within the digestive system, including the stomach and intestinal lining as well as the liver, gall bladder, spleen and pancreas. Intestinal pockets, ulcerations, and inflamed intestinal valves that block passages (often associated with stress-related or autoimmune-based colic) have also responded well to yucca supplementation.

- *Daily Boost* helps reduce intestinal gas, cramping, and colic, prevents fatty deposits, repairs digestive tissue ulcerations, and fights infection. This is an excellent daily tonic for the colon, liver and gall bladder. Stimulates resistance against food or reactive allergies that may trigger colic episode. Helps to relieve gas and cramping while stimulating proper digestion and peristalsis. Chinese Mushrooms, included in Daily Boost's formula, have been used by the Chinese for centuries to prevent and treat cancers associated with the digestive system. Colon cancer in particular responds well to their incredible healing properties. A dramatic reduction in food sensitivities is often the result of long-term supplementation.

- *Herbal Wormer* cleans out the intestinal tract and reverses constipation. A detoxified colon is fundamental to rebalancing the digestive system and increasing assimilation of nutrients necessary for proper health and colic prevention. These herbs can also prevent or reverse intestinal parasitic infestation.

Colitis or Irritable Bowel Syndrome

COLITIS OR IRRITABLE BOWEL SYNDROME is commonly from symptoms associated with stress. This can be environmental stress from pesticides found on the ground and licked off the feet and coat or genetically-based tissue stress from an autoimmune dis-ease. Emotional pets create stress on the immune system and digestive tract beginning their dysfunction. Often more so than food allergies, bacterial infection, infestation or metabolic disease, other factors in developing colitis, "high-strung" pets succumb. However, constant stress of any chronic condition, especially combined with a toxic lifestyle, can also result in diarrhea, constipation (or alternating between the two), mucous covered stools, flatulence and even slight blood in the stool. Animals with a history of poor diets and chemical treatments may shed old fecal material during periods of detoxification resulting in deep internal colon cleansing. This can be combined with dried blood from old intestinal irritations or fresh red blood from recently exposed tissue free of caked on debris. This type of irritation only lasts a few days.

Recommended Remedies

- D'Toxifier contains homeopathic *Arsenicum* with complementary remedies which reduce symptoms of colitis and IBS through improved nutrient utilization and waste elimination; reduces chronic conditions of a toxic lifestyle. Acts as a general restorative. Good combination to use initially as it covers many symptoms associated with bowel and digestive problems.

- Yucca Intensive is a wonderfully soothing and anti-inflammatory herbal remedy. It has been proven as effective as steroids. Yucca Intensive can eliminate the need for drug therapy and its nasty side-effects.

- Fiber supplementation with NaturFiber——can provide proper evacuation and bowel care. Organic Chinese mushrooms give this product an edge in supporting the reversal of intestinal ulcerations and irritations. Psyllium is too harsh when used alone. I combined it with excellent whole grain, fruit and vegetable fibers. Powerful product, combined with Yucca Intensive, has completely reversed and kept the pet free of symptoms in a high number of cases.

- DigestZymez can also be appropriate, but I recommend that you limit their use to a few weeks at a time. The overuse of digestive enzymes can imbalance digestion further.

- Calcium with Boron-3 promotes proper peristalsis to relieve chronic constipation and tones the colon when spasms are common, as in the case of chronic diarrhea. Helps prevent colon cancer from developing in severe cases of colitis.

- Calming products with herbs, such as Azmira®'s Calm & Relax are also helpful with high-strung or pained animals.

- Daily Boost is an herbal supplement for the digestive tract, improves over-all colon and liver performance. This is a good general supplement to prevent reoccurrence.

(see Constipation and Diarrhea)

Colorado River Toad Poison

COLORADO RIVER TOAD POISON can have serious long-term side-effects, and can be fatal. In very young, sick or old pets their condition can deteriorate quickly. Symptoms include foaming at the mouth, fearful whining and your pet will shake his head violently trying to escape the burning, bitter slime released by the toad where it was licked or mouthed. Breathing can become labored due to the inflammatory response. Toads are prominent during monsoons. It is impossible to avoid the toads so do not allow your pet to wander unattended, especially in the evening hours.

- Using a garden hose rinse the mouth out thoroughly. Be careful not to point the hose directly to the back of the throat by rinsing from side to side. Do this step first!

- Tell your vet you're addressing this situation at home but to stand by should respiratory symptoms worsen. The veterinarian can best advise you regarding the severity of the situation.

- Start a crisis dose (every five to fifteen minutes for the first hour then every hour after until stable) of homeopathic *Mercurius Corrosivus* (for the venom's symptoms, including respiratory distress) and *Hypericum* 6X (for the burning pain).

- Follow a twice per day maintenance dose of D'Toxifier for one week following the crisis. This helps to prevent any side-effects from the encounter to occur.

- For a tumultuous, violent heart beat with labored breathing give a crisis dose of homeopathic *Belladonna* and/or *Aconite*.

- Feed herbal Yucca Intensive, a natural steroid alternative, to reduce swelling and pain of mucous membranes. An oral feeding may be required for the first dose, as the slime can severely irritate tissue in the mouth rendering it too sensitive for eating. Simply mix Yucca Intensive with one tablespoon or so of apple juice or broth. Use Azmira® feeding syringe.

Confusion (and Senility)

CONFUSION (AND SENILITY) are classic secondary symptoms of a toxic lifestyle and premature aging. A by-product of strokes, seizures or infection, confusion can also be a side-effect of vaccinosis. Chemicals on the brain, such as ammonia (a natural catabolic waste), can interfere with proper thinking functions creating a state of confusion for the pet. So can a blood sugar imbalance from diabetes, hunger or malabsorption. These triggers can lead to anxiety or behavioral issues; confusion is counter productive to learning and retaining information.

I have personally had several dogs (ages up to sixteen for Rottweilers), a thirty two year old Quarter Horse and cats (aged up to twenty two years) that lived well into their senior years with never a day's confusion. A toxic lifestyle stresses the body's systems and results in premature aging and senility. Feed and care well for the body and the brain will be well!

- A dose every five minutes apart of homeopathically-potentized flower remedy **R&R Essence** will help clear up most cases of acute confusion in short order, regardless of the cause.

- Homeopathic **D'Toxifier**, as part of your maintenance protocol, can help prevent symptoms from occurring.

(see Behavioral Problems, Nervous System Disorders)

Conjunctivitis

(see Eye Problems: *Infection*)

Constipation

CONSTIPATION is a common symptom associated with dehydration, stress and/or dietary toxicity. Constipation can be harmful to the body and weaken it further, due to improper elimination of waste products. These toxins continue to be reabsorbed, through the colon, into the blood.

Several factors can contribute to bowel upsets and constipation, including medications often used during crisis such as antibiotics, steroids and antihistamines, so first eliminate any possible culprits:

- Inadequate amounts of fluids being taken in (add water to food if needed to increase intake).

- Hard to digest commercial pet food ingredients, such as "plant cellulose", which is often soy castings, peanut shells or recycled paper pulp and "flours" including potato or rice flour—that are used as filler/fiber.

- Poor sources of dietary fiber—remember the paper pulp… where's the whole grain?

- Lack of exercise—especially with 6 hours or more of prolonged confinement daily.

- Recent increase in therapeutic levels of Iron can cause constipation and dark stools.

- Excessive ingestion of fur—due to licking and chewing of self or another.

To Promote Bowel Evacuation

- D'Toxifier contains *Arsenicum* with complementary remedies which help the digestive and eliminatory system through improved nutrient utilization and waste elimination; give every five to fifteen minutes apart for one hour to help stimulate evacuation. Reduces chronic conditions of a toxic lifestyle to prevent constipation; general restorative to help regulate the bowels and improve colon health.

- Be sure to increase fluids and lubrication; feed chicken broth and add vegetable oil or canola oil for horses and dogs. Use olive oil for cats, vegetable oil if they are very finicky. Repeat twice a day. <u>For cats and small dogs:</u> give four ounces broth with one tablespoon of oil. <u>For medium to large dogs</u>: give double these amounts or more as needed. <u>For horses</u>: use one-fourth cup oil only in well soaked pellets and/or bran mash.

- *Psyllium seed or husk* is the most commonly used fiber to help regulate bowel movement, but often can be too harsh on the digestive tract when used alone. I highly recommend NaturFiber which combines Psyllium with other fruit and vegetable fiber sources such as *carrots, apple fiber and pectin, guar gum* (a misunderstood, but excellent, source of natural fiber that swells to retain water which helps stool pass), *and bran. Chinese mushrooms,* such as *Shiitake and Reishi,* have long been noted for their fiber content as well as their curative potential in reversing chronic colon conditions, including pre-cancerous growths.

- Yucca Intensive helps soothe irritated intestinal tissues and repairs damage done by straining or impaction; reduces inflammation so evacuation is easier. Proven as effective as steroid medications for reducing inflammation.

- **Herbal Wormer** will help gently evacuate the bowels, usually overnight, when used as needed with or without fasting. Use <u>with</u> fasting for severe cases.

- Cooked *oatmeal,* added to meals or given alone with vegetable, fish or meat broth, provides an excellent source of fiber as well as detoxifying properties to help eliminate old fecal material from the bowels. A short, one meal fast can work wonders. Add oil and supplements chosen (see above) plus one tablespoon per ten pounds of body weight of canned pumpkin (optional) to help encourage evacuation of the bowels.

- Homeopathic *Phosphorus* can help expel hard, dry stools

(see Chapter 4: **Step One**; Detoxification & Nutrition)

Corneal Ulcers

CORNEAL ULCERS often occur in pets that have suffered from chronic inhaled, ingested or environmental allergies. Lack of tears, scratching and rubbing of the eyes, especially for pets who are rarely cleaned of their crusty eye discharge, as well as those suffering nutritional deficiencies, also contribute to the development of ulcers on the outer protective layer of the eyeball. Sometimes, a scratch from a fight or a branch that has not healed well can develop into an ulcer, remaining unnoticeable for months, even years.

Once your veterinarian has diagnosed this problem, it can often be quickly reversed:

- To make a natural eye cleanser: u*se* Azmira® Goldenseal Extract (addresses infection) and Calendula Extract (soothing), separately or in combination. These herbs can help fight infection, unblock the tear duct and soothe the eyes when applied as eye wash prior to applying the vitamin E. Simply dilute six drops each extract to two ounces of filtered or distilled water in a clean dropper bottle (available at pharmacies or health food stores) and apply a few drops.

- Applications, twice daily of natural *vitamin E* (d-Alpha, *not* dL-Alpha) such as our VitaE200, promote tissue repair. Prick the capsule with a clean pin to avoid contaminating the oil and apply directly to the inner eye lid, so blinking can spread it over the entire eye. This can be a little sticky, but it will not interfere with your pet's eyesight. It will help reverse inflammation and irritation and prevent permanent damage. Use one-half capsule per eye daily, applying half in the morning and the other half at night.

- Feed *vitamin E,* 100 IU's per day for cats and small dogs, up to 200 IU's for larger dogs as found in Mega Pet Daily. Add Vita E 200 for more serious or poorly responsive cases.

- Supplement with herbs such as Yucca Intensive (for inflammation and irritation) and Eyebright (strengthens the eye)

- Feed sulfur through MSM which supplies this tissue repairing nutrient.

- Use D'Toxifier which contains homeopathic *Arsenicum* and complementary remedies which help the eyes through improved nutrient utilization and waste elimination. They reduce chronic eye inflammation and stimulate a general restorative process to prevent scarring.

- Homeopathic *Euphrasia* is an excellent general remedy for the eyes. Benefits the pet whose eyes are irritated, inflamed and itchy. May have excessive tearing. Stimulates the reversal of ulceration or blisters on the cornea.

(see Eye Problems.)

Coronavirus

CORONAVIRUS is a highly contagious viral infection which is very similar in clinical symptoms to the parvovirus, and the two are often diagnosed together. Although the coronavirus is not as fatal, it will increase the fatality rate of a parvovirus infection. By itself, it causes tremendous gastrointestinal distress which can lead to chronic problems of the digestive system and general poor condition. Vaccination is highly recommended by traditional veterinary minds—but infection is still possible and the rate of vaccinosis too great to risk; especially when a naturopathic LifeStyle™ prevents infection or symptom development very successfully.

- Please note: A dilution of 1:30 of bleach can kill the virus on contact. It is recommended that you wash your shoe soles, floors and kennel runs (or other sources of contamination) with this when there is any sign of the virus.

- D'Toxifier contains *Arsenicum* with complementary remedies which help the immune system through improved nutrient utilization and waste elimination; promotes an immune response. Reverses nausea, diarrhea, soreness and irritability associated with coronavirus infection. Helps balance the appetite. Reduces chronic conditions of a toxic lifestyle; general restorative. Give every fifteen minutes to control diarrhea or vomiting, then every hour or so for the first day.

- Follow detailed instructions for parvo regarding prevention and addressing colon-specific infection, inflammation and fever.

(see Parvovirus, Infections and other Symptom-specific subjects)

Coughing

COUGHING can indicate a host of problems. It is best with a generalized symptom, such as coughing, to eliminate the most obvious trigger and systematically track down the culprit. Whatever remedies you choose to give for general cough symptoms, prior to a specific diagnosis, will benefit the condition of your pet's respiratory system in any event.

Common cough sources and general herbal remedies

(see specific topics such as ALLERGIES or HEART CONDITIONS for details)

- Dust or dried mold *(clean the house and wet down the yard, use* Aller'g Free, *increase* Super C 2000 *then add* Aller'G: Grass & Pollen *if cough is slow to improve within a week).*

- Chronic allergies *(use* Aller'G Free, Yucca Intensive *and* MSM*).*

- Fungal mycosis such as Valley Fever or heavy mold infestation around the pet's area or in your home *(use* Yeast & Fungal D'Tox *and* Yucca Intensive*).*

- Heart problems (after diagnosis use Yucca Intensive for inflammation *and* MSM to repair heart tissue).

Homeopathic Remedies for Coughs

- D'Toxifier contains *Arsenicum* with complementary remedies which help the lungs and respiratory system through improved nutrient utilization and waste elimination; reduces chronic conditions of a toxic lifestyle; general restorative. *Arsenicum* relieves the general dry cough with wheezing.

- *Belladonna* is for a barking or whooping cough. Dry coughs worse at night. Nose is noticeably dry. This animal may take shallow breaths.

- *Cantharis* is for a frequent, dry cough. A short hacking cough with blood streaked mucous.

- *Carbo Veg.* is for the animal who suffers a spasmodic cough with gagging and vomiting of mucous. Wheezing and rattling of mucous in the chest. Worse in the evening and in the open air. Can bring up bloody mucous.

- *Phosphorus* addresses the cough with lung congestion or a hard, dry cough.

Cribbing

CRIBBING is an obsessive behavior where the horse will pull its teeth against a pipe or board, sucking in air. It is believed that the horse is producing "feel good" changes in its brain through this repetitive motion. Some horses are so badly "hooked" on this that they will forgo feed, preferring instead to participate in this behavior.

Collars are available to curb this behavior although I have had success with remedies alone.

(see Obsessive Behavior)

Cruciate

CRUCIATE ligament damage, general tearing or severe sprain occurs in many pets which have not been fed the best diet and supplemented with therapeutic levels of Super C 2000 (minimum 1000 mg. per day for small pets, 4000 mg. per day for larger dogs). Poor tissue growth due to a lack of nutrition is common. This ligament is vital to the proper function of the knee.

- Super C 2000 repairs and strengthens the cruciate ligament, often eliminating the need for surgery. Vitamin C promotes the production of collagen, the building blocks of ligaments.

- MSM promotes further strengthening of connective tissue in more severe cases, and after surgery when needed.

- Yucca Intensive is as effective as steroids in reducing inflammation. Promotes circulation to fuel nutrient rich cells which repair tissue. Addressing inflammation is vital to recovery.

- Homeopathic cruciate repair is stimulated by dosing with low potency *Ruta*.

- D'Toxifier contains homeopathic *Arsenicum* with complementary remedies which help cruciate repair and strengthening through improved nutrient utilization and waste elimination; reduces chronic conditions of a toxic lifestyle; general restorative.

- Excessive weight puts pressure on the ligament. An overweight pet is more likely to damage the cruciate. Maintaining proper weight is vital to protecting the knee joint.

- Gentle exercise, especially swimming, strengthens the ligament. A lack of exercise puts a pet in danger of chronic strains and torn ligaments.

- Genetics and injury can play a part in ligament damage, but the likelihood is lessened through the LifeStyle™ approach.

(see Arthritis)

Curative Responses

CURATIVE RESPONSES are periods of symptom aggravation while the body is responding to nutritional, homeopathic and herbal changes.

(see Aggravations)

Cushing's Disease

CUSHING'S DISEASE is a serious malfunction of the adrenal gland, requiring a veterinarian's diagnosis.

Symptoms can include fatigue, hair color loss or poor coat growth, excessive shedding, slow tissue repair, and a droopy belly. The skin may be gray/black and leathery, resembling an elephant's skin. Within six months of natural support, this skin condition, which is generally believed to be irreversible, has actually been reduced in severity by up to eighty percent.

(see Adrenal Malfunction)

Cystitis

(see Bladder & Kidney Problems)

Deafness

DEAFNESS can be inherited or caused by a severe reaction to an organism (parasitic, fungal, bacterial or viral), an allergen or toxin. Cases of drug reaction, interaction or vaccinosis have also occurred. Often, in the course of addressing a different chronic health condition through the LifeStyle™ protocol, the owner will report back in as soon as six weeks (the time needed for a healthy cell to replace the dis-eased one) that their animal's hearing is also improving. This is due to the fact that deafness can be a primary side-effect in the degenerative, prematurely-aging process a toxic lifestyle creates.

I have had my own Rottweilers live to be an average of fifteen years old (one was sixteen and he was a "mess-rescue" at twelve years old when I got him). Only one ever became deaf in her final years and she was from a line of deafness genes. But the LifeStyle™ kept her from going deaf as early as her litter mates, who were deaf at five years old, whereas she only went deaf around her fourteenth birthday. When I realized Zaezar's hearing was diminishing the year before—through her uncharacteristic anxiety, and lack of excitement at hearing a baby cry—I taught her more hand signals beginning with "good girl" so I could validate for her when she got the other lessons correct. She already knew the ones from obedience training; *sit, down, stay, come, back* and *up.* I had also, prior to her loss of hearing, taught her to recognize over one hundred objects and their names so it was easy to now teach her "look there" to get her attention on something and "go get it!" She loved the challenge of learning. Her new hand signals included questions I could ask her when she obviously wanted something from me: "ball/toy?", "cookie?," "walk?," "eat?," "drink?" and "outside?" These commands helped her to communicate with me much as she had done with her hearing and eliminated her anxiety.

Apart from reversing deafness through the daily foundation nutritional supplements of **Step Two** and detoxification, try:

Homeopathic Remedies

- D'Toxifier contains *Arsenicum* with complementary remedies which help the ears function through improved nutrient utilization and waste elimination; reduces chronic conditions of a toxic lifestyle; general restorative.

- *Hepar Sulph.* reverses deafness which is the result of chronic infections.

- *Lycopodium* is good for general hard of hearing symptoms.

- *Thuja,* another ingredient in D'Toxifier, benefits the pet whose deafness came on as a result of a vaccine.

Herbal and Nutritional Remedies

- Grape Seed Extract is a powerful antioxidant which reduces free radicals known to interfere with hearing or which encourage the degenerative process in the ear.

- Immuno Stim'R, for the pet who has suffered a toxic lifestyle, helps reduce catabolic waste which can interfere with hearing and inner-ear function.

- MSM promotes the repair and strengthening of inner ear tissue.

- Skin & Liv-A-Plex promotes the detoxification of sensitive inner ear tissues and circulation of nutrient-rich blood to weakened 'hearing' cells.

- Yucca Intensive benefits the pet whose hearing loss is due to trauma and inflammation.

Degenerative Disc Disease

DEGENERATIVE DISC DISEASE is characterized by a slow deterioration of the cushiony disc in between the vertebrae. This can be caused by a toxic lifestyle, whereas the discs do not receive adequate nutrition as metabolic waste builds up. Disc tissues become weak and the gelatinous interior (the shock absorber) compresses and can even calcify. Over exertion can lead to the disc rupturing and putting pressure on the spinal cord. Paralysis can be the end result, especially in long back breeds such as the Dachshund, and even Poodles, Pekingeses and Lhasas. Neck ruptures are common in Beagles and Cocker Spaniels. Horses with a history of hard jumping or rodeo are often diagnosed.

Prevention is the best cure and proper nutrition is the best bet. Second best thing is keeping your animal at a healthy weight as obesity can be a leading contributor to degenerative disc disorders.

Nutritional Supplementation

- **Super C 2000**, in high therapeutic doses (to bowel tolerance). Vitamin C will provide the building blocks to regenerate and strengthen connective and disc tissues, eliminate toxins that inflame and stimulate circulation to promote superior nutrient utilization.

- **Calcium with Boron-3** provides calcium to prevent the body from storing calcium through such processes as calcifying deteriorating discs. Boron improves assimilation and tissue repair to strengthen the fibrous outer protective coating of the disc.

  When the body is lacking in minerals (or leeching them from bone tissue due to dis-ease), it attempts to store this mineral to ward off *starvation,* or total loss. Unfortunately, where the body chooses to store minerals (resulting in bladder stones, bone spurs and calcified joints) can be detrimental in the long run. Although traditional veterinary logic is to reduce minerals when this occurs—I saw the connection over twenty years ago and began working with the therapeutic levels of calcium and magnesium to reverse arthritis and bladder stones with great success. Recently, Harvard Medical School published reports that recommended mineral supplementation for bladder stones, based on the same principle.

- **MSM** repairs and strengthens connective tissue to stabilize the intervertebral discs, reducing the sway-back effect, and helps maintain the spinal disc tissue itself by improving the "cushion" affect.

- **MegaOmega-3** greatly benefits tissue repair and softening of the cushioning disc. Protecting it from further damage especially when combined with an additional *(to Mega Pet Daily)* 100 mg. for smaller pets and 200 mg. for larger animals of **VitaE200** (d-Alpha vitamin E). Prevents inflammation and pain during the maintenance phase; use Yucca Intensive to first eliminate the severe chronic or acute pain. Omega-3 fatty acids should be introduced to *aid* in reversing the inflammatory response and in the *least severe cases,* they can take the place of Yucca to help maintain inflammation-free tissues.

Homeopathic Remedies

- D'Toxifier contains *Arsenicum* with complementary remedies which slows the degenerative process through improved nutrient utilization and waste elimination; reduces chronic conditions of a toxic lifestyle. Stimulates an anti-inflammatory response. General restorative.

- *Arnica* for muscular pain, especially marked by heat (inflammation). Sore and lame is the picture of this remedy. This is an excellent acute remedy, especially following any trauma to the area (i.e. chiropractic adjustment, fall, stress from travel, hard play-day).

- *Colchicum* benefits chronic pain and numbness resulting from muscular tension, particularly aching in the lumbar and lumbo-sacral regions; common side-effects of poor shock absorbency. Reduces sharp pains in extremities (chewing on feet and legs with no signs of allergies or parasites indicates nerve involvement). Pet seems to be receiving "shocks" from time to time where they may jump suddenly and look at their body in confusion. Symptoms improve with rest and pressure and/or massage.

- *Dulcamara* is particularly recommended for intervertebral disc conditions of the neck. Addresses rheumatic-type pains which are made worse by cold, damp weather. Spasms, even mild paralysis, are markers for this remedy. Rheumatism can alternate with chronic diarrhea or worsen after acute skin eruptions. I rescued a Rottie at twelve years old who was slated to be euthanized he was in so much pain. This remedy combined with Yucca Intensive saved Gucci and returned him to full pain-free function for the last four years of his life.

- *Hypericum* relieves the pain associated with a pinched nerve. Helps the nerve regenerate, reverse paralysis and strengthen to return optimum function. Dose as needed for acute pain, then dose once a week for one month with the lower potency. After the symptoms are under control dose once a week for three months with a 200C (during the strengthening period), and then continue once or twice a month for maintenance.

- *Ruta* reduces disc calcification while it acts upon the cartilage and muscles to reduce tension and pain. A noted remedy for lameness in both horses and dogs. Pain worse in morning before getting up and improves with massage or pressure applied to area.

Herbal Remedies

- **Yucca Intensive** is the number one herbal remedy for inflammation of the disc. Reduces the trauma of inflamed tissues; the longer tissue is allowed to remain inflamed, the more damage (breakdown) occurs, weakening the affected tissue and leaving it vulnerable to additional injury, tearing or permanent deterioration. As potent as steroid medication—with none of the dangerous side-effects. Safe to use for severe acute pain (even in double dose), or as a long-term supplement for maintenance.

- **Calm & Relax** provides physically-relaxing compounds which reduce muscular tension or spasm, helps promote needed sleep (for tissue repair process) and provides exceptional pain relief when extra support is needed to augment Yucca Intensive. Especially benefits the animal who has become irritable due to fighting chronic pain and discomfort.

- **ImmunoStim'R** promotes metabolic waste removal from the blood and tissues of the intervertebral spaces. These wastes, and other toxins in the blood stream, feed the inflammatory response creating more heat and discomfort, hastening the deterioration of these sensitive tissues. Promotes circulation which encourages tissue repairing nutrients to nourish these areas instead.

Dehydration

DEHYDRATION can be the result of excessive vomiting or diarrhea and will quickly shut down bodily functions, especially detoxification, when an imbalance of nutrients and electrolytes occur. Other causes include commercial diets high in fiber, lack of potable water, excessive exercise, high fever and anxiety.

To check for dehydration

- in little dogs, cats and ferrets, grab skin from the back of the neck between your forefinger and thumb, pulling it gently upwards and releasing it.

- in medium to large sized dogs, you can also press the side of the lip up and release it.

- for horses, grab a pinch of skin off the side of their neck between your forefinger and thumb, pulling it upwards and releasing it.

- all pulled skin should return to normal within a second or two. If the skin snap test takes longer, then dehydration is a problem.

To reverse dehydration

- If the skin remains in a peak and doesn't snap back (in very rare instances), you will need to consult with your veterinarian immediately for subcutaneous fluid replacement therapy.

- In all other instances you can easily rehydrate your pet orally with a feeding syringe or encouraging fluid intake. **Provide one ounce of water per one pound of body weight, per day. This will allow for some spillage during oral feeding. Give horses a minimum of seven to ten gallons per day.**

- Electrolyte solutions can be added to the water if the animal seems weakened by the dehydration or has been constitutionally weak to begin with. Store bought solutions are also available but be careful to avoid heavily chemical or sugar-based ones. A home remedy I have used in a pinch is one-half teaspoon of Morton®'s Lite salt mixed in a quart of water. One teaspoon of honey can be added if pet is very weak. Give this instead of plain water for the first few hours.

- D'Toxifier contains *Arsenicum* and complementary remedies which help relieve the symptoms of dehydration and rebalance the body. This formula reduces chronic conditions of a toxic lifestyle which can include dehydration, when used weekly; general restorative.

- Keep a dehydrated pet quiet, in a cool dark area—avoid harsh lights and noise.

Demodectic Mange

(See Skin Parasites)

Dental Problems

DENTAL PROBLEMS are often overlooked and should not be. They will weaken the body's defenses against disease and premature aging. It is essential that you keep your pet's teeth and gums clean and free of infection. Do consult with your veterinarian immediately if you ever suspect a serious gum infection or find loose or broken teeth.

(see Teeth, Infections)

Depression

DEPRESSION can be more common than you would think, especially in animals whose caregivers are depressed themselves. Long-term illness, the loss of routine or a close pal, human or animal, can trigger a sense of hopelessness in an animal. Anyone who has had a dog who lost his life-long "human child companion" to college knows how sad and withdrawn they can get. Some of the older or weakened pets actually give up and die from grief. The use of certain medications, especially steroids, can trigger a depressive episode.

The symptoms of depression are the same in pets as they are in humans: lack of appetite, weight loss, withdrawal, sleeping all the time and change in routine (ie. won't go out to play by themselves).

To help alleviate symptoms of depression

- Homeopathic D'Toxifier, which contains *Arsenicum* and complementary remedies that improve mood through nutrient utilization and waste elimination, is effective in stimulating the reduction of symptoms.

- Herbal Calm & Relax will help regulate brain activity and lift the depressive state.

- R&R Essence flower remedy helps the pet cope with negative attitudes and feelings.

- For nutritional augmentation try L-Trypto Pet which stimulates seratonin levels in the brain.

- In addition to foundation supplements including Mega Pet Daily, feed 25 mg. to 50 mg. of B-Complex 50 to help restore the nervous system and reduce stress.

- Mega Omega-3 contains fish oils which are considered beneficial to reversing mood disorders.

Dermatitis

DERMATITIS is a common diagnosis describing a chronic skin condition. Manifesting in pets suffering from poor health and toxicity, the skin develops symptoms including pimples and hot spots. Flea or tick bites are also a common source of dermatitis. When the skin becomes irritated, inflamed and itchy, pets begin to scratch, rub, chew and lick themselves, and the skin becomes so irritated and inflamed that other problems arise: hair loss, dandruff, greasy skin, and open sores. A ***hot spot*** is an irritated, open area of skin caused by licking, scratching or biting, and can result in infection. If a pet has chronic dermatitis and has been exposed to many cycles of antibiotics, a staph infection may arise that becomes difficult to treat through standard medical treatment. Naturopathy is the best way to reverse dermatitis.

(see Infections, Skin and Coat Problems)

Diabetes

DIABETES is another disease frequently associated with a history of poor health problems and toxic lifestyles. I believe that there is a strong relationship between blood sugar stabilization (or lack of it) and the chronic weaknesses so frequently diagnosed including allergies, arthritis, organ dysfunction and behavioral problems. Blood sugar stabilization provides improved nutrient utilization and allows the immune system to receive stable fuel throughout the day, increasing resistance to toxins. For instance, many pets suffering from allergies responded *finally* to medical treatment *for their allergy symptoms* when, later in life, they were diagnosed with diabetes, and their blood sugar stabilized through insulin and diet! Therefore I feel the opposite is true that pets whose blood sugar is not maintained stable are more likely to exhibit "allergic" reactions to their toxic lifestyles.

When chronic symptoms, regardless of the diagnosis, present themselves early in your pet's life adhere to The Holistic Animal Care LifeStyle™ to help prevent a diabetic condition, or worse, from developing. Feeding at least twice per day, even three to four smaller meals per day as needed during stressful times, will support the body's resistance to symptoms/ toxic reactions.

For diabetic animals, Herbal Remedies in addition to proper diet and supplementation can help reduce the amount of insulin needed:

- Panc'rse & GlucoBalance can eliminate the need for insulin in many pets. This clinically-proven standardized herbal formula strengthens the pancreas, promoting better production and utilization of insulin, and also normalizes and restores the organs and glands associated with carbohydrate and sugar metabolism. Re-synthesis of glycogen promotes greater balance of glucose and is indicated in both hyper and hypoglycemia. Reduces insulin need.

- *Daily Boost* helps reduce digestive malfunctions which may encourage a diabetic predisposition. This is also an excellent daily tonic for the colon, liver and gall bladder. Stimulates resistance against food or reactive allergies that may trigger diabetic episode. A dramatic reduction in insulin need is often the result of long-term supplementation.

Homeopathic Remedies

- *D'Toxifier* contains *Arsenicum* with complementary remedies which help the digestive and eliminatory system through improved nutrient utilization and waste elimination. Reduces chronic conditions of a toxic lifestyle to prevent symptoms of diabetes; general restorative to help regulate blood sugar in pets.

- *Calcarea Carb.* is good for an animal who has suffered malnutrition resulting in a poor coat and skin condition. Excellent remedy or for any small wound that won't heal readily. A weekly maintenance dose of 200C improves digestion in diabetics resulting in a better skin condition.

- *Nux Vomica* stabilizes many of the digestive imbalances associated with diabetes. Do not use with D'Toxifier as Arsenicum and Nux antidote each other.

- *Phosphorus* is for animals whose diabetic symptoms came on suddenly and aggressively. These cases have not responded well to insulin therapy; it exacerbated their condition.

(see Digestive Disorders, Weight Problems)

Diarrhea

DIARRHEA is often associated with over-eating, toxic reactions, viral infection and food sensitivities. I have seen it manifested in pets suffering from other stress, such as fear and anxiety, especially during the constant scratching and biting associated with allergies. Suffering any irritating chronic symptom can trigger it; all that nervous energy just churns up the bowel.

General Recommendations

- Use cooked *oatmeal,* added to daily diet or given alone to help firm up the stool and soothe the intestinal tract. A meal of oatmeal alone, with fish or meat broth, is not only an excellent source of fiber, but also has detoxifying properties that can help eliminate old fecal material from the bowels which may have triggered the bout of diarrhea. Old fecal material can become toxic (especially with bacterial infection) and trigger the body's attempt to eliminate the irritation. Oatmeal water (soak a handful of oatmeal in two cups of cool purified water overnight) can be given strained and fed during fasting to help soothe and cleanse the digestive tract.

- Feed NaturFiber: Psyllium seed or husk is the most commonly used fiber to help regulate bowel movement, but often can be too harsh on the digestive tract, when used alone. I highly recommend feeding it as Azmira® has combined it: with other fruit and vegetable fiber sources such as *carrots, apple fiber and pectin, guar gum* (a misunderstood, but excellent, source of natural fiber that swells to retain water), and *bran. In addition,* NaturFiber contains *Chinese mushrooms, such as Shiitake and Reishi,* which have long been noted for their fiber content as well as their curative potential in reversing chronic colon conditions, including pre-cancerous growths—which may be irritating the colon and triggering the diarrhea.

Homeopathic Remedies are effective in relieving diarrhea and associated symptoms.

- D'Toxifier contains *Arsenicum* with complementary remedies which help the digestive and eliminatory system through improved nutrient utilization and waste elimination; given every five minutes apart for one hour D'Toxifier will help control diarrhea. Reduces chronic conditions of a toxic lifestyle which trigger loose stools; general restorative to help regulate the bowels.
- *China* is used for debilitating fluid loss.

Herbal Remedies

- Yucca Intensive (a proven natural steroid alternative) *and/or* Calendula Extract soothe irritated and inflamed intestinal tissues. Be sure that fluid intake is maintained, as diarrhea can quickly dehydrate your pet.
- Remember to double the use of Garlic Daily Aid (1000 mg. to 2000 mg. per day for small dogs and cats, and up to 4000 mg. for

medium to large sized dogs). This regimen is antiseptic: will give your pet natural antibiotic support and rebalance the digestive system. Slows the rate and severity of diarrhea.

- Add one-half teaspoon of *raw honey* per twenty pounds of body weight per day to fluids or herbal preparations. Honey is not only soothing to an irritated colon; it is an antiseptic and provides energy for a weakened pet.

Fasting With Fluids During Severe Diarrhea (result of viral infection, etc.)

- Fast the symptomatic pet while force-feeding fluids to prevent dehydration; make a solution of two ounces each of apple juice and purified water. Add one tablespoon of raw honey (for energy and intestinal repair) and one teaspoon of fresh lemon juice (antiseptic, if needed for bloody diarrhea or parasitic infestations). Use a syringe (without the needle) and place towards the back of the pet's mouth, in the corners, to get the fluid on the back of the tongue. Give one ounce of solution per pound of body weight per day. This will compensate for spillage. It is best to give some fluid every couple of hours during the height of symptoms when accompanying fever, vomiting, bloody diarrhea, or exhaustion to ward off dehydration and keep up the pet's energy needed for healing. Daily supplements and herbal remedies can be added to fresh fluid solution to be used within the next twenty four hours.

- As symptoms improve <u>oatmeal water</u> can also be used in this solution instead of plain water, eventually thickening it up to a soup once the fever has ended. To make oatmeal water soak overnight two handfuls of oatmeal in a pint of water and strain.

- Once the diarrhea has stopped, chicken broth can be substituted for plain water to make the oatmeal water. This will provide easily digestible fats and encourage the digestive tract to function.

- Feed cooked oatmeal as appetite and digestion stabilizes to help break the fever-fasting period. Give four small meals the first few days. A tablespoon or two of yogurt can be added for acidophilus and use Azmira®'s Acidophilus. Tuna can water or meat-based baby food can be added for flavor. Oatmeal is soothing to irritated intestinal tissues and will help eliminate dis-eased tissue from the colon.

- Chicken & Beef or Ocean Fish canned formulas can be later added to the oatmeal as stools firm up and appetite is strong. These are the easiest to digest and given in three smaller daily meals, they will help bring digestion back on line. After a week of recovery, return to normal daily schedule and meal planning for the pet's age.

(see Dehydration, Digestive Disorders, Infections)

Digestive Disorders

DIGESTIVE DISORDERS are very common to overly emotional and/ or physically stressed pets; most naturally associated with toxic foods, environments and conditions including allergies and vaccinosis. The second most common complaint I hear (skin problems is number one) is a digestive disorder: lack of appetite, vomiting, stool changes, colic or hairballs. Difficulty with weight loss or gain and poor assimilation of diet often indicates the need for enzymes. The use of digestive enzymes such as DigestZymez with meat-eating pets can be beneficial in the short term. You will still have to address the actual imbalance for long-term symptom reversal. When digestive enzymes are overused, the potential loss of the body's own ability to digest and assimilate foods increases. Therefore, alternatives to the sole use of digestive enzymes are recommended.

Acute reactions of digestive imbalance can be successfully "suppressed" with a few doses of *homeopathy*, given five to fifteen minutes apart in lower potencies (3X to 30C).

Homeopathy is very effective in reversing acute stomach aches, liver inflammation (especially due to vaccines, toxic diets or pesticides), stool changes, intestinal spasms and underlying stress that often accompanies these digestive disorders.

Homeopathic Remedies for Digestive Disorders

*part of Azmira®'s D'Toxifier

- D'Toxifier contains *Arsenicum* with complementary remedies which help the digestive and eliminatory system through improved nutrient utilization and waste elimination; given every five minutes apart for one hour will stimulate symptom suppression. Reduces chronic conditions of a toxic lifestyle to prevent digestive problems; general restorative to help regulate the bowels.

- **Arsenicum* is used for digestive imbalances from poor quality diets or general toxicity and will alleviate most digestive disorders, especially if there is liver or spleen involvement. This remedy is especially effective when the disorder has been triggered by a season of ingesting monthly flea and tick control medications or other drugs. Alternate weekly doses of Arsenicum 200C with daily doses of D'Toxifier for severe cases of digestive problems and toxic reactions.

- *Belladonna* is for the sudden onset of gastrointestinal symptoms. After initial use, should be tapered off slowly and then followed by a more specific remedy. Belladonna is indicated for "fatty" stools and lack of appetite resulting from pancreatic imbalances. Acute colic and excessive flatulence are also markers for this remedy.

- **Berberis Vulg.* stimulates liver function, reduces uric acid and regulates anal glands.

- *Bryonia* addresses those pets that are also cramping or whose stomach rumble, but they avoid hard surfaces or respond in pain when their stomachs are rubbed. They may also exhibit arthritic pains as a result of an allergic or infectious reaction.

- *Carbo Veg* is helpful when the pet is also overweight, has chronic stool problems, seems to have trouble digesting well, and burps soon after eating. Is extremely beneficial when used with Nux Vomica. This is a good senior pet tonic.

- *China* supports pets that have chronic liver involvement with digestive imbalances who are very sensitive to touch and open air. They chill easily and seek to hide, especially after meals. Although they may crave cold water, it will cause them to burp up partially digested food.

- *Colocynthis* is indicated for pets who are cramping or whose stomachs are rumbling. There may be other symptoms. They want to lie on a hard surface or they will respond too positively when you rub their belly. Movement, drinking or eating will aggravate symptoms.

- **Iris* benefits glandular function, primarily the thyroid, pancreas, and liver. Also improves digestion.

- *Nux Vomica* also addresses the majority of digestive imbalances, including gas, vomiting, lack of appetite or stool problems (especially alternating between constipation and diarrhea). Use this when D'Toxifier is not available.

- *Phosphorous* is indicated if the digestive problems include great debilitation, fluid loss or frequent vomiting or diarrhea soon after meals. Partially digested food often comes up immediately. Pet has difficulty in expelling stools. Phosphorous quickly eliminates blood (from old fecal material, viral or bacterial detoxification) or fatty mucous (from pancreatic imbalance) in the stool.

- *Podophyllum* can be used when profuse, offensive-smelling stools occur. Color may be yellowish or greenish, is often completely liquid or begins formed and turns loose as the bowel movement progresses, and can also be accompanied by dry heaves or gagging.

- *Pulsatilla* aids diarrhea or mucous covered stools, which are often greenish in color. This stool will frequently change in character or color, even during the bowel movement. Diarrhea is likely to be worse at night or aggravated by warmth. Symptoms, such as nausea, vomiting or diarrhea, are not too severe. Food is often the culprit, especially if it is high in animal fats or rancid ingredients. The offending food might be vomited up partially digested. The tongue may become coated with a thick white or yellowish material.

- **Taraxacum* stimulates liver function and proper bowel evacuation. Promotes general rest and recovery of the digestive system.

- *Urtica Urens* addresses a lack of appetite often accompanied by extensive itchy eruptions, hives or serious welts. These afflictions which are not responsive to Apis or Sulphur often appear in conjunction with digestive or eliminatory problems, and dry skin aggravated by warmth or bathing. Digestive problems may also be associated with profuse discharges from mucous membranes, ears and eyes. Symptoms may be localized to the right side of the body.

- *Ipecac* can quickly subdue vomiting, especially when it is related to food or ingested chemical allergies.

- *Mercurius* benefits pets who have marked upper digestive tract and liver involvement, especially when they feel pain when they are touched or lying on the right side. Stools may be whitish-gray or yellowish green. Often, these pets are very irritable with swollen gums that bleed easily, and their tongue may be slightly swollen and coated with a yeast-like substance.

- *Lycopodium* is another excellent liver remedy, especially with back pain, gas, bloating, discomfort and rumbling of the stomach soon after meals. These pets seem to fill up quickly after only a few bites of solid food. A dose of Lycopodium fifteen minutes prior to meals can help the pet eat their whole meal, given that they are fed a reasonable amount for their individual need at the moment.

Herbal remedies can support reversal of many symptoms associated with digestive disorders. They can increase digestion or assimilation, and stabilize appetite. Many pets cannot tolerate herbs on an empty stomach. In fact, they may create some of the digestive stress. When pets have digestive upsets, it is best to give herbs with a little food, until they are better tolerated, or you might try to obtain better quality herbs such as found in Azmira®, proven to reduce digestive difficulties.

- Yucca Intensive extract provides natural steroidal saponins, which effectively reduce inflammation within the digestive system, including the stomach and intestinal lining as well as the liver, gall bladder, spleen and pancreas. A reduction in excessive peristalsis—a squeezing response of the intestines, to process and move digested material toward the colon—can help relieve diarrhea due to allergic or other inflammatory responses, including that from emotional stress. Intestinal pockets, ulcerations, and inflamed intestinal valves that block passages (often associated with stress-related colitis) have also responded well to yucca supplementation.

- Garlic Daily Aid is excellent for digestive complaints. Not only is it antiseptic and a natural antibiotic, it effectively supports proper digestion and colon health through its anti-parasitic and anti-yeast properties. Higher allicin contents are beneficial in reversing general diarrhea, flatulence and fatty stool deposits.

- *Daily Boost* helps reduce intestinal gas, cramping, and colic, prevents fatty deposits, repairs digestive tissue ulcerations, and fights infection. This is an excellent tonic for the liver and gall bladder. Stimulates resistance against food or reactive allergies. Helps to relieve gas, cramping, and mucous while stimulating proper digestion and peristalsis. Chinese Mushrooms, included in

Daily Boost's formula, have been used by the Chinese for centuries to prevent and treat cancers associated with the digestive system. Colon cancer in particular responds well to their incredible healing properties. A dramatic reduction in food sensitivities is often the result of long-term supplementation.

- **Milk Thistle Seed** supports proper liver function and helps promote basic liver detoxification.

- **Calendula Extract** contains therapeutic components that soothe sensitive and irritated digestive tissues, including the stomach and intestinal lining, as well as the liver, gall bladder, spleen and pancreas.

- **Panc'rse & GlucoBalance** reduces the occurrence of soft, fatty, off-colored stools. (see Diabetes)

- *Herbal Wormer* cleans out the intestinal tract. A detoxified colon is fundamental to rebalancing the digestive system and increasing assimilation of nutrients necessary for proper health. These herbs can also prevent or reverse intestinal parasitic infestation.

(see Appetite Problems, Constipation, Colitis, Diarrhea, Vomiting)

Distemper

DISTEMPER is a viral infection which produces a multitude of symptoms—with twenty-five percent of cases fatal. It can affect the respiratory, digestive (gastrointestinal) or nervous systems. The most notable difference in this viral disease is related seizures, sometimes called "chewing gum fits" for the way the animal looks as if he is chewing gum at those moments. These seizures can predispose a pet to a future of epilepsy, especially if the initial fits are treated with a veterinary-prescribed anticonvulsant medication.

Early signs of this infection include a fever, loss of appetite and eye inflammation (conjunctivitis). These markers can be short-term and transitory—easily missed by the owner—allowing the dis-ease to progress and take hold of the body. Secondary symptoms are more obvious as coughing, respiratory distress, vomiting and diarrhea with nasal and eye discharge become more extensive. Seizures and paralysis are the end results of this progression and can come on suddenly in an untreated animal.

The veterinary community does not have high expectations for an infected animal. They believe twenty-five percent will die, twenty-five percent will survive with no lasting side effects, twenty-five percent will survive with non-life-threatening side effects such as hard pad (a condition where the pad of the feet harden and thicken) and another twenty-five percent will survive with life-threatening side-effects such as nervous system deterioration, over a few years, ending in paralysis or debilitating seizures. But many veterinarians admit that the number is closer to fifty percent of pets who recover from infection will suffer some type of life-long neurological dysfunction.

Another rule of thumb I have read they use is that fifty percent of severely ill pets die despite "good" supportive veterinary care such as fluids, antibiotics and anticonvulsants. This is why they push prevention through vaccination, although the distemper vaccine has a high number of complaints, such as fever, vomiting and even seizures that accompany the shot (especially when given to older animals). Vaccination is recommended to start as early as six weeks of age. This is such as tender young age for a body that is still adjusting to *being*. No wonder we see cases of vaccinosis in puppies and kittens shortly after they begin their "routine" vaccinations.

Of course, the odds of both these outcomes (preventing vaccinosis and reversing infection) are better with the LifeStyle™ approach. Not only can this naturopathic approach reverse severe symptoms related to infection but the outcome of its general preventative program is to build up the immune system response to these (and all) invading organisms— killing them off before they have a chance to "infect." No need to sicken the body first through vaccination. In addition, the use of homeopathic nosodes (made from actual distemper dis-eased tissue) is a wonderful preventative to both infection and vaccinosis. This is available from Newton's Homeopathic Labs.®

(See Infection—*for related symptom support*)

Dry Eyed

(see Eye Problems)

Dying

DYING is the inevitable conclusion to living. All things must come to an end. Even with the best veterinary or naturopathic care, some bodies just don't have the vitality (or will) to live on. There must be a spark of life available to be flamed into wellness. If this spark is not there, the process has become a destructive one (rather than curative) and the conclusion can only be death—regardless of what you have tried, wished or paid for.

Dying is a process which does not have to be one of suffering or anguish. Many pets will simply "give up" and slip away silently in the night—although many will fight (for you) to stay alive despite their pain and suffering. My own Rottweiler Zaezar, bless her heart, actually came back from the dead, having had her heart stopped for at least three minutes, in order to say good-bye to my ex who drove up shortly after Zaezar had died of a heart attack. Having been raised as a pup by us both and spent many a summer vacation or long weekend there, their connection was still strong. Death shudders and no pulse later; I saw my ex drive onto my ranch's access road and cried out in grief that Zaezar had missed that last visit; darn if that ornery old dog (at fifteen years old she certainly had her due to stay dead) didn't open her eyes, lift up onto her elbows and wagged her tail—no small feat in itself considering she had awakened paralyzed in her rear end that morning.

They shared their good-byes and fifteen minutes later the vet showed up, as I had called her earlier that morning to come in the afternoon and euthanize Zaezar. Like everything else in our life together—she had beaten me to the punch by dying first and gave me one final incredible Zaezar story to boot. Oh, I could fill another book with her life's adventures. When the vet administered the valium (a common method of preparing the pet for the final heart injection) she simply passed again from the relaxant. The vet had never seen a dog pass on from the valium itself and when we explained her condition just minutes earlier, the vet felt Zaezar had simply been ready to let go this time (again). It was a most touching reminder of the tremendous bond Zaezar had shared with us all. What love!

When we woke up that morning and saw her condition, having spent six weeks in a steady decline, we knew that it was time to be strong for her and to help her pass. Her heart, lungs and digestive system, we had been told, was that of a young dog so I knew she would not go on her own easily. The heart attack had taken us by surprise and was due to the extraordinary stress her body was under that morning as she had held her bladder, probably due to the paralysis, for over eighteen hours and she died finally passing urine.

An early rabies vaccinosis (prior to my current knowledge of the dangers) had given her a cancerous spinal tumor between her shoulder blades (the vaccine's site). She was then two years of age. This tumor had partially paralyzed her back then, but all symptoms had been reversed (through my desperate development of the LifeStyle™ vaccinosis and cancer protocols) and stayed symptom-free until shortly before her fifteenth birthday.

Our vet explained that she conceivably could have stayed alive another few years but at what expense. She could not have gotten around on her own even with the help of wheels, we could see her grief in her expression, as her front legs had recently developed degenerative arthritis in genetically-prone elbows. We had already been helping all 90 lbs. of her to stand up and to get around, for six months; she wasn't very mobile those last weeks and she was getting more frustrated and irritable at times. At fifteen years old she was also still clear-eyed, vibrant and quite the sassy gal she had always been, eating everything she could. Just days earlier, still keeping an eye out each morning for the coyotes and warning them off—okay, so she couldn't hear that well and couldn't go from zero to sixty anymore—but she still ran fast for twenty seconds when she saw something that she wanted.

It was not an easy decision to make. The vet had already come out earlier but saw that neither I nor Zaezar were ready to let go (hence, the importance of a good relationship with your vet is that they know you and can advise you better). She prescribed steroid injections which I gave to Zaezar in those final six weeks to help keep her comfortable and mobile. We knew we were ready when she woke completely paralyzed that morning.

You will know as well when the time comes. I have never worked with anyone who did not say later, "It was <u>then</u> that I knew." If you are not sure now whether you should selflessly allow your beloved pet to pass, then honor that, but ask yourself some hard questions: Is their quality of life still good? Are they in unmanageable pain? Has this condition become nonreversible and the body in a permanent phase of degeneration? Ask the veterinarian if he or she would keep their own animal alive in this condition.

Euthanasia Is a Gentle Release

Certainly, some people euthanize their animals out of selfishness or it's easier than taking the pet with them when they move. I am not condoning that. What I am encouraging you to think about is the fact that your pet may hang on past their time to keep you from grieving for them and feeling the pain of their loss—they love you that much. This is not fair to them *if they are suffering and no longer have a quality to their life.* It is time to say good-bye when their bad days way outnumber their good.

Today's euthanasia is a process of gentle release. The animal feels no pain. Once the relaxant is given there is no suffering or anxiety. Then a final shot is given directly into the heart or vein to stop the heart's function. It's over in a matter of minutes. We should only be so lucky when our time comes.

Remedies To Help The Process Of Dying

- Homeopathic *Arsenicum*, in the 200C potency, gives peace to an animal in the final moments of life. If a pet is prepared to pass on, this remedy will help it occur. Dose every fifteen minutes for the first hour, then give one dose per hour. The animal (or human) will pass on their own generally within twelve hours if it is their time.

  If not, the remedy *Arsenicum* is a potent purifier and immune stimulant. This is why it is included in Azmira®'s D'Toxifier. It is a primary remedy of choice for detoxification—the animal will experience a sparking of their life force, if at all possible. You may instead find your pet begins to recover from this episode.

- R&R Essence is a homeopathically-potentized flower remedy which helps bring balance and clarity to the emotions. Reduces negative, stressful emotions experienced in the final moments preceding death. This remedy helps lessen the anxiety associated with crisis or stressful situations. Be sure to partake in this remedy with your pet (its human-grade) as it will also help your own sorrow and anxiety as well; paramount to making clear-headed decisions for your friend's final hours.

Ear Mites

EAR MITES or *Otodectes* are tiny, white spider-like pests. They are practically impossible to see with the naked eye. They leave a trail of digested blood and debris in the ear, which resembles finely ground pepper and results in a gritty discharge. Long-term infestation or serious ear infections can lead to deafness and despondency.

To dissolve a suspected infestation *that is not creating severe pain or bleeding:*

- Warm up two tablespoons of light clear oil (soybean, canola, vegetable) and add a capsule of Garlic Daily Aid extract to it—

which will help discourage bacterial growth and soothe any minor inflammation.

- For infected or seriously irritated ears use an additional six drops of **Goldenseal Extract**, one drop of **Yucca Intensive** and the contents of one **Vita E 200**.

- If a serious infestation has occurred—one that has been non-responsive to previous oil applications—add four drops of **Neem Dip** to the solution.

- Apply with a dropper, spoon or cotton ball, dripping it down into the ear. Allow it to set for as long as your pet will tolerate, at least one-half hour, if possible. *The object is to suffocate the mites.*

- Finish by massaging the base of the ear to loosen any mite/dirt debris further before flushing the ear out with a solution of two ounces of **Rejuva Spray**, two ounces warm purified water and 4 drops of alcohol (to help remove the oil). A child's ear bulb, available at any drugstore, works well for flushing the ear. Allow the animal to shake its head well to eliminate this solution and the collected debris; it is messy so it is best done inside your shower or outdoors. You can then use an absorbent tissue (do not use the ones coated with aloe or creams) to dab out the ear and remove the dirty solution.

- Wipe out the ear last with a cotton ball soaked in **Rejuva Spray**.

- If infestation is accompanied by a great deal of head shaking and/or anxiety use **R&R Essence** and homeopathic *Apis* to help minimize symptoms.

Be sure that you remove all the loose oil and debris or this can become clogged down in the base of the canal creating an infection. A Q-tip can be used to clean out the crevices of the ear—be careful not to stick the tip down into the ear canal or you may damage the ear drum. Repeat several times per day until all the mites are removed, usually within a day or two.

(see Ear Problems, Infections)

Ear Problems

EAR PROBLEMS commonly occur in animals suffering toxic lifestyles. The liver, a primary organ often affected by allergens, metabolic waste and chemicals, has a special relationship to the ears and eyes. As the liver becomes burdened the ears begin to exhibit symptoms associated with toxic reactions. They become more prone to irritation (waxy built-up, pustules, rashes, etc.) from grasses, pollen, mold, urea, yeast, sugar, vaccinations, parasites, bacterial or viral organisms, pesticides, food stabilizers and various other chemicals—just to name a few of the possible assaults the body suffers daily. Therefore, a clean body (liver) is vital to the reversal of ear problems—this is why chronic ear conditions do not clear up long-term with the use of medicated ear drops and antibiotics.

Ear conditions often occur during warmer weather when dogs might have allergic sensitivities (note again the liver connection), are bathed and swim more. Water may become trapped in the ear canal, encouraging bacteria and yeast to grow there, followed by an ear infection. Foxtails and other foreign bodies may also become lodged in the ear. Always check first to see if you can find anything in the ear and remove it prior to treatment. If needed, seek proper removal by a veterinarian.

How To Clean Ears

- Use a saturated cotton ball to squeeze a little **Rejuva Spray** solution into the ear.

- Rub the outer base of the ear to massage the solution into any debris that needs to be removed (you may hear a slight suction-like noise inside the ear).

- Allow your pet to shake out their ears then wipe out the rest of debris and fluid with a soft tissue wrapped around your finger (avoid aloe or conditioner-impregnated tissues).

- To avoid damage, do not insert anything down into the inner ear, but rather let the tissue absorb up any impurities.

- Follow cleanings with an application of **Rejuva Spray** around the flap and ear opening, especially to help address infection or **Rejuva Gel**, if pain is present.

  For dogs with ear flaps in the down position, tie them up over the head with an elastic hair band to encourage air circulation. As little as one hour a day after cleaning can reduce bacterial or yeast growth and encourage healing.

  Be careful not to use heavy, oil-based ingredients or vegetable oils, unless you are attempting to dissolve a foreign body or kill ear mites (see Ear Mites). Although such oils may seem to be conditioning the ear and reducing irritation, they may also be nurturing a bacterial or yeast infection, by providing a warm, moist, oxygen-less environment.

To dissolve a suspected foreign body *that is not creating severe pain or bleeding*:

- Make a solution by warming up two tablespoons of light clear oil (soybean, canola, vegetable) and adding a capsule of Garlic Daily Aid extract to it—which will help discourage bacterial growth and soothe any minor inflammation.

- For infected or seriously irritated ears use an additional six drops of Goldenseal Extract, one drop of Yucca Intensive and the contents of one Vita E 200.

    Keep the dissolving oil solution you have made in the ear for as long as your pet will tolerate it, and massage the base of the ear to loosen the object further before *flushing the ear out* with a cleaning solution or Rejuva Spray. A child's ear bulb, available at any drugstore, works well for flushing the ear. Repeat several times per day until the object is removed, usually within a day or two. This will dissolve or dislodge hardened debris as well as many plant particles. Never force fluid into the ear with pressure, or you may drive the object further in, making it harder to remove it safely yourself. This is the only thing I use.

- *Rejuva Spray* is excellent for cleaning the ear in between deeper veterinary prescribed cleanings or home flushing, to fight bacterial or yeast infections while it also soothes irritated and infected ears.

Avoid alcohol based products, which can irritate the ears further—unless you suspect water or oil is trapped in the ear canal; a few drops of pure alcohol can dry up the fluid residue. Don't worry about the alcohol found in herbal extracts if you make your own ear drops—very little alcohol remains by the final dilution.

Proper grooming is also beneficial in keeping ears free of infection or waxy build-up. Many breeds, such as Poodles, Terriers and Cocker Spaniels, grow hair close around the ear, and sometimes, even in it. You must pull the hair from in the ear and clip the outer areas close, to help air circulate. Ask a groomer to show you how to maintain your dog's ears or have it done professionally. Many dog breeds who are prone to ear infections have a closed flap ear, rather than a standing flap ear. A standing ear allows additional air to circulate, drying ears quickly and thoroughly, thus avoiding infection.

Proper ear care is of utmost importance to an animal's wellness. Long-term ear problems can lead to deafness and despondency. I have had several cases where after years of deafness, a build-up of old debris (some even from previously untreated mite infestations) was finally reversed and the body built-up through the LifeStyle™ process. There was a full recovery of the hearing within three months to six months.

Nutritional supplements for ear conditions:

- MSM helps repair and strengthen the sensitive tissues in the ear, especially tissue which has been chronically ravaged by allergies or fungal infections for years.

- Grape Seed Extract is a powerful antioxidant which provides exceptional immune support and reversal in chronic ear conditions. Excellent preventative during maintenance years as it also helps prevent so many other dis-eases, including cancer.

Herbal remedies for ear problems:

- Garlic Daily Aid is vital to eliminating ear problems. Use this high potency supplement for antibacterial or antifungal support. Because it is high in natural sulfur, garlic helps heal irritated tissue and reverse eruptions and irritations. Double your normal LifeStyle™ recommended dose until infection is not noticeable for two weeks.

- Yucca Intensive works as well as steroids, in reducing inflammatory responses. (See Allergic Reactions.)

- Yeast & Fungal D'Tox is an herbal formula which works well together for more serious or chronic yeast and/or fungal infections. Can be used internally as well as adding eight drops to your cleaning solution when needed.

- Aller'G Skin & Pimple helps soothe irritated tissue, often seen in chronic and/or severely itchy ears with rashes or tiny pimples inside and around the ear. Give as a supplement to support skin health. It also acts as a diuretic to help eliminate the waste that feeds ear rashes and infections. One bottle each spring as a preventative detox protocol will help reduce the occurrence of ear infections that spring/summer.

- **Aller'G Skin & Digestive** works the magic of several herbs in a combination that protects the liver from circulating antigens and allergens, thereby reducing ear infections and irritations associated with air-borne (including secondary cough) and food related allergies. Helps promote blood sugar balance and liver function to maintain proper nutrient assimilation and detoxification. Ear problems, particularly those accompanied by digestive disorders, respond well to this combination.

- **Aller'G Grass & Pollen** is an excellent formula to address ear infections directly related to grass or pollen sensitivities, often accompanied by eye irritation or discharge. Symptoms include very itchy, blotchy, infected ear tissue, often visibly swollen.

- **Blood & Lymph D'Tox** cleanses the blood and lymphatic systems, and activates the body's immune response. This combination is beneficial when the ear condition is associated with autoimmune dysfunction, which is chronic and difficult to address. Other symptoms that respond well to this herbal combination include ear flap hematoma, or blood blisters, which are often the result of trauma due to scratching.

- **Immuno Stim'R** is often the key to chronic symptom reversal through daily catabolic waste cleansing of the blood and immune stimulation. This herbal extract supplement can be the key to permanent symptom reversal in some severely chronically-affected pets when given for the remainder of their lives. Over many years of chronic symptoms (weakness) the body is so compromised that it needs life-long support or will rapidly regress back into its former condition, regardless of the LifeStyle™ supplements and diets fed. (See Immune System Dysfunction.)

While nutritional and herbal supplementation works to reverse systemic weaknesses and reduces symptom reoccurrence, homeopathic remedies can quickly reverse acute symptoms associated with ear-related allergies or irritation, giving the body the chance to build-up the fuel to reverse the underlying weakness associated with the symptom.

Homeopathic remedies for ear problems:

- D'Toxifier contains *Arsenicum* with complementary remedies which help the ears through improved nutrient utilization and waste elimination; given every five minutes apart for up to one hour will help stimulate suppression of most ear irritations. Reduces chronic conditions of a toxic lifestyle to prevent waxy discharge and infection; general restorative to help improve hearing.

- *R&R Essence and/or Aconite* support the pet who becomes overly sensitive about being petted on the head during or after being treated for ear problems.

- *Apis* is effective for sensitivities resulting in itchy ears.

- *Graphites* works well for foul smelling discharge.

- *Hepar Sulph* helps control sensitive, inflamed ears with discharge.

- *Hypericum* can be used if ears are extremely sensitive to touch.

- *Mercurius* relieves boils and hematoma found on the external canal, and is good for reversing thick, yellow discharge that is often foul smelling and bloody.

- *Rhus Tox* is indicated in chronic ear infections. It works well with Arsenicum.

- *Silicea and Arnica* combined are effective when a hematoma (large blood blister) has formed on the ear flap. The Silicea expels the blister, while the arnica helps it heal pain-free. Arnica can be used in a topical gel as well. (See Abscesses.)

If the ear seems more irritated, begins to bleed profusely, becomes unbearably painful, or develops a severe discharge, and is non-responsive to home treatment within a few days, then seek out veterinarian care immediately. Do not take ear problems lightly, as chronic inflammation and infections can lead to permanent damage, resulting in deafness. Reliance on a chemically-based, medicated ear wash or drops can also permanently damage the sensitive tissues of the ear.

(see Infections, Skin & Coat Problems, and Skin Parasites)

Eczema

(see Skin & Coat Problems)

Ehrlichiosis

(see Tick Fever)

Emotional Problems

(see Behavioral Problems, *specific behaviors are also listed, i.e.* Fearful, Shock)

Encephalitis

ENCEPHALITIS is retention of fluid on the brain and/or brain stem which causes pressure and dysfunction in the nervous system resulting in coordination problems, respiratory distress, vomiting and irritability, even aggression. It is generally caused by viral, fungal or bacterial infection or injury to the head. This is a symptom which needs veterinary diagnosis and support, although the remedies I am going to share with you have worked as well as the medical treatments, with less toxic side-effects, in the long-term. Acute, severe swelling may need to be handled with a medical steroid for the first twenty-four hours of injury but can be supported naturopathically once the life-threatening phase is over. Chronic brain swelling is best reversed naturopathically as the long-term use of medications can cause liver dis-ease and additional damage to the sensitive brain tissues.

Encephalitis may trigger seizures, stiffness about the head and aversion to being touched. Symptoms are similar to pets thought to have suffered from a STROKE, and the recommendations are the same.

(see Infections, Stroke)

Epilepsy

(See Seizure Disorders.)

Eye Problems

EYE PROBLEMS are almost always involved in toxic responses internally as well as topically, resulting in tearing (staining), redness or matter build-up and can accompany ear symptoms, as both the eyes and ears are indicative of liver function. Toxins, allergens and antigens can overwhelm the liver. Resistance to air-borne sensitivities, in particular, is compromised. Check your pet's eyes daily, and wipe away any matter present. Always address eye problems quickly as chronic irritation or infection can permanently damage the eye, possibly leading to corneal ulceration, cataract formation and even blindness.

To clean and condition the eyes and tear ducts:

- *To clean away slight discharge,* use a warm, damp cotton cloth. Always use distilled or purified water on the cloth, not chlorinated tap water. Wipe in the direction of the eyelashes to avoid further irritating the eye. Start in the inside corner; allow your pet to close the eye before gently wiping lightly downwards towards the outside corner.

- *To remove heavy matter or copious discharge,* in and around the eye, use a warm, wet cotton pad or ultra-soft cotton paper towel. Hold it gently against the eye, allowing it time to soften any hardened matter. Gently wipe the inside of the lid to remove discharge on the eyeball, being careful not to introduce any dirt or crust into the eye. Then remove the remaining matter on the outside lashes. Repeat as often as needed. Do not allow the eye to remain crusted-over and shut. This will encourage infection and can damage the eye or tear duct permanently.

- *Follow cleaning with an application of natural eye drops* made from a dilution of 6 drops of Calendula Extract into a couple of ounces of distilled water. An empty eye dropper is often available for sale at health food stores, or through Azmira®.

- If infection is present, six drops of Goldenseal Extract can also be added to eye drops, this will also help to open up tear ducts and encourage natural lubrication.

- For very irritated or dry eyes, apply a few drops of natural Vita E 200 oil, every other day, directly to the inside of the lower eye lid. Be careful not to scratch the eye. Blinking will disperse the vitamin E.

Herbal Supplements for eye problems

Always supplement with herbs to strengthen and cleanse the eye, increase resistance to allergens and infections, and support anti-inflammatory and antihistamine action. Proper nutritional and herbal supplementation can prevent and even reverse cataracts, a common side effect of chronic eye irritation.

- *Yucca Intensive* works as well as steroids in reducing inflammatory responses responsible for red, itchy eyes, swollen eyes, Cherry Eye and blocked tear ducts. This works well on symptoms of autoimmune and inflammatory dis-eases which render the animal blind.

- **Aller'G Free** is a natural antihistamine combination which quickly reduces acute responses resulting in itchy eyes and tearing. It is an excellent, short-term symptom suppresser, allowing other herbs and nutrients a chance to build up the body.

- **Aller'G Grass & Pollen** addresses symptoms that include very itchy, dry eyes, often visibly swollen, or weepy with infection.

- *Aller'G Skin & Pimple D'Tox* soothes irritated tissue which can manifest as severely inflamed, itchy eyes, with rashes or tiny pimples around the eyes, face and ears. It can help prevent and eliminate tiny eyelid cysts and is excellent for mange-reactive eye sensitivities.

- *Blood & Lymph D'Tox* cleans the blood and lymphatic systems and activates the body's immune response. This combination is beneficial when the eye condition may be associated with autoimmune dysfunction and can be difficult to address. This has been a wonderful therapeutic agent for the reversal of many types of blindness due to a reaction to a chemical, allergen or viral infection. Other symptoms that respond well to this combination include tiny blood blisters, or cysts around the lids, often the result of trauma due to scratching.

- *Immuno Stim'R* is often the key to chronic symptom reversal through daily cleansing and immune stimulation. This supplement can be the key to permanent symptom reversal in some severely, chronically-affected pets when given for the remainder of their lives. Over many years of chronic symptoms (weakness), the body can become so compromised that it needs life-long support or will rapidly regress back into its former condition. The LifeStyle™ supplements and diets help fuel wellness but the body seems so prone to regressing that the slightest catabolic waste builds up and the immune system falters. This remedy can help prevent, when given as daily support, and maintain reversal of some forms of blindness associated with a reaction to a substance.

Homeopathic remedies for eye problems

- D'Toxifier contains *Arsenicum* with complementary remedies for corneal ulceration and external inflammation. Great remedy for Cherry Eye. Lids are red, scabby, scaly and ulcerated. Hates to be in the sunlight or in bright lights. This formula helps the eyes through improved nutrient utilization and waste elimination. Reduces chronic conditions of a toxic lifestyle to prevent degenerative eye conditions; general restorative.

- *Aconite* is beneficial when the eyes are severely inflamed and red, with hard, swollen lids. Eyes seem aggravated by wind and sunlight, and tend to tear profusely.

- *Apis* is great for sensitivities to air-borne allergens or a toxic lifestyle, especially resulting in swollen, itchy, runny eyes. Helps slow the progression of reactive blindness.

- *Euphrasia* reduces excessive tearing, inflammation of lids and thick, sticky discharges. Ulceration of the cornea.

- *Hypericum and Arnica* should be used if there is injury and pain, due to a puncture, scratching or heavy rubbing of the eyes.

- *Hypericum and Silicea* work together to help unblock tear ducts. Also follow directions for abscesses, if needed.

- *Lycopodium* is for degenerative blindness. Eyes half open during sleep. Red, ulcerated lids.

- *Pulsatilla* is indicated for creamy, profuse eye discharges.

(See Corneal Ulcers, Immune System Dysfunction, Allergic Reactions, Infections)

Exhaustion

(see Lethargy)

Failure to Thrive

FAILURE TO THRIVE is often seen in pets with chronic disease after heavy doses of drugs have left them depleted and overwhelmed with toxins. This robs the body of vital nutrients, imbalances digestion and prohibits proper assimilation of future nutrition. Some autoimmune dis-eases and long term struggles with cancer lead to the breakdown of muscular tissues resulting in a "wasting away" condition.

Baby animals born of unwell mothers or too small to compete with their litter mates begin life depleted. If they cannot get enough nutrition, they too will soon fail to thrive. I've even seen babies weaned before their eating capabilities have fully matured, leaving them to a slow death from starvation and dehydration. They will attempt to eat and drink but slowly lose vitality. Shotgun medications are also suspect. Vaccinations given during a medical crisis or dental cleanings can often trigger, from the toxic overload, a failure-to-thrive condition particularly leading to anorexia and wasting disease. Therefore, detoxification and supplementation is paramount. Be sure to use homeopathic D'Toxifier which can stimulate reversal of many symptoms related to a failure to thrive.

Oral feedings may be warranted with Dairy & Egg Protein Powder. Mix three to six tablespoons of this nutritional powder with eight ounces of goat's milk for a mother's milk replacer or meal substitute. Increase thickness as appetite improves. The B-Complex in Mega Pet Daily should stimulate appetite. If not; add an additional 50 to 100 mg. of B-Complex 50 daily for a few days until the appetite improves. Supplements and herbal extracts can be added into the dairy and egg formula.

Fatty Tumors

(see Skin & Coat Problems)

Fearful Animals

FEARFUL ANIMALS, or those with vague fears and anxieties, are common. Many animals today do not understand what is expected of them or have homes where trust and routine are non-existent. They can be scared from trauma during their first experiences in another home but still see the world from that perspective, regardless of the love you give. Symptoms in the pet that lives with apprehension are varied. These pets react with overtly submissive behaviors that can be very frustrating to the owner or trainer. Submission is only second to hyperactivity as a deterrent to learning. Submissive urination is a prime example of this.

Fearful pets will shy away from your actions and are troubled, easy to panic. They will repeatedly perform poorly due to these worries interfering with their ability to pay attention and retain information learned, becoming easily discouraged. Lacking self-confidence and being fearful of known things is characteristic of these pets.

Fearful and overly anxious types may often also be diagnosed with some form of autoimmune or neurological dysfunction, including cancer, allergies, diabetes, arthritis, paralysis, seizures and general organ failure. Fear creates constant stress in the body disrupting the normal function of the digestive system which reduces nutrient assimilation and a build up of metabolic wastes causing a burden on the liver and kidneys, and so forth.

- Flower remedy—Fear—often does the trick when used both as needed and as a preventative. For known or vague fears.

Herbal Remedies

- Herbal Calm is a good supplement to give prior to a fearful situation.
- Calm & Relax can be given on a continuous basis for the severely fearful pet.

Homeopathic Remedies

- D'Toxifier contains *Arsenicum* with complementary remedies which help a fearful animal with chronic illness adjust, or after having suffered a toxic lifestyle. This formula aids the mind and body through improved nutrient utilization and waste elimination. Reduces chronic conditions of a toxic lifestyle to prevent fearful behavior; general restorative to help regulate the emotions.
- *Aconite* reduces the effects of any shock, resulting in a known fear.
- *Ignatia* comforts the grieving pet who now acts fearful.
- *Phosphorus* addresses fear triggered by the sudden onset of disease.

Nutritional Supplement

- B Complex-50 protects the nervous system in a chronically fearful pet and helps calm fear-induced anxiety.

Behavioral Guidance

Fearful pets need reassurance that you are non-threatening. They prefer things to be calm and hide from conflict, literally backing down or away from any perceived threat. They crumble under pressure or discipline; therefore it is best to focus on only positive reinforcement and easily obtainable goals. Try easy-to-complete exercises, such as retrieving a toy from the toy box. Give the command "get your toy" and praise when they return. Make it easy and fun.

This is an appropriate time to use treat-based training if needed. "Come" and "sit" for a cookie; it doesn't get any easier or more rewarding than that! Be a pal and a safe harbor and soon you'll see a new, more self assured animal at your side.

A Note on Fourth of July Fireworks, Thunder and Lightning

Dogs especially, are so fearful of loud noises that they can tear through doors and windows trying to escape thunder and lightning. Every Fourth of July the rescue, animal control and humane society shelters are filled to capacity due to the large stampede of dogs, cats and even a few horses, etc. that get lost trying to escape the light show and booms. They suffer through a night of summer storms, shivering under the bed. Unfortunately, there is no way to teach an animal what or where these noises are—but you can teach them (change their filters) to accept the noise and not fear it.

Calm & Relax should be given during the storm season. This will quiet the animal's nervous system rendering them less reactive to the noise. A few doses of Fear remedy in the water (in case you are not home when the storm hits) and a dose given every five minutes at the start of the storm will dramatically change their reaction. Following the recommended trust building exercises will help the animal "trust" you when you give them the command that it is, "Okay." Having you by their side, calm and collected and talking to them in a soothing voice will help them desensitize to the situation. There are sound recordings of thunder and lightning storms that can be purchased and used to help desensitize your pet to the sounds. Simply expose your pet to the recording a few minutes each day until they no longer react. This should also be done with the Fear flower remedy. If you can't be home and they are still fearful of the noise, then be sure to have a safe area (your bedroom is best) with their bed in it that they can get to for comfort. Close all the window shades to minimize the sounds. For severe cases, use an inside room with no windows.

During fireworks, be sure to have your animal restrained properly in a safe, quiet room and not left outside where they can get hurt in their panic. Have all windows properly secured so they can not get out and some soothing music playing. Give Calm & Relax (an herbal extract which affects the nervous system in a sedative way) three times a day for two days prior to the fireworks and R&R Essence the evening of the show, or more frequently if needed. If you have not had the time to build-up a therapeutic level in the body over a couple of days, then give a double dose of the extract as soon as you are aware that there will be fireworks that evening and rely heavily (every five minutes) on the R&R Essence. This has made a significant difference in animals of all ages, even those who suffered for years (increases the likelihood of a learned phobia) with fear of fireworks and now can rest through the night.

Feline Hyperesthesia Syndrome

FELINE HYPERESTHESIA SYNDROME or *Twitchy Skin Syndrome* is a condition characterized by a rippling of the skin on a cat's back, especially when they lick or are petted in the lower back region. Some veterinarians feel that it is a form of mild epilepsy—a theory I hold true as I highly suspect food additives and chemicals to be a primary culprit. I have also seen several cases develop following vaccination. Because this "weird behavior" is most often seen in high-strung cats such as Siamese and Himilayans—it is widely considered to simply be a behavioral disorder. Regardless of the cause, it can be very frustrating behavior to witness. A cat might chew or lick their rear end obsessively—often appearing spaced out or withdrawn from the family; jump and twitch in mid-air for no apparent reason or spontaneously dart about—attacking imaginary or real objects, including the owners or other pets. Drug sedatives or progestin compounds are the medical routes—often unsuccessful. The Holistic Animal Care LifeStyle™ can quickly reverse these behaviors through the use of calming and hormonal balancing remedies as described for EPILEPSY.

Feline Infectious Peritonitis or F.I.P.

FELINE INFECTIOUS PERITONITIS OR F.I.P. is a viral infection in the same family as the coronavirus which affects dogs. There are two types of coronavirus: one which is easy for the cat's body to shed, causing brief digestive upset, and the F.I.P.-causing virus. This highly contagious form is passed from cat to cat through the inhalation or ingestion of infected secretions or excretions.

Symptoms usually show up within weeks of exposure although it can take months or years for some cats to become symptomatic. Even then, the cat can often allow this potentially deadly virus to multiply and take hold before any outward symptoms appear—then symptoms can hit with a vengeance. Initial signs include upper respiratory problems which can subside quickly with no other signs until the body begins to fall apart. Unfortunately, the most common time to discover the cat has F.I.P. is during an examination and blood work-up for feline leukemia, as the two seem to often happen together. *This protocol is good for both feline leukemia and peritonitis infections.*

The scary part of F.I.P. is that the virus itself does little specific damage to the body. It is the body's exaggerated immune response to the virus that destroys the body's tissues, organs and blood vessels (and leaves it vulnerable to other dis-ease). This leads to two types of F.I.P. infection:

Wet (or effusive) F.I.P. —the immune system attacks blood vessels in response to the spreading virus. Fluid leaks out of damaged vessels and accumulates in the chest and/or abdomen, causing breathing difficulties or a distended belly which is often not painful.

Dry F.I.P. —inflammation appears all over the body and a wide variety of symptoms are suffered including coughing, vomiting, diarrhea, appetite loss, seizures, renal failure, coordination problems and even blindness.

The traditional veterinary mind-set on this disease (and many others) is that there are no effective treatments aimed at eliminating the virus from the body. Reducing the immune response with steroids and chemotherapy drugs might help temporarily with the clinical signs but cannot cure the dis-ease. Drug suppression of the symptoms at times only seems to cause the viral load to spread and the damage to be greater in effect. A vaccine has been available but it seems to create a great deal of vaccinosis and is one that I highly recommend against especially for isolated, in-door cats. Remember, it takes exposure to a carrier *plus* a depressed immune system to sicken the cat.

The most outstanding protocol I have ever followed for the reversal of F.I.P. infection is the use of herbs and homeopathy. It is amazing how quickly the LifeStyle™ naturopathic approach reverses the weakness caused by the body's attack on infected tissues, slows the viral load and eventually kills off the virus.

Herbal Remedies Proven to Help:

- Viral D'tox is used in the initial stages of infection and has been used successfully as a preventative to ward off any infection after known exposure.

- Blood & Lymph D'Tox benefits the body by halting the spread of inflammation in response to the viral load and removing damaged cells (keeping them from weakening the body further) during the more chronic cases especially involving wet FIP. This allows the body to repair itself faster.

- Immuno Stim'R is important to maintain wellness, after crisis has passed, and avoid a relapse.

Homeopathic and Nutritional Remedies: should be chosen to stimulate and support reversal of the specific symptom.

- D'Toxifier contains *Arsenicum* with complementary remedies which help the immune system through improved nutrient utilization and waste elimination. Reduces chronic conditions of a toxic lifestyle to prevent symptoms of FIP; general restorative.

(see Infections and Symptom-specific subjects)

Feline Immunodeficiency Virus (FIV or feline AIDS)

FELINE IMMUNODEFICIENCY VIRUS **(FIV or feline AIDS)** was discovered in the late 1980's. Until then the feline leukemia virus was considered the only trigger of immunodeficiency syndrome in cats. It is now widespread among cats. FIV is commonly transmitted through a bite which introduces virus-rich saliva deep into the tissues where it quickly spreads infecting the body. This results in symptoms similar to human AIDS. Wasting dis-ease (with or without anorexia), fever, diarrhea, chronic skin, bladder or respiratory infections and behavioral changes are common. Oral or lip lesions, lymph node engorgement, anemia, cancerous growths and edema are also noted.

Address prevention of FIV or viral load elimination and symptom reversal through recommendations listed for FELINE LEUKEMIA **(FeLV)** prevention and reversal.

Feline Leukemia or FeLV

FELINE LEUKEMIA OR **FeLV** is a devastating and fatal retrovirus infection, highly contagious and shares similarities with the human AIDS virus. It is spread through close contact between cats. The veterinarians recommend heavy vaccination against the virus despite the fact that Cornell University proved that over sixty percent of cats got FeLV from the vaccine. The clinical trial results were reported in the New York Times! Besides, I have found that an inordinate amount of vaccinosis diagnosis follows a history of FeLV vaccination. This is as deadly as the disease itself.

FeLV can be acquired and lay dormant for years until the right (or wrong) immune response triggers the virus' spread and damage to the surrounding tissues. This results in an overall suppression of the immune system, leading to chronic dis-eases which eventually kill the cat. That is if a drug-suppressive attitude is behind treatment.

Cancer (especially leukemia and lymphosarcoma), chronic anemia, lethargy, weight loss, oral lesions and even gingivitis can be symptoms of infection. The inability to fight off allergies or heal minor wounds is another symptom of immune suppression. Queens can pass the virus on to offspring through milk or the birthing process and kittens can be born failing to thrive or suffer poor reproductive success in general. These are simply symptoms of a toxic body, triggered by a virus instead of a chemical, allergen or other organism—the same applies in any case. I have had tremendous success with the reversal of feline leukemia itself and the variety of symptoms which accompany it. A naturopathic approach quickly addresses the body's weaknesses and brings the right fuel and tools for the body to heal itself.

First, let's discuss prevention, Isolation is detrimental to the emotional wellness of a cat, so in case of exposure, the cat must be protected from allowing the virus to take hold of the body before it can suppress the immune system. Since very few owners have ever been able to pinpoint a source or date of infection, I recommend that a cat be given one bottle (lasts approximately six weeks) of Viral D'Tox at least once a year as a way of killing off any traces of the virus that might have infected the cat recently—before it can develop into a serious organ weakness.

To address an active infection

- Viral D'Tox has been clinically proven effective in reducing the viral load, possibly eliminating the virus completely. Allopathic veterinary medicine sees no cure but I witness it everyday. We have cats return from the brink of death, after taking this product, and with the addition of symptom-specific remedies they fully recovered their health and lived out the remainder of their natural lives in wellness (as long as the LifeStyle™ was followed).

- Blood & Lymph D'Tox benefits the body by halting the spread of infection and inflammation in response to the viral load. It removes damaged cells (keeping them from weakening the body further) and promotes healthy tissue growth. This allows the body to repair itself faster and reverse wasting dis-ease, so common to FeLV cats.

- Immuno Stim'R is important to maintain wellness, after crisis has passed, and avoid a relapse. Can give an additional boost to the process of detoxification and strengthening in more severe cases.

Homeopathic and Nutritional Remedies

In addition to those listed here; others should be chosen to stimulate and support reversal of the specific symptoms suffered.

- D'Toxifier contains *Arsenicum* with complementary remedies which help the immune system through improved nutrient utilization and waste elimination. Reduces chronic conditions of a toxic lifestyle to prevent many symptoms of FeLV; general restorative.

- B-Complex 50 provides additional B vitamins which can promote appetite and energy, often lost when suffering from leukemia, anemia and wasting dis-ease.

(see Infections, Inflamation and other Symptom-specific subjects)

Feline Urological Syndrome or FUS

FELINE UROLOGICAL SYNDROME or **FUS** is often seen in cats with chronic health symptoms, especially after months of chemical therapies (steroids, antibiotics and even pest control products). As the body attempts to eliminate these toxins, the urinary tract can become alkaline and irritated, even blocked with bacteria or mineral crystallization. Detoxification can often clear up this chronic condition, but additional support may be needed.

- Daily nutrients provided in Mega Pet Daily and Super C 2000 should maintain acidic urine, if not, increase vitamin C by 500 mg. for cats. Acidic urine helps prevent crystals from forming and bacteria from growing into an infection. Vitamin A, E, Zinc and Selenium, included in Mega Pet Daily, also aid in repairing damaged tissue.

Herbal Remedies for FUS:

Herbal care can strengthen and tone the bladder and kidneys, encourage urine output and elimination of blockages and infection. These remedies can be used separately as needed or in combination with one another. ***Do note:*** failure to pass urine for twelve hours, regardless of remedy use, is a symptom which requires immediate veterinary intervention.

- *Kidni Flow* will stimulate proper urine production and elimination, reduce obstruction or crystal and stone formation, and soothe irritated membranes. Its disinfecting properties help reduce infection.

- *Kidni Biotic* acts as a natural antibiotic to kill off any bacterial organisms infecting your animal. Supports immune response function.

- *Yucca Intensive* acts as a general anti-inflammatory and alternative to steroids to support the urinary tract.

Homeopathic Remedies for Acute Symptoms of FUS:

- ***Thlaspi Bursa* is for the most urgent, emergency need without urine presenting; frequent F.U.S. with blockages.** Use every five minutes until urine passes, then every hour for four hours until pet is resting well. Use twice a day to promote full reversal of the blockage.

- D'Toxifier contains *Arsenicum* and is indicated for chronic urinary blockages to help eliminate toxins and organ wastes responsible for creating debris, crystals and stones in the urinary tract; given every five to fifteen minutes apart for one hour will help stimulate reversal of many acute symptoms. This is a good maintenance remedy for general FUS symptoms. A weekly, low potency dose is a wonderful detoxifier and urinary tract "toner" helping to keep things flowing smoothly. Complementary remedies also help the urinary system through improved nutrient utilization and waste elimination.

- *Aconite* or *Cantharis* reduces irritation and pain during urination

- R&R Essence helps relieve the tension and anxiety associated with painful urination. Works well when experienced discomfort has created a reluctance to urinate, even after the crisis has passed.

- *Uva Ursi* also helps urine pass freely past blockages when given every five minutes, usually in four to six doses. It is a lifeline for owners whose cats are still periodically blocking up despite the best diet, remedies and supplementation available.

(see Bladder and Kidney Problems)

Fever

FEVER is often a good sign, indicating that the body's immune system is responding to an imbalance through detoxification; destroying foreign objects (i.e. splinters), cancerous tissue or parasitic, bacterial and viral organisms which are weakening their host. The body is literally "burning up" these invaders in order to shed them. Same holds true for the cleansing of blood, organs or eliminatory wastes. Unfortunately, when the body breaks down its own muscle and organ tissues during anorexia/wasting or autoimmune disease as found in particular with kidney disease and cancers such as FIP, or the body's joints are too rapidly growing damaging new bone tissue, ligaments and muscles, this also produces fever and indicates an immune system imbalance.

Normal body temperature readings

DOGS: 100° to 101.5° The smaller dogs may run higher normally

CATS: 100° to 102° Breeds who are more energetic, like the Siamese, might have the highest normal readings, even up to 102.2° due to their higher metabolism.

HORSES: 100° to 102°

Temperature is best taken with a digital ear unit for dogs and cats. If this is not the case, be sure to use a non-petroleum jelly to lubricate a rectal thermometer prior to inserting it. For horses, be sure to hold on or attach the rectal thermometer to the tail to avoid losing it.

When we treat a fever with an OTC anti-inflammatory such as aspirin, or worse, steroids, we reduce the fever yet do nothing to eliminate the source. The fever often returns as soon as the suppressor is no longer working. Fever is best *supported* during infection, to more quickly eliminate the source of illness, rather than be suppressed.

Homeopathic Fever Remedies

- D'Toxifier contains *Arsenicum* with complementary remedies which help stimulate the immune system through improved nutrient utilization and waste elimination; given every fifteen minutes apart for one hour will help reduce a fever and resulting symptoms. Reduces chronic conditions of a toxic lifestyle to prevent a degenerative process.

- *Phosphorous* is excellent in reducing a fever without eliminating the goal of that fever; to eliminate the source of irritation. Often brings on a deep sleep which helps the process of detoxification.

- Calendula, when given as a supplement four times a day in the herbal extract form, helps lessen chronic fevers.

(see Infection, Cancer and Symptom-specific subjects)

Fleabite Dermatitis

(See Skin & Coat Problems)

Fleas

FLEAS can multiply to the hundreds just within the time it took me to write this sentence. They scared me; once an infestation began inside the home and yard, it took cans of chemical foggers and toxic dips to eradicate them. I saw many pets, especially cats, get very sick from the chemical warfare. But not today!

First, I have learned in twenty years of fighting these ancient vermin that a holistically-raised animal simply does not attract pests. I can't remember the last time I suffered an infestation despite the fact that my neighbors (on both sides) do not keep their dogs and cats flea-free. I have even had company bring over infested dogs to play with mine, yet still my own dogs remained free of parasites.

The biggest myth I wish to dispel is the fact that yeast is a preventative; this is so not true! Yeast can become a toxic substance to the liver, congesting this vital detoxifying organ and supplying metabolic waste in the blood to be exuded through the skin (the largest eliminatory organ the body has other than the liver). This exuded metabolic waste product actually attracts and feeds parasites such as fleas and ticks! Eliminate their dinner bell through detoxification. If the body is clean (inside and out) then it will never attract these pests. Prevention is the best cure!

Topical Solutions

- Groom daily to help spot (prevention) or remove pests, dead skin and coat. This also will make skin treatments easier.

- Form a protective barrier between invading pests and your home. Pick up the yard, clean the bedding and your pet well with a natural insecticide shampoo which can be made with Neem Dip mixed with Organic Shampoo, and followed with Neem Dip as a final rinse.

- Diatomaceous Earth can be an effective barrier between your home or yard and the pests. It is ground-up fossils which, when the dust coats the body of the flea, dehydrate and kills the pest with no dangers to the environment, children, beneficial pests or other animals. This can easily be spread around the yard and inside the house. It is economical and also effective against ticks, ants, cockroaches, silverfish and fly larva (spread it on your manure piles). It can be applied directly to the pet if needed, although some drying of the skin will occur.

  Azmira® only sells Food-Grade DE, so it is safe if ingested or laid in. Pool-grade DE is toxic to all living beings.

- Organic Shampoo is a wonderful shampoo. Safe for debilitated, very young or older pets. Gentle enough to use for regular preventative coat and skin cleaning. Can be used to kill off a small infestation when a half-teaspoon of Neem Dip is added to eight ounces of shampoo. Use neem with care on very young or weakened pets and rinse well; it is very powerful.

- Organic Neem Spray provides immediate protection for those trips to the park or other areas where fleas may infest your pet. Is also protective against ticks, flies, chiggers and heart worm-infected mosquitoes.

- Organic Neem Dip is the powerhouse of our arsenal against skin parasites. This is a very strong, "knock-down" product which kills fleas on contact. Use for heavy infestations, followed by the Organic Neem Shampoo. Can also be sprayed directly around the house and yard—as you would any flea spray—to kill those hiding in the carpet, furniture and baseboard cracks. First, be sure to test your fabrics for color-fastness.

This product can also be used as a preventative. Dip at the beginning of your rainy season (fall and spring) or anytime you hear that the fleas are on the rise—for year-round protection. Also good for mites and ticks.

Herbal Remedies

- Garlic Daily Aid provides therapeutic doses of sulfur which is good for tissue repair and strengthening and Thiamine (B_1)—a natural flea and tick repellent. Studies have shown that garlic is much more effective by itself than when combined with yeast.

- Blood & Lymph D'Tox is an organ and blood detoxifier which removes waste from the body and promotes optimum resistance against parasites. This is a good remedy to use for the severely debilitated and infested pet.

- Immuno Stim'R promotes catabolic waste removal on a maintenance basis, helping to keep the body clean and resilient against infestation. Especially benefits the weakened pet (suffering chronic dis-ease), to keep resistance high and avoid infestation.

- Stress & A'drenal Plex promotes vitality, restoring integrity to the adrenal glands when the flea infestation has exhausted the animal. As an adaptogenic formula, these herbs reduce the stress on a body that is constantly exposed to excessive physical or emotional conditions preventing or reversing a severe loss of energy, with anemia, low blood pressure and anxiety.

Homeopathic Remedy

- D'Toxifier contains *Arsenicum* with complementary remedies which when given weekly as a maintenance dose help the pet's resistance to parasitic infestation through improved nutrient utilization and waste elimination; given every five to fifteen minutes apart for one hour will help stimulate suppression of most skin irritations.

(see Allergies, Skin Conditions)

Food Allergies

FOOD ALLERGIES are often seen in pets with other chronic weaknesses as secondary symptoms. Poor digestion, combined with low-quality food ingredients, are most likely the culprits. The majority of *diagnosed* food allergies disappear soon after the animal is properly detoxified and is fed a high quality diet like Azmira®. (see Allergies, Digestive Problems; read Chapter 4: **Step One** and Chapter 5: **Step Two**)

Fractures

FRACTURES can occur due to trauma but are common in pets with nutritionally depleted and frail skeletal structures. These conditions may be due to metabolic bone disease or cancer. Symptoms will include non-weight-bearing lameness, with noticeable swelling and pain. Broken bones may present themselves through the skin or a grinding may be heard.

- Seek to immobilize the fractured area immediately and get to the emergency veterinary clinic.

- Emergency care can benefit from homeopathic support; use R&R Essence for emotional trauma and shock with *Arnica* and *Hypericum* for pain and physical trauma respectively.

- Utilize herbal Yucca Intensive to reduce inflammation and pain.

- Supplement with Calm & Relax if there is much pain or to help keep the pet quiet to protect the cast and rest the limb.

- Follow up with increased minerals, as found in Calcium with Boron-3 (*boron* 1 to 3 mg. and *calcium* 250 mg. to 500 mg. per day) supplementation for the first six weeks.

Fungal Infection or Mycosis

FUNGAL INFECTION OR MYCOSIS is both preventable and reversible through the use of The Holistic Animal Care LifeStyle™, homeopathic D'Toxifier and herbal Yeast & Fungal D'Tox.

(see Valley Fever, Ear Problems and other Symptom-specific subjects)

GastroIntestinal Disorders

(see Digestive Disorders)

Giardia

GIARDIA is often seen in pets who drink from puddles or dirty water buckets where this protozoa thrives. Bird baths can be a particularly difficult source of infestation to control, as many large dogs love to drink from these. It creates mild to severe intestinal distress resulting in diarrhea, even weight loss. Chronic infestation can lead to irritable bowel disorders. These secondary symptoms should be addressed as needed while the parasitic infestation is eliminated and the intestinal tract re-established.

Due to the wide-spread cases of giardia and the severe intestinal infestations that can accompany them, I created an herbal formula to eliminate this pest. This combined with the LifeStyle™ approach has quickly reversed cases of Giardia and strengthened the digestive tract.

Recommended Remedies

- **Giardia & Parasitic D'Tox** controls the spread of infestation as well as eliminates the organism through bitter compounds which activate digestive secretions, elimination of the parasite and blood cleansing. This herbal formula can be safely used with an irritated colon or severely weakened pet. This remedy can be used as a preventative, given for two to six weeks anytime you fear your pet may have been drinking out of puddles or exposed in any other way.

- **Yucca Intensive** will reduce bowel inflammation (a common secondary symptom) in severe or chronic cases. This herb contains steroidal saponins proven as effective as medical steroids.

- Homeopathic **D'Toxifier** contains *Arsenicum* with complementary remedies which help the intestinal tract through improved nutrient utilization and waste elimination; given every fifteen minutes apart for one hour will help stimulate suppression of most symptoms. Reduces chronic conditions of a toxic lifestyle to prevent infection. *Arsenicum* is very helpful in controlling many of the symptoms of bowel irritation, diarrhea and disrupted nutrition assimilation associated with giardia infestation.

- To help with recovery, Azmira®'s **Acidophilus** contains powdered Lactobacillus to replace friendly bacteria (needed for proper food absorption) in the intestinal tract when compromised by parasitic infestation or chemical deworming; a two to four week course is sufficient to re-establish a healthy environment.

- **NaturFiber** is an herbal product which helps repair intestinal distress and return proper bowel function when fed as a dietary supplement. This can also be given for a short term course, minimum of a month, or long-term to help provide and maintain a healthy digestive tract.

(see Symptom-specific subjects)

Gingivitis (Gum Disease)

GINGIVITIS (GUM DISEASE) is the sign of an unhealthy lifestyle and diet resulting in a toxic, weakened immune system. The body lacks nutrients to nourish healthy gums and the diet contains chemicals, sugars and by-products which are not only plaque-producing and bacteria-feeding but also nutrient-robbing in nature. It's a vicious cycle but one easily broken through the Holistic Animal Care LifeStyle™. I have never had dogs or cats develop major tartar or gum disease while on my protocols and I am still amazed how quickly the gums improve after beginning the LifeStyle™. Any broken or missing teeth should be examined immediately and dealt with through your veterinarian.

In addition to the LifeStyle™'s **Three Steps**, a healthy mouth requires routine brushing and dental care at home, as described for: TEETH. I highly recommend you engage in regular home dental care because the alternatives are scary. Dental cleanings are not only expensive but can be dangerous; your pet is put on a respirator during the cleaning and fully unconscious.

Herbal Mouthwash and Supplements: Rinse the mouth twice a day or more as needed

- Topically, a mouthwash can easily be made from two ounces of purified water with a half-dropper-full (approximately fifteen drops) of Goldenseal Extract or for a small pet use six drops in two tablespoons of water. Add fifteen drops of Calendula Extract if the gums are ulcerated or very angry. Some pets may object to the slight foaming that may occur. Reduce the number of drops used if this is a problem.

- Supplement with Yucca Intensive for very painful, irritated and inflamed gums.

- Blood & Lymph D'Tox addresses chronic, infected gum disease.

- Feed MSM to help strengthen gum tissue and tighten the teeth in gums.

- Grape Seed Extract is a powerful antioxidant which helps increase gum health.

- Vita E 200 helps provide additional vitamin E which is helpful in gum tissue repair; feed half a capsule a day (in addition to Mega Pet Daily) for cats and small dogs and one capsule per day for medium to large dogs and horses.

- Coenzyme Q10 is another excellent supplement for reversing gum disease and maintaining healthy teeth and gums. Use with MSM for severe cases.

Homeopathic Remedies for Gum Dis-ease

- D'Toxifier contains *Arsenicum* with complementary remedies which help prevent gum dis-ease through improved nutrient utilization and waste elimination. Reduces chronic conditions of a toxic lifestyle to prevent degeneration and infection; general restorative helps improve mouth health. Stimulates reversal of symptoms associated with irritation and infection.

- *Apis* addresses gums which are bright red and swollen.

- *Mercurius* is for gums affected by tooth decay (especially around the crowns) that are sore, painful to touch while eating and/or bleeding heavily.

- *Phosphorus* reduces bleeding and tender gums. Minimizes blood loss during oral surgery and tooth extraction when given prior to and during procedure.

(see Infections and/or Teeth for dis-ease and cleaning recommendations)

Granulomas

GRANULOMAS can develop from a penetration of an injurious agent (an imbedded foreign substance, allergen or infectious organism) that the body has "walled off" and created a small, hard raised mass of inflammatory cells on the skin. This hard knot slowly develops and can become the primary spot for a pet's focus of licking and chewing, which inflames the area more. Therefore, it is commonly thought to be simply part of an allergic reaction or obsessive behavior, and the condition is not addressed until the granuloma appears. Once the licking has become chronic, *it has also become obsessive behavior* and this is not addressed during traditional treatment. Although the "culprit" itself has been suppressed or eliminated, compulsive licking of the area will help continue the symptom cycle by re-irritating the skin. Azmira®'s homeopathically potentized remedy Obsessive is an excellent preventative to future obsessive licking.

Although surgical removal of the granuloma is often the suggested course of veterinary treatment, I discourage it because it can return with a vengeance and is then more likely to become cancerous.

Recommendations

- Homeopathic *Graphites* is a remedy of the highest caliber for the reversal of granulomas. Begin with a low potency dose, four times per day for the first two weeks, two times per day for another two weeks, then switch to a 200C dose once a day for four more weeks. This can be done in conjunction with D'Toxifier for the best results.

- D'Toxifier contains *Arsenicum* with complementary remedies which help the skin and immune system through improved nutrient utilization and waste elimination. Reduces chronic conditions of a toxic lifestyle to prevent development of growth of granulomas; general restorative to help tissue repair. It also contains *Thuja* for more stubborn cases; especially pets who have had a history of vaccinations as this seems to be more common.

- There should be noticeable improvement during detoxification and ongoing remedy use, with complete elimination of the growth possible. A life-long maintenance dose may be needed if the growth returns—give a *Graphites* 200C dose once a month after the symptoms are under control to prevent recurrence. Use this in addition to the recommended weekly dose of D'Toxifer.

(see Skin Disorders, Infections)

Grief

(see Shock)

Hairballs

HAIRBALLS can be a great source of frustration for the cat owner (and even a few dog owners). Unfortunately, one finally knows their cat has hairballs due to the vomited evidence left all over the rug. Some animals are automatically prone to ingesting hair as they groom themselves and others. Poor quality nutrition also encourages hair balls to develop. Diets heavy in fillers and animal fat promotes the collection of hair in the intestinal tract and stomach. Hair is not digestible, it must be moved through the digestive tract. Prescription diets aimed at prevention are actually detrimental to digestive health in the long run as the heavy fibrous content (often from harsh ingredients such as ground peanut shells or recycled cardboard and even sawdust can cause irritable bowel syndrome.

Most hairball remedies have petroleum jelly as the base or carrier for other ingredients and it is even a veterinary recommendation to put a dab of petroleum jelly on the cat's paws so they can lick it off, ingest it and pass the hairball with it lubricating the way. But, petroleum jelly is a toxic substance which can create liver inflammation, kidney disease and intestinal distress! For those who like this quick fix, there is a natural product available in the health food stores, that works in the same manner called **Un-Petroleum Jelly®**.

Following **Steps One** and **Two** is often all that is needed to reverse chronic hairball conditions. Azmira® diets contain whole ground grains and oatmeal, which help promote a properly functioning digestive tract, assuring passage of any collected hair or fur. A healthy body on a quality diet simply processes and eliminates ingested fur rather than vomit it back up. It is by-products and chemicals in the diet, plus a sluggish digestive tract, which leads to hairballs.

Topical Suggestions

- Increase daily fluid intake; add un-salted chicken broth to the diet or give as a treat.

- Give free access to potty and provide daily walks to promote proper elimination.

- Fast for twenty four-hours and feed Azmira® canned food exclusively for two weeks to help regulate bowel.

- Be sure to feed a minimum of two meals per day.

- Feed Mega Omega-3 (fish oil) which helps lubricate the colon and reduce inflammation.

Hairball Remedies

- NaturFiber is a great preventative supplement as well as therapeutic agent. This formula contains Chinese mushrooms, vegetable and fruit fiber. Optimal stool evacuation comes from moisture; guar gum and psyllium (which when used alone may be too harsh on the colon) are included for their moisture-retaining fiber, which helps form healthy stools.

- Herbal Wormer helps relieve intestinal blockage, constipation and minor irritation regardless of whether the symptoms are caused by intestinal worms or clogged hair. This is a good product to use in between fasting to help cleanse the colon of old fecal matter (which may be prohibiting the proper passage of ingested fur).

- **Acidophilus** helps promote the proper balance of friendly bacteria to aid in intestinal function. This should be given for two weeks after fasting and cleansing of hairballs. Can be given weekly as a preventative, to maintain proper intestinal wellness.

- **DigestZymez** aids digestion by providing enzymes, especially for protein digestion involved in breaking down and eliminating hairballs. Can help re-establish digestion in a chronically ill cat or dog.

- **MSM** provides tissue-toning nutritional sulfur to strengthen intestinal tissues and repair damage from chronic hairball conditions.

- **Calcium with Boron-3** provides minerals which help regulate (muscular) peristalsis; the intestinal "squeezing" which aids in moving food or hair matter through the intestines. Some older pets lose the ability to properly move bulk through their intestinal tract and need regulation. This product also provides the additional minerals older pets need for optimum structural strength and muscular function.

- **Herbal Wormer** has stool-softening properties and will help eliminate a hairball blockage resulting in constipation.

- *Bryonia* is an exceptional homeopathic remedy for hairballs. It can be used both as needed for acute upsets relating to the passage of hairballs (vomiting or constipation), or as a preventative. Give one low potency dose weekly.

- **D'Toxifier** contains *Arsenicum* with complementary remedies which help the bowel through improved nutrient utilization and waste elimination. Reduces chronic conditions of a toxic lifestyle to prevent hairballs; general restorative to help peristalsis (intestinal movement which passes hair through). Helps reverse numerous symptoms associated with hairballs.

Hair Loss

(See Skin & Coat Problems.)

Heart Ailments

HEART AILMENTS, such as a rapid heartbeat, can accompany chronic health conditions, such as allergies which stress this organ due to powerful surges of histamine and adrenaline. Acute symptoms from viral infection, poisoning or environmental triggers are commonly the basis for future chronic heart ailments if not addressed holistically. Genetic dysfunction such as heart murmurs and poorly developed chambers can also be aided through naturopathic care. Even congenital heart disease, in advanced stages, can be greatly improved through these recommendations. Most heart conditions can be prevented or reversed.

Genetic conditions are more common today but toxic, injured organs place an additional burden on the heart. I have even seen severe symptoms improve once the animal was placed on the LifeStyle™.

Since the heart is such an important organ, responsible for pumping all nutrients and oxygen through the blood and aiding in the elimination of cellular waste, it is vital for wellness that it functions properly. When heart problems are secondary symptoms primarily affected by a toxic lifestyle, then condition-specific remedies listed under the specific subjects should quickly address them. Excessive panting can mistakenly be attributed to pain associated with another condition, yet possibly indicate a more serious heart ailment. Be sure to report any changes in breathing patterns or weakness with exercise to your veterinarian. If your veterinarian has diagnosed a heart condition, and you need more support, consider the LifeStyle™ approach before relying on life-long medications.

Nutritional Supplements for Heart Problems

- Yucca Intensive, a steroid alternative, reduces acute heart inflammation.

- GLA 125 helps prevent inflammation, regulates heart function and repairs tissue. Improves elasticity and strengthening of heart muscle. Supports glandular functions, especially thyroid and adrenal needs.

- L-Carnitine helps strengthen the heart muscle. Minimizes heart murmurs and reverses heart dis-ease. Improves cardio / respiratory functions.

- Co-Q 10 aids circulation, respiration and the heart. Particularly beneficial with older, more debilitated pets. Supports the heart in better utilizing vitamins, minerals and amino acids for repairs and strengthening.

- MSM and Vita E 200 provide sulfur and vitamin E for tissue repair and strengthening.
- Calcium with Boron-3 helps regulate the heartbeat.

Homeopathic Remedies for Heart Problems

- D'Toxifier contains *Arsenicum* with complementary remedies which help the heart through improved nutrient utilization and waste elimination; given every five to fifteen minutes for one hour will help stimulate suppression of most heart irregularities such as a rapid or labored heart beat. Reduces chronic conditions of a toxic lifestyle to prevent heart dis-ease; general restorative to help improve the circulatory system. D'Toxifier is indicated when weakness is triggered by a chemical reaction, particularly by vaccination, topical skin treatment or pest control products. The heart may experience wild fluctuations. This formula also contains *Iberis* which helps to regulate a generally irregular heartbeat and reduce acute palpitations.

- *Aconite* is beneficial when labored breathing and tumultuous heart action follows allergic response, trauma, accident or when heart inflammation is suspected.

- *Digitalis* promotes a balanced, regular heartbeat (pulse) in cases of mitral dis-ease. This is an excellent chronic heart condition remedy. Improves the dilated heart, tired, irregular, with slow and feeble pulse where the least movement causes great distress with violent palpitations. For cardiac failure following fevers. For cardiac dropsy and hypertrophy with dilatation.

- *Phosphorus* is indicated for an inflammatory response due to viral or bacterial infection.

Herbal Remedies

- Yucca Intensive is a steroid alternative which quickly decreases heart tissue inflammation. Any time the heart is enlarged or inflamed this herbal remedy promotes the flow of nutrient-rich blood. This helps repair and strengthen heart tissue.

- **Stress & A'drenal Plex** promotes vitality, restoring integrity to the adrenal glands when heart dis-ease has exhausted the animal. As an adaptogenic formula, these herbs reduce the stress on a body that is constantly exposed to excessive physical or emotional conditions preventing or reversing a severe loss of energy, with anemia, low blood pressure and anxiety.

- **Calm & Relax** promotes relaxation, including relaxation for a trembling or thumping heart beat. Helps control high blood pressure when given as a daily supplement.

Heartworm

HEARTWORM has become a topic of great debate. On one hand, heartworm infestation can result in a painful death. On the other hand, the likelihood of your animal being bitten and infested is minimal in most parts of the country—and only during the rainy seasons. Therefore, why are <u>year-long, monthly doses</u> of heartworm prevention medication recommended? Why poison your pet with the hopes that a mosquito will then bite them and poison themselves? All this poison going through your pet's blood is also flooding its organ systems and burdening its immune system. This weakens the body and can result in cancer.

One hundred percent of dogs surveyed in 2003 through Azmira®'s customer service center had been on heartworm prevention drugs for at least three months prior to their first symptom leading to a lymphosarcoma diagnosis (cancer of the lymph nodes which had filtered blood carrying the heartworm medication's poison). We are now tracking the percentages that took heartworm medications and now suffer hemolytic anemia—it seems as bleak. Any chemical pesticide is dangerous and the side-effects are numerous. I highly recommend using natural heartworm prevention as we have had great results, including in Florida and other heavily mosquito-infested and heartworm prone areas.

Heartworm Prevention

- Newton's Homeopathic Lab® manufactures a heartworm nosode with which we have also documented great results preventing heartworm among Azmira®'s customers for years. This nosode is a must when attempting to prevent or reverse heartworm infestation. Follow the manufacturer's recommendations. Nosodes are homeopathic remedies made from diseased tissue that help stimulate an immune response.

- Follow a twice yearly protocol of **Giardia & Parasitic Cleanse.** Give it for a minimum of six weeks in the spring and repeat beginning in the last month of mosquito season. If concern is high, then give this supplement all season long plus an additional six weeks, in addition to doubling the **Garlic Daily Aid** supplement in your animal's diet.

Heartworm Reversal

- To kill the heartworm, cleanse and strengthen the heart: products listed above are also effective, but be sure to use under veterinary supervision as dying heartworms may block blood flow and proper heart function (as with the medical heartworm treatment with arsenic-based poisoning). May double the recommended dose for severe cases.

- **MSM** and **Vita E 200** will help repair and strengthen the heart muscles and surrounding tissues after infection has occurred.

- **Yucca Intensive** and **GLA 125** are valuable for reducing heart inflammation and discomfort. This may protect the heart from blockage as the worms are dying off but I have not been able to prove it clinically... yet.

- **Daily Boost** is a blood purifier and red blood cell builder to counter the effects of heartworm infestation. Reduces fatigue. Improves the function of the heart by encouraging better nutrient utilization. This is a general supplement which also works well in a preventative program, to help keep the body strong.

- **Blood & Lymph D'Tox** should be used with heavy infestations to help the body eliminate dead heartworms that have been killed with **Giardia & Parasitic Cleanse.** Use with very debilitated pets who need the extra boost.

For Topical Pest Control

- To repel mosquitoes that carry heartworm use **Organic Neem Spray** and/or **Organic Neem Dip** when exposure is high.

- **Diatomaceous Earth** works great at killing off mosquitoes by drying out the eggs. Sprinkle over wet areas to control mosquito hatching until the area is dried.

- Be sure to avoid having any stagnant water, such as unused bird baths or chronic puddles, on your property. This is where they breed and hatch.

(see Symptom-specific subjects)

Hepatitis

HEPATITIS is a serious, and at times, a life-threatening condition involving inflammation of the liver. This can be the result of an acute chemical, drug or allergic reaction, a symptom of parasitic, viral or bacterial infection, vaccinosis or even brought on by diabetes, heart disease, starvation, cancer, or simply a sluggish metabolism due to a poor quality diet and toxic lifestyle. Hepatitis can also develop with serious effects on chronic conditions including arthritis, allergies (poor skin & coat symptoms), nervous conditions and aggression, or digestive, eliminatory and immune system dysfunction. Not all cases of hepatitis are contagious in nature. Those that are contagious should be addressed as you would any other infectious disease such as parvovirus.

There are numerous diagnoses which have hepatitis as the root cause; the names are not important. Find out from your veterinarian HOW the liver is involved so you can apply homeopathic remedies (to stimulate) and herbs (to support) its healing. Is an infection the culprit, or vaccinosis? Then the appropriate remedies should be given to eliminate the injurious trigger. In each symptom-specific section you will see numerous references to liver involvement, especially within each product description—the liver is as vital an organ as the heart—Azmira® formulas always address this fact.

When the liver is in crisis the body immediately shows us there's an imbalance through digestive upsets: diarrhea, fever, vomiting, and loss of appetite. Therefore, most symptoms involve the liver to some degree, either as a side-effect or cause.

The liver filters your animal's blood of harmful toxins, drugs and organisms, promotes proper assimilation of nutrients through the intestines and maintains the pet's wellness. Unfortunately, the liver is such a resilient organ that liver inflammation usually doesn't show itself until the condition has become severe.

Since most veterinarians and owners suppress symptoms of gastrointestinal distress rather than support the liver in rebalancing and therefore reversing the symptom, it is no surprise that liver conditions are so numerous. Chronic use of anti-inflammatory drugs and antibiotics, diarrhea medications and diet changes (from one poor quality brand to another) to suppress gastrointestinal symptoms only hasten the demise of this incredible organ. Advanced hepatitis results in a yellowing of the eyes, skin, and mucous membranes, called jaundice, and is caused by elevated bile pigments in the bloodstream.

Reversing Hepatitis

- No matter what symptom progression you have witnessed, remember: **this organ is resilient and powerful given the proper three steps of The Holistic Animal Care LifeStyle™.** Detoxification and proper nutrition *to clean the liver and the body,* supplementation that *provides the "fuel" to heal,* and remedy use *to stimulate and support that healing,* will quickly promote proper liver function.

- D'Toxifier contains *Arsenicum* with complementary homeopathic remedies which help the liver through improved nutrient utilization and waste elimination; given every five minutes for fifteen minutes then every hour will help stimulate suppression of most liver-related symptoms. Reduces chronic conditions of a toxic lifestyle to prevent degenerative processes including hepatitis; general liver restorative.

- Skin & Liv-a-plex helps detoxify, decongest and repair liver tissue. This is an incredible herbal remedy for hepatitis and other liver-related conditions.

(see Liver Problems and Symptom-specific subjects)

Hip Dysplasia

HIP DYSPLASIA is a partial dislocation of the hip joints and is genetically passed down in many popular dog breeds today including German Shepherds, Dobermans, Rottweilers, Labs, Golden Retrievers, Mastiffs and St. Bernards. The genetic trait has become so dominant that in several breeds, particularly the Shepherds—as many as eight out of every ten pups born will develop symptoms before their second birthday! Cats can also pass this on genetically although injury is the most common trigger for their dysplasia, as it is with horses. Severe trauma, from a car accident, excessive exercise or jumping can also dislocate the hips.

Most symptoms occur in animals, especially dogs, within the first six to twelve months of age. I believe this is due to owners pushing their young pups who *look* grown due to their large size, but have not matured. A similar situation occurs when yearlings are pushed too hard and under saddle by two years of age. These young bone, ligament, tendon and muscle tissues are sensitive to trauma. Once your animal has been diagnosed—common symptoms are walking with a rear-end stagger and sway (wiggle) or a bunny hop with discomfort or trouble getting up and down—you must limit exercise to a few short walks per day. If the joint is pushed too far, to the point of fatigue, the tissue will begin to degenerate resulting in inflammation and pain.

Surgery is often sought out to stabilize the hip, yet I have found that it is not as effective in the long run, unless total dislocation and tearing of supportive tissue has occurred. Nutritional, herbal and homeopathic remedies have provided so much more support and recovery—in a high number of severe cases—than I have seen through surgery. If surgery is your only option, then these recommendations will also serve you well.

Topical Suggestions

- Avoid encouraging your pet to overexert him or herself—allowing pets to run or jump about too wildly could trigger inflammation and pain. Jumping up too high, especially straight up and down often, or excessive rotation of the limb can damage the joint and tear ligaments. Flying disc games are responsible for many a case of hip dysplasia in dogs.

- Never pull your young pet by the legs, and provide gentle exercise until they reach twelve months of age for dogs and cats or two years old for foals. This is the time needed for proper growth and strengthening of the structural and muscular systems. Long, hard hikes, jumps or rides are a major stressor to young joints.

- Swimming is an excellent way to exercise your dog or horse while strengthening the ligaments. High-end equine centers have long lap pools that accommodate horses. Cats will exercise themselves mostly, although be sure to encourage movement when needed. The stronger you can build the connective tissue, the more stable the hip will remain within the joint—reducing the very damage which leads to mobility difficulties, joint degeneration, calcification (from chronic bone repair) and pain.

Nutritional Supplements for Hip Dysplasia

- High doses of **Super C 2000**: up to bowel tolerance, or at least 2000 mg. for cats and smaller dogs to 4000 mg. for medium and large breeds, 4000 mg. for horses—can help prevent hip dysplasia—or at least slow down the degeneration and help relieve pain by strengthening connective tissue in existing cases.

- **Calcium with Boron-3** aids in the assimilation of calcium to prevent storage, through bone spurs or calcification of the joint (often associated with advanced dysplasia), and improves the tissue repairing capabilities of the body. Calcium is also an excellent tension reliever in the lower back and leg muscles, reducing spasms.

(see Arthritis for additional suggestions, remedies and nutritional support)

Hissing

HISSING between cats can strike fear into an owner's heart. There is no other sound like it. Luckily, there are several things that can be done about it without having to resort to giving away one of the cats. The homeopathic flower remedy **R&R Essence** is a wonderful place to start. Give it orally and put a few drops of it in a dish of clean water. Be sure that each cat has a safe place to retreat to or other behaviors and symptoms of stress might crop up. If needed, have someone handle the other cat while you take one in your arms (wrapping them in a towel for an added sense of safety: for them as well as you) and bring them close together with loving tones in your voices. Do this for thirty seconds at first and each step away praising the cat and soothing it. Wait a few moments until the cats have relaxed (giving them a shot of remedy if needed) and bring them together again for a minute, retreating and repeating the process over until you can have each cat face the other for longer periods of time.

Repeat this every day if they refuse to get together on their own. This will help to desensitize them to one another. Generally within a few weeks the cats should become acclimated to one another.

If the hissing is clearly a response of fear or aggression, then consider using the remedy **Fear** or **Aggression** instead. The herbal remedy **Calm & Relax** can be added for very difficult cases. Give for a minimum of two days before attempting desensitization.

(see Behavioral Problems)

Hot Spots

(See Skin & Coat Problems.)

House Training Problems

HOUSE TRAINING PROBLEMS can be very frustrating, especially when there seems to be no good reason for it—but there always is. First thing you need to do is rule out the obvious:

- Is there a physical cause for the animal's house training problem? Urinary tract infection or digestive upsets, even pain spasms, can cause "accidents." Seek to address this problem first.

- Does the animal have free access to potty areas or are its scheduled times too far between? Very young or old pets cannot "hold it" for longer than a few hours at a time. Chronic fecal or urine retention past comfort hour in a healthy pet (ten hours maximum) will create a weakness in the eliminatory system leading to retention problems. They can not hold it day after day without damage. Support proper elimination by providing proper potty areas and access.

- Has something threatened the animal's territory or routine? A new arrival or change in routine will often create stress in a pet that may result in house training accidents. Use the appropriate homeopathic flower remedies, i.e. Abandonment, Aggression, Fear or Spraying (marking territory).

If you are dealing with a new puppy, you can teach this puppy to piddle on command with approximately seventy-five repetitions of the same command (I use "pee-pee" as dog's respond best to two-syllable words). It eliminates the standing around waiting and begging them to go. I have taught all my dogs this command, including the older ones I acquired. This usually only takes a few days to accomplish; repetition is the key to success. You bring the puppy or dog outside to the same spot or to the paper each time after they eat, sleep or play, prime times when the urge naturally hits, especially after meals and nap time. *As they are sniffing around*, give them your command; softly repeating it until they make good. Then you praise them with lots of love and a favorite toy. After a few days the pup or dog will begin to sniff when you give the command. This is a great way to train a puppy so as a dog they are easy to introduce to a new potty area or to hurry up when you need them to go on command—for instance, during a storm or a car trip.

Kittens just need a clean litter box, out of the way as they need their privacy. Too much commotion and they will shy from using it. Be sure that the kitten is placed in the box after they eat, sleep and play. After a few times the kitten will associate the box but may still need reminders to go until they are three months old. A word of caution: Do not use clumping cat litter as it has been traced to severe gastrointestinal and respiratory symptoms, since the litter clumps when in contact with *any* moisture. Cedar shavings are too strong aromatically for cats and especially kittens to endure. Newsprint can be toxic to some cats and does not absorb well or provide any odor control, therefore, many cats simply stop using it. Plant-based (corn cob, wheat, etc.) and pine litters are most effective, economical and safe. Avoid using strong solutions or chemicals to clean a litter box; it may cause your cat to stop using the box.

Do not use chemicals or ammonia to clean your carpets or floors. Not only is this harmful to your pets, it enhances the urine signal left by previous accidents. Try applying vinegar to the spot to neutralize the odor, after first removing stool and blotting away all the urine moisture. Sprinkle baking soda over a smelly wet spot, left behind after stool removal, and it will absorb moisture and odor from the spot. This is easily vacuumed up the next day, leaving behind a fresher smell. An open dish or more with two ounces each of cheap vanilla extract (not imitation vanilla), left for a day or two in the room is also a wonderful smell neutralizer as it absorbs odors quickly and permanently.

Hyperactivity

HYPERACTIVITY is exhausting to both the animal and the caregiver. Certainly it can lead an owner to want to tear their hair out but it is far worse for the pet. Hyperactivity can lead to, or be a secondary symptom to stress-related conditions including diarrhea, cancer, allergies, kidney dis-ease, seizures and liver disorders. It certainly is a great detriment to responding appropriately to behavior guidance.

This emotional condition often has physical triggers at its source. Diets and treats high in sugar, beet pulp (even with the "sugar removed" there remains enough sugar to create an imbalance), artificial sweeteners or flavors and colors can leave a pet susceptible to hyperactivity. Some chemical preservatives may also alter brain chemistry or at the very least create a toxic environment for it as ammonia easily builds around the brain. Ammonia is a natural by-product of cellular processes, particularly elimination. Yeast and mold (found on poor quality grain by-products used in pet food or treats) are other injurious agents. Even the side-effects of vaccinosis or some medications such as steroids can leave an animal high strung. These should be addressed as well when suspected.

Behavior Modification Recommendations

- Allow your animal plenty of routine exercise and play time to help reduce anxiety.

- Choose one trick that they can learn well and consistently complete (i.e. fetching a toy). Use this to "distract" them during moments of hyperactive outbursts. It will have a grounding effect on them.

- Avoid situations which will trigger an outburst. For example, when company comes over, rather than allow the animal to run around crazy and escalate, simply put them away in a quiet room for a few minutes until they calm down and then lead them out to say hello. Return them to this room if they begin to get out of control. Don't fight the stimulation; avoid it until your pet can experience a different reaction through desensitizing exercises (see Behavioral Problems).

- Always maintain a calming voice—hyper animals escalate quickly with the escalation of excitement, fear or frustration in the owner's voice.

- Spay and neuter your pets. Unaltered animals tend to be high strung, although it can become a learned behavior as older pets do not seem to be as influenced by surgery and do not receive as much relief. But beware: if altered too early, before three months of age, they may become high strung from hormonal imbalances and trauma related to the experience.

Nutritional Supplements for the Hyperactive Animal

- B-Complex 50 provides vital B vitamins, needed to help soothe, tone or repair the nervous system. Mega Pet Daily already provides a good foundation but, in this case, the *addition* of another 25 mg. per cat and small dog to 50 mg. for large dogs and horses is recommended. This level can also be doubled as needed for severe cases.

- L-TryptoPet is a powerful amino acid which has beneficial effects on the hyperactive pet. It can help change and regulate brain chemistry—returning the brain to a calmer state. Some animals with severe hyperactivity require this supplement for life.

- **L-PhenyPet** is another powerful amino acid which has beneficial effects on the hyperactive pet. One trainer I know of uses this with great success to boost the benefits of L-TryptoPet in severely hyper and aggressive dogs. It can help change and regulate brain chemistry—returning the brain to a calmer state through an opiate-like reaction.

Herbal Remedies

- **Herbal Calm** promotes a rapid reduction in hyperactive behavior, used as needed for situational triggers (i.e. given an hour prior to company arriving).

- **Calm & Relax** benefits the ongoing protocol aimed at reversal of hyperactive behaviors. Promotes a deeper sense of relaxation, regulating brain chemistry and returning balance. Should be used for no less then six weeks, regardless of initial benefit, for optimum effect.

- **Stress & A'Drenal Plex** promotes vitality, restoring integrity to the adrenal glands when hyperactive behavior has exhausted the animal. As an adaptogenic formula, these herbs reduce the stress on a body that is constantly exposed to excessive physical or emotional conditions preventing or reversing a severe loss of energy, with anemia, low blood pressure and anxiety.

Homeopathic Remedy

- **D'Toxifier** contains *Arsenicum* with complementary remedies which help lessen hyperactive behaviors through improved nutrient utilization and waste elimination. Given every fifteen minutes for one hour will help stimulate suppression of most outbursts and lessen hyperactivity in general. Given as a weekly maintenance dose, it reduces chronic conditions of a toxic lifestyle to prevent negative behavior. It is a general restorative to help improve the nervous system.

I.B.S. or Irritable Bowel Syndrome

(See Colitis, Digestive Disorders)

Immune System Dysfunction

IMMUNE SYSTEM DYSFUNCTION is often the root of severe chronic conditions. It is vital that you address and support proper immune function regardless of your diagnosis. Unfortunately, it is common to see pets develop more serious dis-ease, such as cancer, after struggling years with digestive conditions, arthritis or allergy-related symptoms that have been suppressed. Each suppressive therapy has further weakened an already toxic immune system.

Many people have also reported an increase or sudden development of allergy-like symptoms after the pet has been treated medically for another condition (through suppression), such as kidney problems. This is because the immune system (or rather the organs which support it) can only take so much. It is a delicate balance between how many harmful agents these organs can filter and when their burden exceeds their manufacture of healthy immune cells.

Organs and Glands of the Immune System

- **The liver and kidneys** improve nutrient utilization and cleanse the blood.

- **The spleen** filters blood/lymph tissue, is a storehouse for white blood cells.

- **Bone marrow and thymus** is where cells of the immune system are manufactured.

- **Lymph nodes** provide frontline immune response.

Two Types of Immune System Disorders

- **Immunosuppression** is a condition where the immune system has been suppressed through an injurious agent: viral (such as parvovirus or canine distemper), drug therapy (especially steroids), vaccinosis, disorders of the bone marrow and/or severe stress. A suppressed immune system leaves the body open to all types of invading foreign organisms, allergens and cancer cells.

  Animals can inherit poorly functioning immune systems but the majority are created by a toxic lifestyle. A new trend, monthly pest control medications, has grave implications in creating a suppressed immune system. One hundred percent of all dogs with lymphosarcoma (a fatal cancer of the lymph system) have a history of being fed flea, tick and/or heartworm preventative drugs monthly. I suspect cats suffer the same on flea and tick preventative medications, although we have not studied this yet.

- **Autoimmune Dis-ease** is characterized by an overactive immune system that can damage (or inflame) the body's own tissues in response to an injurious agent. Reactive arthritis, lupus and atopic dermatitis (result of an overactive response to inhaled pollen) are prime examples. In autoimmune hemolytic anemia the body is destroying its own red blood cells and even some cases of hypothyroidism are thought to be an autoimmune response. As a side note, hemolytic anemia is currently being studied at Azmira® and heartworm medications are being considered as a common cause. The traditional veterinary therapy is high doses of corticosteroids—which suppress the immune system, leading to further complications with profound side-effects.

  In whichever case you address, the underlying weakness is an imbalance of the immune system's organs (function), and the best way to reverse most symptoms and health conditions is to detoxify, rebalance and strengthen the immune system first. This is the goal of The Holistic Animal Care LifeStye™'s **Three Step** approach.

Nutritional Supplements for Strong Immune Function

Vitamin C, A, B-complex and *E* cannot be surpassed for their immune-enhancing capabilities. Several other vitamins and minerals such as *Zinc, Selenium,* and *Chromium* can stimulate the capability of these nutrients, so a properly balanced and therapeutically-potent multiple supplement is essential, like Mega Pet Daily. To augment these vital nutrients, consider:

- Immune Factor Colostrum provides first-hour collected colostrum, the natural antibiotic-rich mother's milk that passes along a strong immune response. Helps to stimulate and support proper immune function.

- Co-Q 10 is referred to as a coenzyme which supports the body to assimilate various other nutrients. Promotes cellular detoxification and energy production, while aiding circulation. Benefits aging and ill pets; slows premature aging and reverses dis-ease by acting as an antioxidant and immune stimulator.

- **GLA 125 - Borage Seed Oil** maintains proper glandular function and thyroid support. Provides essential fatty acids and additional nutrients to fuel the body. Especially beneficial to pets who have severe skin problems or allergies, in addition to other immunosuppressive tendencies.

- **MSM** promotes tissue repair, especially in organs of the immune system.

Herbal Remedies for Immune Dysfunction

- **ImmunoStim'R** is an old tribal herbal remedy to eliminate catabolic waste (burdens the immune maintaining organs) and stimulate the immune system into rebalance. This remedy is a general one regardless of auto immune or immunosuppressive dysfunctions. Chronic cases often need this foundation for continued cellular detoxification and increased resistance. Several dog breeds such as Dalmatians, Cockers, and German Shepherds and Siamese or Persian cats, who genetically suffer chronic immune weaknesses such as infections, often fail to recover until this combination is introduced. A good preventative herbal remedy, this is beneficial for long-term use.

- **Goldenseal Extract** is one of Nature's antibiotics. Effective in fighting off viral, bacterial, yeast, and fungal infection while stimulating the immune system in general. This natural antibiotic cleanses the blood, lymph system, liver and kidneys. It can be used topically for the reversal of abscesses, gangrene, and pus discharge, and also as an eye wash to open up blocked tear ducts or as an ear wash to counter ear infections.

- **Viral D'Tox** promotes strong anti-viral **(and antibacterial)** activity and has immune-enhancing properties. These herbs enhance cellular immunity and liver function to protect healthy cells from antigens and infection. They are indicated in cases of chronic infections that have not responded well to medications, or where the liver may be inflamed. Can be used with **Immuno Stim'R** for debilitating or chronic infections, including Feline Leukemia, parvovirus and distemper.

- **Blood & Lymph D'Tox** acts as a blood and lymphatic drainer while activating the body's immune response. Symptoms that respond well to this combination include these and other conditions associated with a breakdown of the autoimmune system and catabolic waste build-up: cancer, general infections, chronic staph infection, tiny blood blisters, pimples / acne, skin ulcerations, lymphatic engorgement, tumor growth, cysts, fluid cysts, reactive arthritis and wasting disease.

- **Yucca Intensive** addresses the inflammatory response that accompanies autoimmune dysfunction.

- **Pau d' Arco** is beneficial for the whole body. Stimulates the immune system, heals wounds and combats infections. Kills viruses, effective against cancers (including lupus and leukemia), cysts, and tumors. Use both internally and topically for ringworm, hot spots, eczema, psoriasis and staph infections. Minor antifungal benefits. Excellent general support and reversal of cystitis, colitis, gastritis, diabetes, liver and kidney weaknesses. Relieves reactive arthritic pain and is easier on very sick, weakened or older pets to tolerate, than Goldenseal Root.

- **Yeast & Fungal D'Tox** formula combines herbs which are very powerful anti-fungal and anti-yeast agents. This combination is beneficial in reducing Valley Fever spore infestation and other fungal mycoses which are opportunistic of a suppressed immune system. It helps the immune system eliminate yeast overgrowth, vaginal infection, penis discharge and ringworm.

- **Stress & A'drenal Plex** promotes vitality, restoring integrity to the adrenal glands when illness has exhausted the animal. As an adaptogenic formula, these herbs reduce the stress on a body that is constantly exposed to excessive physical or emotional conditions preventing or reversing a severe loss of energy, with anemia, low blood pressure and anxiety.

- **Daily Boost** is an herbal blend which purifies the blood, replenishes red blood cells and improves digestion and assimilation to feed immune function. This is an excellent daily supplement for all pets to prevent immune problems and stabilize or strengthen a weak immune response. This is a must for older pets who are slowing down and more prone to dis-ease.

Homeopathic Remedies for Immune Dysfunction

Homeopathic remedies can facilitate the immune system's response to a specific toxin, allergen/antigen, bacterial, viral, yeast infection, or parasitic infestation, although they should never be relied upon *solely* to address immune imbalance. Homeopathy stimulates the body into responding by relying on the fuel and compounds available in the body. Therefore, you must supplement! If an animal is so debilitated, you have no choice but to use a homeopathic remedy *along with* nutritional and herbal supplementation.

- D'Toxifier contains *Arsenicum* with complementary remedies which help the immune system through improved nutrient utilization and waste elimination. Reduces chronic conditions of a toxic lifestyle to prevent dis-ease; general restorative which quickly triggers detoxification and elimination through the liver and kidneys. Helps your protocol work more effectively. Address a variety of symptoms associated with immune dysfunction.

- *Gelsemium* is an outstanding remedy for the first signs of disease, especially fever. Use this remedy for pets who seem very needy and want to be held when they begin to feel poorly, or have had a relapse after a long, debilitating illness and weak recovery.

- *Echinacea* is good for recurring boils, intolerance of insect bites, and lymphatic engorgement. It helps address fatigue often experienced during immune problems.

- R&R Essence is a flower remedy combination that addresses deep despair and anguish often experienced by a pet during and after a long illness.

(see Symptom-specific topics, i.e. Cancer)

Infections

INFECTIONS are generally a symptom of a depressed immune system which allowed viral, bacterial, parasitic or fungal organisms to establish themselves on a weakened host and are very responsive to naturopathic care. Some viral infections, such as parvovirus, actually suppress the host's immune system upon attack which is why the LifeStyle™ approach is so important for prevention as well. Once the organism attacks, it quickly gains control of the immune system's cells, often causing grave damage before any notable symptoms appear (i.e. severe fever and bloody diarrhea). Therefore it is vital that the protective, natural antibiotic compounds and nutrients are already there, in case of exposure. The same holds true after the introduction of a foreign object, such as a deep splinter.

Many lesser infections have completely reversed with only **Steps One** and **Two** before the host became weakened to any degree. Many foreign objects or organisms have simply been shed during detoxification. For the more difficult conditions, Azmira® has a full line of immune enhancing and infection-fighting herbal remedies (blood purifiers, natural antibiotics, antiparasitic and antifungals) and nutritional supplements.

There is one exception to addressing infections naturopathically: *Homeopathic support has never been, in my opinion, very effective in fighting infection by itself (there is no physical compound available to actually "kill" the offending organism) but should be used instead to address acute secondary symptoms (i.e. fever).*

(See Abscesses, Fever, Immune System Dysfunction and other Symptom-specific subjects)

Inflammation

INFLAMMATION is the leading symptom of dis-ease in general. When the body has been exposed to an injurious agent, such as an allergen or chemical (even metabolic waste), or sustained actual physical trauma, it causes congestion in the tissues. Congested blood and lymph fluids cause swelling and discomfort. This pain is the body's way of letting the host know that there has been an injury and resulting imbalance.

There are also dis-eases which are solely characterized by an inflammatory condition including myositis (inflammation of the muscles), hepatitis (inflammation of the liver) and pancreatitis (inflammation of the pancreas).

You will see Yucca Intensive listed in most of the subject-specific recommendations I have described in this chapter. This incredible herbal product contains *steroidal saponins*; compounds which are as effective as steroid medications—without the side-effects. Azmira® has conducted extensive research and clinical studies to prove its effectiveness in reducing inflammation and improving circulation, vital to detoxification. Azmira®'s ingredient is obtained from the concentrated extract, not the waste by-product powders the other manufacturers use due to their inexpensive cost. In addition I formulated Blood & Lymph D'Tox, and other antibiotic, antiviral and antifungal remedies, to help detoxify the tissues of congested fluids and eliminate the injurious agent.

Numerous homeopathic remedies are also listed by subject and quite effective in stimulating the body to reduce the inflammation by utilizing the available herbal and nutritional tools available to their fullest abilities. D'Toxifier contains *Arsenicum* with complementary remedies which help reverse inflammation through improved nutrient utilization and waste elimination; given every five minutes apart for one hour will help stimulate suppression of most inflammatory reactions.

(see Symptom-specific subjects such as Arthritis, Fever, Viral Infection, etc.)

InterVertebral Disc Disorder

INTERVERTEBRAL DISC DISORDER or *Spondylosis deformans* is a degenerative bone condition related to aging. It seems to have the greatest effect on large dogs, long backed animals or excessive jumpers (especially too high, too hard jumps). Pets that have suffered hard play (pups or small dogs pounced on by older, larger dogs) and cats and horses that have suffered back trauma are also susceptible. A sway-back is a predominant marker that this animal is susceptible to developing intervertebral disc disorders. Early notice of this structural weakness with chiropractic adjustment plus nutritional augmentation can help prevent the disorder.

It promotes the development of bony spurs that originate from the intervertebral discs and grow to bridge the gap between adjacent vertebrae. Pain and pressure on nerves from these growths can cause prominent hind-end weakness, interfere with digestion and elimination, and can progress into paralysis if left untreated. Homeopathic and herbal remedies are excellent for controlling secondary symptoms while these nutritional recommendations will help regenerate nerves and stabilize bone tissue.

Nutritional Supplementation

- Super C 2000, in high therapeutic doses (to bowel tolerance or a minimum of 2000 mg. for cats and small dogs, 4000 mg. for large dogs and horses); vitamin C will provide the building blocks to regenerate and strengthen connective tissues, eliminate toxins that inflame and stimulate circulation to promote superior nutrient utilization.

- Calcium with Boron-3 provides calcium to prevent the body from storing calcium through such processes as building bone spurs. Boron improves assimilation and tissue repair. When the body is lacking in minerals (or leeching them from bone tissue due to disease), it attempts to store this mineral to ward off *starvation* or total loss. Unfortunately, where the body chooses to store minerals (resulting in bladder stones, bone spurs and calcified joints) can be detrimental in the long run. Although traditional veterinary

237

logic is to reduce minerals when this occurs, I saw the connection over twenty years ago and began working with the therapeutic levels of calcium and magnesium to reverse arthritis and bladder stones with great success. Recently, Harvard Medical School published reports that backed up my beliefs and recommended mineral supplementation for bladder stones.

- MSM repairs and strengthens connective tissue to stabilize the intervertebral discs, reducing the sway-back effect, and helps maintain the spinal disc tissue itself by improving the "cushion" affect.

- Glucosamine also repairs and strengthens connective tissue to stabilize the intervertebral discs, reducing the sway-back effect. Should be added with MSM for severe cases.

- MegaOmega-3 greatly benefits tissue repair and softening of the cushioning disc. Protecting it from further damage especially when combined with an additional *(to* Mega Pet Daily*)* 100 mg. for smaller pets and 200 mg. for larger animals of VitaE200 (d-Alpha vitamin E). Prevents inflammation and pain during the maintenance phase; use Yucca Intensive to first eliminate the severe chronic or acute pain. Omega-3 fatty acids should be introduced to *aid* in reversing the inflammatory response and in the *least severe cases,* they can take the place of Yucca Intensive to help maintain inflammation-free tissues.

Homeopathic Remedies

- D'Toxifier contains *Arsenicum* with complementary remedies which help the discs through improved nutrient utilization and waste elimination. Reduces chronic conditions of a toxic lifestyle to prevent inflammation. General restorative to help improve disc health and elasticity.

- *Arnica* for muscular pain, especially marked by heat (sign of inflammation). Sore and lame is the picture of this remedy. This is an excellent acute remedy, especially following any trauma to the area (i.e. difficult chiropractic adjustment, fall, stress from travel, hard play-day).

- *Colchicum* benefits chronic pain and numbness resulting from muscular tension, particularly aching in the lumbar and lumbo-sacral regions. Sharp pains or numbness in extremities (chewing on feet and legs with no signs of allergies or parasites). Pet seems to be receiving "shocks" from time to time; may jump and then stare at their body with no apparent cause for this behavior. Symptoms improve with rest and pressure and/or massage.

- *Dulcamara* is particularly recommended for intervertebral disc conditions of the neck. Addresses rheumatic-type pains which are made worse by cold, damp weather. Spasms, even mild paralysis, are markers for this remedy. Rheumatism can alternate with chronic diarrhea or worsen after acute skin eruptions.

- *Hypericum* relieves the pain associated with a pinched nerve. Helps the nerve regenerate, reverse paralysis and strengthen to return optimum function. Dose as needed for acute pain, then dose once a week for one month with the lower potency. After the symptoms are under control, dose once a week for three months with a 200C (during the strengthening period), and then continue once or twice a month for maintenance.

- *Ruta* reduces formation of bone spurs while it acts upon the cartilage and muscles to reduce tension and pain. A noted remedy for lameness. Pain worse in morning before getting up and improves with massage or pressure applied to area.

- R&R Essence promotes a sense of well being, reducing stress associated with pain.

Herbal Remedies

- Yucca Intensive is the number one herbal remedy for inflammation. Reduces the trauma of inflamed tissues; the longer the disc and nerves are allowed to remain inflamed the more damage (breakdown) occurs, weakening the affected tissue and leaving it vulnerable to additional injury, tearing or permanent deterioration. As potent as steroid medication with none of the dangerous side-effects. Safe to use (even in double dose) for severe acute pain, or as a long-term supplement for maintenance.

- Calm & Relax provides physically-relaxing compounds which provide exceptional pain relief, reduce muscular tension and help promote a deeper sleep (for tissue repair process) when extra support is needed to augment Yucca Intensive. Especially benefits the animal who has become irritable due to fighting chronic pain and discomfort.

239

- ImmunoStim'R promotes metabolic waste removal from the blood and tissues of the intervertebral spaces. These wastes, and other toxins in the blood stream, feed the inflammatory response which creates more heat and discomfort, hastening the deterioration of these sensitive tissues. Promotes circulation which encourages tissue repairing nutrients to nourish these areas. This is an excellent daily herbal supplement to augment other anti-inflammatory remedies.

Irritable Bowel Syndrome

(see Colitis, Digestive Disorders)

Jealousy

JEALOUSY is a general term used for many behavioral symptoms pets seem to exhibit. For specific resentments and behaviors indicating jealousy or *bitterness*, these recommendations work well. They help stabilize the emotions triggered by another person or pet in the household, and changes in routine or family wellness (one person or pet is now receiving most of the attention due to medical, physical and/or emotional needs). These recommendations reduce negative thoughts and anxieties that can also trigger destructive behaviors (i.e. tearing up the other pet's favorite toy, or your shoe, in retaliation). Physically, jealousy and resentment can cause health reactions similar to fear and anxiety. Emotional stress creates physical stress; these pets seem to suffer an increase in urinary issues such as kidney and bladder stones or digestive symptoms such as diarrhea.

- Homeopathic Flower Remedy—Jealousy
- Behavioral Guidance—these pets need reassurance that you still hold them in high esteem and/or that ongoing changes will not effect them negatively. For instance, the new baby arrives and the pet is introduced as soon as possible (allow them to first sniff the baby's bare feet while you hold the baby and your partner holds the pet). Then the animal is allowed to be a part of the daily routines revolving around the baby (let them watch you changing the diaper and feeding while talking to your baby and pet about what you are doing)—while the pet is still receiving ten minutes of personal time a day with you, alone. Animals do better with a set routine, especially being given individualized attention (even if

only for feeding, training or exercise) in the same place and at the same time each day. They release negative emotions of jealousy the more involved they can become in the new situation, but often have not been allowed to participate due to their negative behavior. It's a vicious circle—only serving to reinforce their feelings of jealousy and promoting the dynamic—resulting in more acting out.

Joint Disease

(see Arthritis, Cancer, Pain, Infection, Inflammation, Hip Dysplasia, Patellar Luxation, Osteochondrosis, Panosteitis)

Kennel Cough

KENNEL COUGH is a problem of great consequence to kenneled dogs, particularly puppies and older, weaker dogs. I believe that a toxic lifestyle leaves the animal more susceptible but it is in the emotional stress of the experience that sends the immune system into suppression allowing the invading bacterial organism to infect seemingly healthy upper respiratory tissues. Therefore, prevention is the best cure! These recommendations can be used as a preventative or applied to reverse the symptoms of infection. Once infected, the symptoms will generally run their course in two weeks with no intervention—but the damage done to the immune and respiratory systems can permanently leave a dog susceptible to other conditions (especially allergies) later in life. With the LifeStyle™ antibacterial protocol, most dogs are completely well in forty-eight hours with no lasting side-effects.

Nutritional Supplements

- Super C 2000 is given at a rate of 1,000 mg. per twenty-pounds of body weight per day to prevent infection or to help eliminate the bacterium and its secondary symptoms (i.e. fever).

- MSM effectively repairs and strengthens respiratory tissue to counter the bacterium damage.

- Acidophilus is given to the dog who has been put on antibiotics for secondary symptoms. Start right after the drugs are completed and continue for two weeks minimum.

> *Avoid antibiotics at all costs! I have seen a high number of these cases linger longer than normal and I saw the drugs as the only contributing factor. Without the drugs, the body responds much more quickly to naturopathic care.*

Herbal Remedies

- Viral D'Tox (also good for bacterial infection as well) has been proven through countless experiences to effectively prevent the onset, or progression, of symptoms. Works on the bacterium that causes the cough. Helps protect the body from circulating bacteria so they can not infect the dog any further, while eliminating the infection itself.

- Stress & A'drenal Plex promotes vitality, restoring integrity to the adrenal glands when long-term kenneling has exhausted the animal. As an adaptogenic formula, these herbs reduce the stress on a body that is constantly exposed to excessive physical or emotional conditions preventing or reversing a severe loss of energy, with anemia, low blood pressure and anxiety.

Homeopathic Remedies

- *Kennel Cough Nosode* by Newton's Homeopathic Labs® is a remedy made from actual bacterium dis-eased tissues. Not only can this be used as a prevention tool, it quickly helps the body "identify" the invading bacteria and mount a defense to it.

- R&R Essence is a flower combination to help reduce the stress of being kenneled. It can simply be placed in the water dish or given orally. Azmira® has many no-kill shelters, adoption kennels and breeders who use it with tremendous results. Most of these organizations have totally eliminated Kennel Cough from their ranks by eliminating the stress!

- D'Toxifier contains *Arsenicum* with complementary remedies which help the immune system through improved nutrient utilization and waste elimination; given every five to fifteen minutes apart for one hour will help stimulate suppression of most symptoms, such as a rattling cough. Reduces chronic conditions of a toxic lifestyle to prevent kennel cough infection.

General Recommendations

- Send your dog off to the kennel with a favorite toy and one of your dirty night shirts (with lots of your scent on it!) to reduce anxiety and a sense of abandonment. Stress suppresses the immune system. Better yet, try to find a house sitter who will stay with your dog and forget the kennel.

- Once infected, provide rest and a fasting period (especially with fever present) of twenty-four to forty-eight hours with plenty of fresh apple and carrot juices available (dilute by half with purified water). Mix recommended supplements and remedies with juice twice a day.

(see Fever, Infections)

Kidney Disease

(see Bladder and Kidney Disorders)

Laminitis

LAMINITIS is a dis-ease of the equine hoof resulting in lameness. The inside of the hoof swells from premature aging, bad shoeing, trauma or infection and becomes congested with blood. Pressure mounts, creating pain. Eventually the hoof can deteriorate if left untreated. Most cases, even those of a severe chronic nature, reversed with the LifeStyle™ approach. I have had the best results with these remedies:

- Yucca Intensive promotes circulation and waste removal. It is an effective anti-inflammatory and pain remedy. You can apply it directly to the frog of the hoof as well as supplement with it. Generally the horse is standing more comfortably within four to six hours of the initial dose, which should be doubled. Give a dose every four hours for the first day or two, then use as directed. Can be safely given long-term.

- Homeopathic D'Toxifier stimulates the hoof into responding quickly and addresses many of the symptoms caused by laminitis. Complementary remedies help the body through improved circulation, nutrient utilization and waste elimination; given every fifteen minutes apart for one hour will help stimulate suppression of many pain symptoms. Reduces chronic conditions of a toxic lifestyle to prevent inflammation; general hoof restorative. Especially beneficial when vaccinosis precedes a bout of laminitis.

- Nutritional sulfur found in MSM helps repair this sensitive tissue and strengthens the internal structure. This nutrient will promote shock-absorbency in the hoof.

- Biotin promotes the growth and strengthening of the hoof wall.

(for other symptoms, i.e. Pain or Infection, see Symptom-specific subjects)

Lethargy

LETHARGY is a secondary symptom of a toxic, reactive organ system. Often the major symptom is fever, inflammation, vomiting, diarrhea, seizure, allergy reaction or arthritic pain. The pet has simply become overwhelmed and the body exhausted with effort in keeping its biological functions in balance. Detoxification and supplementation can often lift the pet out of this state, reinvigorating them. It builds up their nutritional reserves; provides the fuel to heal. With this energy they can apply the extra to their symptom reversal needs and not exhaust their own daily rations.

For some animals this state may be emotionally based, resulting from shock or depression. Stress will also interfere with proper biological functions such as digestion and elimination causing a physical symptom as well. Has there recently been a stressful situation or separation from a loved one? This could cause the animal to withdraw and mope around the house, losing all enthusiasm for life.

General Remedies

- D'Toxifier contains *Arsenicum* with complementary homeopathic remedies which help the body through improved nutrient utilization and waste elimination. Reduces chronic conditions of lethargy; general restorative to help stimulate vitality.

- Stress & A'Drenal Plex promotes vitality, restoring integrity to the adrenal glands when long-term illness or stress has exhausted the animal. As an adaptogenic formula, these herbs reduce the stress on a body that is constantly exposed to excessive physical or emotional conditions preventing or reversing a severe loss of energy, with anemia, low blood pressure and anxiety.

- **Daily Boost** contains herbs which help improve the digestion and assimilation of nutrients, relieving fatigue. Is a mild blood purifier and toner. Excellent daily supplement to prevent lethargy.

- **R&R Essence** reduces chronic conditions of lethargy resulting from chronic stress, especially emotionally based stress; general restorative to help stimulate vitality.

(see Behavioral Problems, Nervous System Dysfunction and Symptom-specific subjects)

Legg-Perthes Disease

LEGG-PERTHES DISEASE is an orthopedic condition involving the hips of smaller breeds, such as Dachshunds, Terriers or miniature Poodles—characterized by the degeneration of the head of the femur—where it fits into the socket to form the hip joint. This results in general lameness and pain with mobility and getting up. Follow recommendations for Hip Dysplasia.

Lick Granulomas

LICK GRANULOMAS can develop on the body, especially around the lower legs and feet, after chronic trauma and infection where licking has occurred.

(see Granulomas)

Licking

LICKING is a serious concern for many pet owners. Excessive licking is not only irritating to the owner, it will quickly exhaust the pet. The pet's vital healing energy is drawn to address this fatigue instead of supporting tissue repair and immune stimulation.

Although normal daily self-grooming includes licking the body clean, obsessive and chronic licking can lead to hairballs, skin eruptions, even growths.

- Homeopathic *Arsenicum* works the best for constant licking, especially when a build-up of urea is involved. D'Toxifier contains

Arsenicum with complementary remedies which help the skin through improved nutrient utilization and waste elimination; given every five to fifteen minutes apart for one hour will help stimulate suppression of most licking. Reduces chronic conditions of a toxic lifestyle to prevent skin irritation; general restorative to help improve tissue condition.

- **R&R Essence** will help reduce the anxiety associated with chronic licking.

- **Obsessive** is used for compulsive licking, especially when the injurious agent has been eliminated. Addresses chronic licking with no known cause.

- **Clam & Relax** helps reduce the anxiety and physical tension associated with severe, excessive licking.

- **Stress & A'drenal Plex** promotes vitality, restoring integrity to the adrenal glands when excessive licking and chewing has exhausted the animal. As an adaptogenic formula, these herbs reduce the stress on a body that is constantly exposed to excessive physical or emotional conditions preventing or reversing a severe loss of energy, with anemia, low blood pressure and anxiety.

When addressing a licking problem that is not responding; consider a chiropractic adjustment. Many pets are suffering from nerve impingement which is causing a tingling sensation in their limbs, resulting in their licking the area for relief. Sometimes the anti-inflammatory protocol addresses this as well as skin inflammation, so we never know the true cause.

(See Abscesses, Allergy Reactions, Chewing, Hairballs, Digestive Disorders, Granulomas, Skin and Coat Problems)

Liver Problems

LIVER PROBLEMS are often at the root of many symptoms. The liver can become additionally burdened (in excess of its daily function filtering the blood) and congested by seemingly innocent things including dietary agents such as yeast or chemical pest control products. Eliminate all yeast at once from your pet's diet, supplements, treats or pest control products if you suspect liver dis-ease. Do not use any chemical agents on or in your animal. If using drugs of any kind, speak to your veterinarian regarding their effects on the liver and alter or eliminate their use whenever possible. Reduce or eliminate all vaccines except those needed for licensing. These are primary culprits in burdening the liver.

Detoxification of the body is the liver's best talent. Protein digestion and fermentation in the intestines produce an ammonia by-product which is detoxified through the liver. The liver buffers toxins so they can be eliminated through the kidneys. The liver eliminates excreted hormones such as adrenaline, insulin and estrogen, after they have performed their slated tasks.

The liver is a vital organ responsible for the secretion of bile, stored in the gall bladder, which aids in digestion of fats and assimilation of fat-soluble vitamins (A, D, E and K) and the mineral, calcium. It promotes intestinal peristalsis, preventing constipation. Following digestion, nutrients are carried through the bloodstream to the liver for storage. These include vitamin A, B_{12}, and D. These are later utilized in daily functions involving tissue repair, immune response and other types of stress. The liver is important for fat metabolism which fuels the production of energy, cholesterol (as an antioxidant!), lipoproteins and phospholipids. It synthesizes fatty acids from sugars and amino acids while creating a substance called glucose tolerance factor (GTF) from chromium and glutathione to act with insulin in regulating blood sugar levels. Glycogen is finally created; sugar not immediately used for energy is stored in the liver and muscles to be later withdrawn and applied. In addition, the liver is also responsible for regulating thyroid function!

Immediately detox and fast your pet at the first sign of liver dysfunction, unless you have a sick horse or bird; then detox homeopathically only with D'Toxifier. Fasting will help the organ rest and detoxify burdensome metabolic waste, allergens, chemicals, drugs and organisms it has filtered. This will allow the liver to focus on itself, rebalancing its functions and strengthening its reserve.

The liver is a primary organ of the digestive, eliminatory and immune systems. All these systems are involved in the proper functioning of the body's defenses against allergens, toxins, organisms and tissue (body) repair capabilities. If you are to be successful in reversing your pet's condition, regardless of the diagnosis, you will have to be truly concerned about the care and support of your pet's liver. Regardless of whether the liver itself is to blame for the condition or an innocent by-stander, these remedies will help improve and return the liver to optimum health and function.

Herbal Remedies for Liver Problems

- Garlic Daily Aid is a wonderful detoxifier of the liver. Helps reduce general inflammation and organ congestion. Nutritional sulfur feeds tissue repair, promotes immune response. I also recommend garlic as a daily foundation supplement to prevent liver dysfunction.

- **Yucca Intensive** addresses liver inflammation (hepatitis) through detoxification and anti-inflammatory steroidal compounds. Promotes the flow of nutrient-rich blood through the liver which carries away toxins to be eliminated while fueling the liver for repairs and strengthening.

- **Skin & Liv-A-Plex** is a formula of standardized extracts which work together to promote optimum liver health and function. These herbs address improper fat and fatty acid metabolism, detoxify the liver and blood, reduce bacterial and hormonal disorders associated with poor liver function, and alleviate chronic skin conditions associated with hepatitis.

- **Viral D'Tox** targets cellular immunity and liver function to protect healthy cells from antigens, viral *and bacterial* infection. This is an excellent preventative as well as antibiotic formula.

- **Blood & Lymph D'Tox** acts as blood and lymphatic cleansers, reducing liver toxicity. This can be added to **Viral D'Tox** for stubborn, chronic infections.

- **ImmunoStim'R** is an old tribal herbal remedy for catabolic waste elimination and liver stimulation for improved immune response. Despite its name, it is also beneficial during dis-ease of an autoimmune nature (where the immune system is over-active and turns on itself) by reducing catabolic waste and *rebalancing* the immune function.

- **Stress & A'drenal Plex** promotes vitality, restoring integrity to the adrenal glands when liver conditions and chronic illness have exhausted the animal. As an adaptogenic formula, these herbs reduce the stress on a body that is constantly exposed to excessive physical or emotional conditions preventing or reversing a severe loss of energy, anemia, low blood pressure and anxiety.

- **Daily Boost** is an excellent supplement for reversing and preventing liver dysfunction. Promotes proper digestive and eliminatory function to feed and detoxify the liver. This is a excellent product for general liver health.

Homeopathic Remedies are very beneficial in the reversal of liver problems. Be sure to check other symptom-specific subjects in this chapter (i.e. Poison Control or Allergies) for a better understanding of what remedies are available.

- D'Toxifier contains *Arsenicum* (a primary liver remedy) with complementary remedies which help the liver through improved nutrient utilization and waste elimination; given every five to fifteen minutes for one hour it will help stimulate suppression of most symptoms related to liver dysfunction (i.e. vomiting, skin conditions, lethargy, aggression, etc.). Reduces chronic conditions of a toxic lifestyle to prevent a degenerative process; general restorative to help improve liver function.

- *Bryonia* benefits the animal who dislikes being carried or fondled, is irritable with chronic constipation, has excessive thirst with vomiting after eating or drinking. Liver is chronically inflamed and fatty in nature.

- *Mercurius* is indicated for jaundice with excessive flatulence creating distention in the abdomen. Stool is greenish, sometimes bloody and slimy. Animal may tremble and have fever.

- *Lachesis* is for the animal who is always hungry but any food causes upsets. Often has secondary symptoms of excessive, hard ear wax. Gums swollen and bleed easily. This pet may withdraw due to illness. This is a good choice of remedy for the pet who has suffered a toxic lifestyle. Constipated, with offensive stool. Old, dried blood may be eliminated with stool.

- *Natrum sulph.* is the remedy of bilious vomiting with flatulence. These animals suffer hepatitis with a tendency to develop skin warts and colic. They also suffer from loose, watery stools with some yellow diarrhea. These pets may exhibit inflammation around the toes and nail beds, with or without gout or allergies.

(See Anemia, Digestive Disorders, Hepatitis, Immune System Dysfunction, Poison Control and other Symptom-specific subjects)

Lumps

(see Skin Conditions: *fatty tumors, etc.*)

Lupus

LUPUS is a dis-ease of autoimmune dysfunction which attacks and destroys healthy tissue cells. It creates cancerous conditions with compromised liver and/or kidney function and is generally involved in the development of severe skin disorders, ulcerations and lesions with painful arthritic or muscular implications. Once you have a diagnosis of Lupus, the best course is to focus on the symptoms it is creating and the organ systems it is affecting. Do ask your vet to elaborate and explain your pet's condition; it will help you decide on the best approach.

- *Hydrastis* is the homeopathic remedy for Lupus, especially presented with ulcers and cancerous formations or skin lesions that are often markers. *For acute phase:* use a lower potency four times a day for a month. Upon improvement, once a day for another month. Switch to a higher potency (200C) for one daily dose for one month, then one dose per week for two to four months. *For maintenance:* give a single 200C dose per month. In addition to nutritional and herbal augmentation, this protocol will generally help to control this degenerative disorder.

(see Immune Dysfunction and Symptom-specific subjects)

Mange

MANGE is *a common condition in toxic, immune-suppressed pets:*

Demodex Mites are vicious skin parasites, who burrow down into the epidermis, causing **Demodectic Mange** with a great deal of discomfort and irritation. Scratching and chewing can quickly lead to infection with discharge. Puppies and chronically ill or elderly pets are particularly susceptible to demodectic mange, especially those who have recently been vaccinated. Puppies or kittens are often infested by the bitch or queen, who may not be symptomatic with mange but have mites herself.

These babies become symptomatic themselves after their young immune systems are compromised. It is common to see the onset of canine mange shortly after the start of puppy shots. Although they may grow out of it as their immune system matures, puppies can be very debilitated by chronic mange. Though it can be wide spread on the body, it is often located on the head and neck where it causes skin inflammation and spreading patterns of rashes and hair loss.

"Scabies" or Sarcoptic mange is seen in weakened or chronically ill pets. These mites can burrow into human flesh as well in order to lay eggs.

It is vital that you treat the whole household if symptoms appear. They can include itchy rashes localized around the ears, elbows and hocks. Scratching can be intense, so herbal Yucca Intensive and homeopathic *Apis* should be given orally to reduce inflammation. For a topical solution, see the advice given for Demodex mites.

Notoedres Mange is the most common form of mange to infest cats. *Notoedres cati* is a microscopic mite and must be diagnosed with a skin scraping. The nature of this mite is to burrow into the skin; mange is categorized by intense and sudden onset of itching. Hair loss and scaly or scabby skin, including severe dandruff can follow.

This is a highly contagious parasitic disorder and all pets who live with the infested one should be treated with an antiparasitic dip and shampoo. This mange can be common to cats with immune problems such as feline leukemia. The chemical dip is only available through veterinary clinics and is highly toxic. Many cats have negative side-effects, including seizures and autoimmune deficiency. Neem Dip is a safer alternative. Follow recommendations for other forms of mange, being sure to include an herbal compound for immune stimulation

Cheyletiella mange is also known as *walking dandruff.* This is manifested as dry, flaky skin with itching, especially when rubbed. This mange responds quickly to **Step One** detoxification and general anti-parasitic recommendations for scabies.

Topically, Treat Mange Daily:

- Make a mange solution of one teaspoon of Organic Neem Dip (kills mites on contact), half-teaspoon of Goldenseal Root extract with three tablespoons fresh-squeezed *lemon juice* (for infection) and six drops of Yucca Intensive (for irritation) diluted in two ounces of *Witch Hazel* and four ounces of distilled water. Saturate mange-infested area well twice a day with mange solution, then let air dry and leave it uncovered. For very young or debilitated pets, use a half-teaspoon of dip in this solution.

- Follow with an application of Rejuva Spray to reverse or prevent infection. Reduces skin inflammation and irritation. Promotes the repair of damaged skin.

- For very poor coat and skin conditions use Organic Shampoo once or twice a week for three weeks, then as needed. Has herbal properties which soothe irritated skin. This is appropriate for debilitated pets or young puppies and kittens. Can apply dip solution following bath.

General Recommendations for Mange and Mite Infestations:

- Skin & Liv-A-Plex is a wonderful herbal supplement for the treatment of mite infestations and their symptoms of skin irritation.

- Immuno Stim'R detoxifies catabolic waste from the blood. If left to congest the liver and weaken the constitution, this waste renders an animal more susceptible to re-infestation.

- Yucca Intensive is a steroid alternative which reduces the itch and inflammation associated with mange.

Homeopathic Remedies

- D'Toxifier contains *Arsenicum* with complementary remedies which help the skin through improved nutrient utilization and waste elimination; given every fifteen minutes apart for one hour will help stimulate suppression of most mange skin irritations. Reduces chronic conditions of a toxic lifestyle to prevent infestation; general restorative to repair skin.

- *Apis* is a homeopathic remedy for intense itching.

- *Graphites* is an excellent mite remedy as it addresses all the major side-effects of infestation from dry, flaky, unhealthy skin, to sticky discharge from pustules; all with intense itching and pain.

- *Sulphur* aids skin that has been ravished by burrowing mites, leaving pustules and large patches of dry, scaly, unhealthy skin.

(See Allergies, Infections, Skin and Coat Conditions)

Metabolic Bone Disorders

METABOLIC BONE DISORDERS result in a thinning and loss of bone tissue. This leaves the pet predisposed to fractures, growth deformities and bone cancer.

A common condition is *hyperparathyroidism,* where a calcium deficiency within the bone leads to abnormal bone growth and tissue loss as the body tries to correct the calcium imbalance. This occurs as the result of a high protein or all meat-based diet (especially the fad raw food diet which is high in raw meat, even harder to digest and assimilate causing imbalance) or secondary to kidney disease—these conditions all increase the likelihood that your pet will suffer from bone cancer.

A common feline condition is *mucopolysaccharidosis,* where an enzyme deficiency leads to abnormal bone growth and tissue loss as the body tries to correct polysaccharide carbohydrate accumulation. This occurs frequently in Siamese cats (genetics); this condition also increases the likelihood that your cat will suffer from bone cancer. Ask your veterinarian to educate you about your particular case's symptomology so you can best decide on your approach.

Recommendations

- Calcium with Boron-3 is a vital supplement for these conditions. Helps the proper absorption and utilization of calcium, prevents and reverses bone tissue loss.

- Blood & Lymph D'Tox formula is a combination of herbs that are helpful in reducing bone tissue loss. They act as a blood and lymph gland purifier encouraging the proper utilization of nutrients, eliminating catabolic waste (lost bone tissue) and minimizing the bone tissue damaging-effects of toxins and catabolic waste in the body.

- Gotu Kola benefits older pets, when given as a daily maintenance herbal supplement, by slowing down the degenerative process.

Mites

(See Mange, Skin Parasites)

Motion Sickness

MOTION SICKNESS is a particularly distressing condition for both the owner and the animal. Travel by car can become a nightmare. Once the animal "knows" that it has been sick before when traveling (a learned behavior develops), behavioral problems of increased anxiety and refusal to travel are common. Therefore, this is a condition that must be considered from both the physical and behavioral aspects.

Recommendations

- Homeopathically speaking, the use of *Petroleum* is highly recommended. This remedy has a marked influence on the physical motion sickness itself.

- D'Toxifier contains *Arsenicum* with complementary remedies which help the pet through improved nutrient utilization and waste elimination; given every five to fifteen minutes apart for one hour will help stimulate suppression of motion sickness. Reduces chronic conditions of a toxic lifestyle to prevent sensitivity to motion.

- R&R Essence or Fear remedy is a wonderful way to focus a pet, reducing anxieties and fear associated with the travel. A few drops orally every five minutes for three doses prior to embarking in the vehicle will significantly reduce stress and the resulting digestive upset. Continue every hour or so during the trip.

- Herbal Calm provides gentle herbal calming effects within thirty minutes for most pets. Can be used as needed. One dose lasts three to four hours—possibly longer when combined with R&R Essence.

- Calm & Relax is another herbal formula that replaces the use of tranquilizers (and their dangerous side-effects). Given as recommended for two days prior to travel, it will build-up maximum relaxing compounds in the brain. Effects last longer than with Herbal Calm alone, and can be gentler on the stomach, so this is a wonderful plane travel remedy. Use it for severe cases.

Myositis

Myositis triggers inflammation of muscle tissue resulting in stiffness, pain, weakness and eventual muscle atrophy. Partial, short-term paralysis is not an uncommon effect of acute bouts. A feline disease, such as *hypokalemia*—which affects the heart muscles and can cause uncoordinated limbs, difficulty eating and weight loss—is a common side effect of potassium deficiency that in turn can trigger overall myositis. Infectious conditions, including some parasitic infestation can also trigger symptoms, which are best treated individually, as symptoms, rather than a disease.

Another autoimmune disease, *masticatory myositis,* which affects the facial muscles and can cause difficulty eating and drinking, is a common hereditary trigger in German Shepherds. Infectious conditions including some parasitic infestation can also trigger symptoms, which are best treated individually *as symptoms,* rather than a disease.

Recommendations

- Yucca Intensive is an herbal steroid alternative, highly effective in reducing inflammation and pain.

- Herbs, especially in Calm & Relax can relax muscular stress and reduce chronic pain. Use with Yucca Intensive for severe cases.

- Stress & A'Drenal Plex promotes vitality, restoring integrity to the adrenal glands when muscular stress and pain has exhausted the animal. As an adaptogenic formula, these herbs reduce the stress on a body that is constantly exposed to excessive physical or emotional conditions preventing or reversing a severe loss of energy, with anemia, low blood pressure and anxiety.

- L-PhenyPet, an amino acid which reduces muscular tension and pain, can be added to Calm & Relax and Yucca Intensive for advanced pain control.

- B-Complex 50 provides additional B vitamins to help rehabilitate muscle nerve endings which have become hypersensitive.

- MegaOmega-3 is a fish oil-based fatty acid supplement known for its anti-inflammatory properties and ability to return softness to stiff muscles.

- Co-Enzyme Q10 is a nutrient which reduces muscular pain and stiffness by improving circulation to the muscles, providing a vast array of other nutrients to support tissue repair and strengthening. This is an especially good supplement for older or more debilitated pets.

- Grape Seed Extract is five hundred times more potent an antioxidant than vitamin E. Antioxidants are important in reducing the free radicals (from toxins, allergens, metabolic or catabolic waste) that irritate the muscular fibers, adding to the condition.

- OxyPro Antioxidant also provides a variety of standard antioxidants, including vitamin E and is a less expensive, but less potent, alternative to Grape Seed Extract. This is better suited for general maintenance once the **Grape Seed Extract** has helped stabilize the condition.

- *Gelsemium* is an outstanding homeopathic remedy indicated for various degrees of muscular weakness and motor paralysis. Try combining or alternating between acute and chronic potency dosages for best results.

- D'Toxifier contains homeopathic *Arsenicum* with complementary remedies which help the muscles through improved nutrient utilization and waste elimination; given every five to fifteen minutes apart for one hour will help stimulate suppression of general discomfort and stiffness. Reduces chronic conditions of a toxic lifestyle to prevent inflammation; general restorative to help improve muscle tone.

- Massage and gentle exercise can also strengthen the muscular system and greatly improve mobility and flexibility in both these conditions. Acupuncture (or acupressure) is also helpful.

(see Pain, Inflammation)

Myopathy

MYOPATHY is the more common term for generalized muscular weakness or dysfunction. Treat as you would Myositis.

Muscle Discomfort

(see Pain, Myositis)

Neediness

NEEDINESS or being over anxious to please the owner *while seeking constant reassurance* is the best way to describe the needy pet. These pets may also have feelings of inadequacy, but are so overly concerned about things, that this creates a lack of attention to detail. Interfering in their judgment or retention of learned behaviors, this behavior results in poor performances that only serve to reinforce their feelings of inadequacies. They can border on pushy and are often vocal pets, needing constant attention from you or they might retaliate by withdrawing from you. Constipation, fur balls or irritable bowel syndrome can often be the physical companion to neediness. Autoimmune disorders, especially allergies, are also not uncommon in these pets' histories.

- Homeopathically-potentized Flower combination—Neediness

Homeopathic Remedies

- *Arsenicum* is for needy and irritable pets in general. D'Toxifier contains *Arsenicum* and other remedies beneficial in reversing needy behavior resulting from a variety of triggers, including chronic illness, allergies, vaccinosis and thyroid imbalance. Promotes proper nutrient utilization and waste elimination.

- *Ignatia* is used when behaviors arise from the loss of something or someone dear to them. Much grief has been involved.

Nutritional Remedies

- Use herbal Calm & Relax, instead of tranquilizers, for severe behavior-induced stress.

- L-TryptoPet contains an amino acid which helps soothe the needy pet, reducing negative behaviors.

Behavioral Guidance—see recommendations for Jealousy and Resentment

Nervous System Dysfunction

NERVOUS SYSTEM DYSFUNCTION can be the most difficult to treat since so many components are involved. Initiating and regulating electrochemical messages to and from the organ systems and the brain is the work of the tiniest neuron where originating and sharing messages happens to the largest bundle of nerves where the message is received. Creating and carrying the impulses of daily functions proceeds from the brain, which is responsible for muscular movement, sensory awareness, memory, and learning—where even a slight imbalance of minerals such as potassium can cause it to falter and misfire. It continues down through the brain stem (regulates the heartbeat, breathing, vision, and hearing), the hypothalamus (responsible for messages to the endocrine system) and spinal cord (major connection between the brain and the body). From there it proceeds to branch out from in-between each vertebrae through two types of spinal nerve fibers which carry somatic messages of conscious thought to and from the structural system and skin or autonomic messages which are reflexes under little control regulating glands, internal organs and functions such as breathing, temperature and hormone secretion.

From nutrient loss (starving the cells and altering their message) to nerve damage (due to trauma, toxins or organisms), the message can get lost or misinterpreted. This can create a great deal of dis-ease for the body. Many training problems and bad behaviors stem from underlying neurological imbalances. Toxicity, from viral infection, metabolic waste or chemical exposure, which is very highly suspected in these cases as irritation to the brain and nervous system can quickly manifest so many symptoms. Damage to the nerves through structural or traumatic impact can result in mobility issues. Brain damage, from accident or blunt trauma, can trigger encephalitis (inflammation) resulting in seizures and pain. Even recovery from a potentially fatal viral infection can have neurological consequences (such as feline leukemia or distemper). Therefore, prevention and reversal—through the use of The Holistic Animal Care LifeStyle™— is fundamental.

First, find out from your veterinarian what is behind the diagnosis. For instance, what part of the brain and nervous system does she or he think is most affected (damage to the brain stem, nerve deterioration or pinch, etc.) and by what (electrolyte imbalance, poison, dehydration, viral infection, or structural and organ inflammation)? Proceed to work with those symptoms. You must address the injurious agent, if known, or relapse is sure to follow. Suppressive therapies, including drugs and surgeries may temporarily give a fix but they will only hasten the deterioration of the nervous system. It is best addressed and reversed naturopathically.

(see Degenerative Disc Disease, Feline Hyperesthesia-*twitchy skin syndrome*, Intervertebral Disc Disorders, Seizures, Strokes, Paralysis, Wobbler's Syndrome, Vestibular Disease)

Nose Conditions

Nose Conditions can be indicative of a severe imbalance (malabsorption, immune system, thyroid or adrenal malfunction) or environmental stress (exposure to fungus, chemicals and excessive sun rays). The Holistic Animal Care LifeStyle™ promotes healthy tissue everywhere, including the nose. The most common symptom I see is loss of pigmentation. A healthy black nose will fade to grey or pink. This will return with **Step Two**, as pigment is created through nutrients. A loss of pigmentation is often caused by drugs that interfere with nutrient assimilation or poor diets to begin with. **Steps One** and **Two's** nutritional programs will foster a stronger immune system which will be evident in a healthy black nose.

The second most common symptom is that of a rough, discolored ridge of tissue forming on the bridge of the nose pad, just where it connects with the fur. Some animals produce this extra tissue in response to the sun's burns; the majority is showing a toxic reaction due to a toxic lifestyle. Some puppies with Distemper or cats with Feline Leukemia or F.I.P. also are prone to developing this secondary symptom.

In general, whenever you address a primary condition (poor organ health, etc.) through detoxification and supplementation to strengthen the body's immune response, these symptoms will probably begin to improve despite a lack of focus on it.

Nose Pad Protocols

- Depending on the age, previous history and condition of the nose, you may have to add, in **Step Three**, Blood & Lymph D'Tox for a few months to deeply cleanse, rebalance and strengthen the body's organ systems and immune response.

- Herbal Yucca Intensive, MSM and Grape Seed Extract combined, along with the recommendations in **Steps One** and **Two**, have reversed a rough pad condition within six months to a year.

- Topical applications of homeopathic Rejuva Gel can help return tissue elasticity and heal sunburn.

- A natural sunscreen for children can be applied to protect against sunburn.

- D'Toxifier contains *Arsenicum* with complementary remedies which help the nose through improved nutrient utilization and waste elimination. Reduces chronic conditions of a toxic lifestyle which cause the deterioration of the nose pad; general restorative to help improve upper respiratory system.

(See Upper Respiratory Problems)

Obesity

(See Weight Problems)

Obsessive Behavior

The most common obsessive behavior described in dogs is often referred to as the "retriever syndrome" due to the fact that this breed is most prone to a specific fixation—most often to a ball. Cats seem most prone to obsess about places like their feeding station. They will return to the empty dish several times a day in an obsessive attempt to make dinner happen, even right after a meal. Birds, due to their confinement issues, may obsess the most—generally on a person. Horses, as far as I know, do not have the tendency to become obsessed as much as other animals even though they are very emotional creatures. Cribbing is the most common form of obsessing I have found in horses. They can become much attached to another animal, such as the barn cat, and exhibit seemingly obsessive behavior.

All pets who obsess about licking themselves or another object or pet; holding something in their mouths, even if food is available; looking out for or barking after "the enemy"; relentlessly or constantly squawking for no apparent reason—repeating whatever negative behavior they fixated on—often seem desperate to act out this behavior. They can be quick to act out, yet are also often over-anxious and shy. These pets may need to always do better, never satisfied with the routine. Extreme moods and/or mood swings are often the result of hormonal imbalances during different life stages, including the process of dying. The obsessive pet may become controlling and pushy. Physical, neurological or digestive dysfunction, arthritis and allergies can be common ailments found in obsessive pets.

Stabilizing the emotions, especially due to hormonal issues such as reproductive cycles that trigger negative behaviors including vocalizations and escaping, is addressed with these recommendations:

- Homeopathically-potentized Flower Remedy—Obsession

Homeopathic remedies

- D'Toxifier contains *Arsenicum* which detoxifies the brain; for great anguish when obsessed-about object is removed. This is formulated with complementary remedies which help the pet's nervous system through improved nutrient utilization and waste elimination; given every fifteen minutes for one hour during fixation can help reduce the need to obsess. This is an especially good remedy for obsessive pets who become aggressive when the object of their affection is taken away.

- *Chamomile* soothes the whiny pet.

- *Gelsemium* is for the pet who wants to be left alone with the beloved object and is taken by surprise when you come near, they are so fixated.

Herbal Remedy

- Use Calm & Relax to quiet the severely obsessed animal. These compounds promote a deep relaxation which can help while using behavioral guidance to lessen the fixation and accompanying anxiety. This is an excellent alternative to tranquilizers.

Behavioral Guidance

- These pets need to be kept busy with a large variety of activities and toys. They need gentle reassurance and set boundaries around how obsessively they can engage in an activity. Some breeds will obsess on the traits that have been bred into them (such as digging or fetching) but with controlled activities to release these urges, they can become more balanced and less destructive.

(see Behavioral Problems for desensitizing exercises)

Odors; Body

(read Chapter 4: **Step One**)

Orphaned Animals

ORPHANED ANIMALS can be a joy to rescue but it is hard work that requires round-the-clock care when they are very young. There are four things to remember when rescuing a baby: Warmth. Water. Food, and of course, Love. If you are not certain that you can give the time and attention needed, there are many organizations that rescue animals both wild and domestic. Your local humane society can give you referrals. Before rescuing a wild animal, be sure that it is truly abandoned and not simply left by mom temporarily so she could go hunting. If you are not certain, then leave it to Mother Nature.

Warmth

The hardest thing for a young puppy, kitten, bird or foal to do is to maintain its body heat. Especially in the first four weeks of life, the body relies on littermates and/or mom for warmth. When this is lost, the stress of fighting the cold can lead to dis-ease and weight loss from shivering. Too much energy is expended trying to stay warm that there is not enough energy to go towards growing healthy and strong. This can be easily remedied by using a low warmth electric pad in the bed, just be sure that it is water proof. If not, wrap a hot water bottle in a towel and place by the puppy or kitten. A heater or heat lamp works well for foals and birds. A ticking clock can also be wrapped up and placed in the bed or hung in the stall. This is soothing to the baby as it mimics the beating heart of a mother.

Water

Water is the most overlooked nutrient when raising a baby. It is assumed that there are enough fluids being consumed in the milk replacer, and there are at first. But the baby needs to be drinking water on their own during the first month and it is easy to forget to make this available to them. Be sure to provide a shallow dish or bucket that is impossible to tip over and to use filtered water. Chlorine is especially harsh on the baby's sensitive digestive tract.

Food

Food can be tricky to provide for those orphaned animals recently on mother's milk. Fortunately, Azmira® has **Dairy & Egg Protein Powder** which makes a great milk replacer. It is a nutritionally fortified powder which provides all the nutrients a growing foal, puppy or kitten would need. Just add three tablespoons of powder to eight ounces of goat's milk and give as much as the baby can consume at each meal, six to eight times a day before one month of age, then four times a day until they are on solids. The milk replacer can be thickened with Azmira® canned food as the appetite grows and the baby's eating abilities improve. This is what is so important about a baby's food: making sure they get enough of it and frequently. Speak to your veterinarian regarding the feeding a very young birds, as they require special handling. Be sure to add a sprinkle of **Mega Pet Daily** and **Super C 2000** to their meals.

For very weakened pets—those failing to thrive—a capsule of **Immune Factor Colostrum** (for antibiotic-rich colostrum usually received in the first milk meal), can be added to the milk replacer, in addition to any other remedies which may be appropriate to reverse their symptoms of dis-ease.

Love

Love and homeopathic R&R Essence or Abandonment can do wonders to minimize the negative side-effects of abandonment.

(see Abandonment)

Osteoarthritis

OSTEOARTHRITIS or *degenerative joint disease* describes a common condition where the cartilage is defective or deteriorating (a common side-effect to a toxic lifestyle). These conditions allow too much rotation or action in the joint capsule, resulting in bone tissue damage. Calcification occurs to repair bone although, more commonly, over-calcification occurs resulting in stiffness, inflammation, muscular tension and pain. Hip dysplasia is a common form of degenerative joint disease. Many cases of arthritis are due to tissue damage more than that are hereditary. Improper nutrition and old injuries from car accidents or physical over-exertion can result in these conditions. Infectious arthritis is joint inflammation and pain due to a bacterial or viral infection.

Fever and fatigue with painfully swollen joints can accompany cases of infectious arthritis. *Limping kitten syndrome* is a prime example where the kitten manifests generalized lameness and pain with hot, swollen joints from a bout of feline upper respiratory virus. *Polyarthritis* (affecting more than one joint) is a common reaction in pets having been infected from various viral, bacterial or fungal sources.

(See Arthritis, Hip Dysplasia, Immune System Dysfunction and other Symptom-specific subjects)

Osteochondrosis

OSTEOCHONDROSIS *(hypertrophic osteodystrophy HOD)* is a common condition characterized by abnormal growth and development of joint cartilage in young, large breed dogs, resulting in lameness and pain. Over-exertion, trauma and too much high protein or high calorie feeding are the most common culprits. Although many parents pass this predisposition along, It can be easily prevented or minimized, during the pup's first year of nutritional augmentation with the LifeStyle™ foundation supplements.

Especially with the vitamin C and balanced calcium recommended for cartilage and bone tissue strengthening. Cartilage repair and strengthening are also the most effective methods to reverse symptoms non-surgically.

(see Hip Dysplasia, Panosteitis)

Osteomyletis

OSTEOMYLETIS is the result of a deep wound, including a bite from another dog or cat, which has infected bony tissue. Open fractures also predispose a pet to infection, while fungal or bacterial organisms can spread from other parts of the body, via the blood. These pets become feverish and lame—often requiring surgery to remove affected bone mass, but a holistically raised pet will most likely reverse infection prior to becoming so serious.

(see Immune System Dysfunction, Infection)

Patellar Luxation

PATELLAR LUXATION is similar to hip dysplasia—but localized within the knee. Genetics and/or improper nutrition has left the ligaments surrounding and stabilizing the kneecap weakened and vulnerable to injury or degeneration. The animal may walk or run fine until they suddenly yelp and pull up lame. Unable to stand on the affected leg for a few moments they seem to just as suddenly be fine again, with no pain. Arthritis of the knee is a common side-effect. A total dislocation of the patella is possible and requires surgery, in which case my protocols to strengthen the joint while decreasing inflammation and pain can help the knee help faster and stronger. Follow the recommendations for Hip Dysplasia.

(see Pain)

Pain

PAIN can create a host of other symptoms such as digestive upsets and anxiety or irritability and should always be a consideration in any symptom reversal protocol. It is important to never underestimate how much pain an animal is suffering; they will never fake it although some may be more stoic than others. Several factors which cause pain, including inflammation, can reverse themselves during **Steps One** and **Two** alone. The others can easily be addressed in **Step Three**—each symptom-specific subject refers to pain control remedies when appropriate.

Additional support can be sought from a veterinary chiropractor, acupuncturist and/ or massage therapist. Massage and acupressure can be done at home as well, in between professional treatments. There are several books available to help you learn how. These modalities can be extremely helpful in fighting chronic or severe, acute pain. The additional expense may save you hundreds of dollars in future supplementation and months of suffering to your animal.

When needed, for excessive pain which is not fully responding to the symptom-specific recommendations, try these additional suggestions:

Herbal Pain Remedies

- Calm & Relax helps provide proven compounds which work on the nervous system, greatly reducing the tension in the body's muscle groups as well as the nerve endings. Promotes sleep and deep rest to allow the body the energy to heal (rather than fight the pain). Reduces anxiety and depression, symptoms which often accompany pain and chronic conditions. This is a great pain eliminator and my first choice, *along with:*

- Yucca Intensive, a steroid alternative, to counter pain-producing inflammation.

- Stress & A'Drenal Plex promotes vitality, restoring integrity to the adrenal glands when pain has exhausted the animal. As an adaptogenic formula, these herbs reduce the stress on a body that is constantly exposed to excessive physical or emotional conditions preventing or reversing a severe loss of energy, with anemia, low blood pressure and/or anxiety.

Homeopathic Remedies

- D'Toxifier contains *Arsenicum* with complementary remedies which help the body through improved nutrient utilization and waste elimination; given every five to fifteen minutes apart for one hour will help stimulate suppression of many pain symptoms. *Arsenicum* is for the animal who responds with irritation and/ or aggressively to being touched. Often, the liver or other deep organ is involved. Reduces chronic conditions of a toxic lifestyle to prevent pain triggers; general restorative.

- R&R Essence promotes an improved sense of self, reducing the need to fight their pain or your handling of them while they are in pain. This homeopathically potentized flower remedy has been proven beneficial in relieving the emotional (and resulting physical) tension associated with a pain condition thereby reducing the pain response. A great complement to Calm & Relax.

- *Aconite* benefits the pet who doesn't want to be touched due to pain and is in a great state of anguish of mind and body. These pets have a sudden and great sinking of strength.

- *Gelsemium* benefits the animal who becomes hysterical when touched. These cases often revolve around the urinary tract disorders, specifically kidney dis-ease.

Nutritional Remedies

- L-PhenyPet is an amino acid which promotes rest and relaxation of the nervous system. It is a powerful non-addictive analgesic. It seems to be responsible for increasing the activity of brain endorphins believed to be involved in the analgesic response. May also help alleviate depression from long-term pain or illness. Often helps animals have superior responses to other pain therapies. There is some evidence that it may help reverse chemical damage to brain tissue from drugs, pesticides and toxins.

- L-TryptoPet is another powerful amino acid long touted for its ability to promote sleep and a fuller relaxation during rest. This is often the key to reducing muscular tension in the body which increases pain and the sensitivity of nerve endings. Essential in regulating the brain's activity responsible for mood disorders caused by excessive pain and long-term illness.

(see Symptom-specific subjects)

Pancreatitis

(See Digestive Disorders.)

Panosteitis

PANOSTEITIS (Enostosis) is a disorder of the leg bones; the elbow/shoulder joint seems to hurt but the entire shaft of the front or rear long bones can be affected. Young, large breed dogs between the ages six and eighteen months of age are prone. Shepherds (highly genetically-prone),

Danes, Retrievers, Dobermans, Rottweilers and Basset Hounds are most likely to become symptomatic.

Lameness is of sudden onset with no known cause of trauma. It may be localized or the pain may originate on one side and seem to shift to another. One day may be painful, the next day not so bad. Some dogs also show secondary symptoms such as fever and an elevated white blood cell count.

Upon X-ray the bones show a thickening of bone tissue and narrowing of the bone marrow since new bone growth forms on the inner and outer layers of the leg bone. Within two to three months the leg will normalize itself and the X-ray will show no abnormalities. Lameness generally occurs for no less than two to three weeks, no longer than five to six weeks. If there is pain and lameness past this point, than your dog is suffering from another disorder.

Prevention is possible; I have had little cause for concern in the thousands of puppies raised on the LifeStyle™ approach. I have raised several litters of Rottweilers and not one ever had any issues. This is because nutrients found in **Mega Pet Daily** provide a well balanced mineral composition which promotes the proper formation of bone and prevents mineral build-up.

Often dogs with low dietary mineral availability develop Panosteitis in response to storing calcium and magnesium to prevent "starvation" of these vital minerals also needed for proper heart and digestive tract function. I believe this can account for large breeds being so susceptible— they demand much more calcium for their faster growing bones than do the smaller, slower growing breeds. Non-digestible sources of calcium in foods and supplements, such as bone meal, oyster or egg shells, are also the cause of improper use and storage of minerals.

(see Arthritis for other Symptom-specific remedies, i.e. Pain and Inflammation)

Paralysis

PARALYSIS or muscular weakness can result from a reaction to an allergen such as yeast, pollen or food by-products, an infection, vaccination, chemical or medication, in addition to physical trauma. After a proper veterinarian diagnosis to identify bacterial, viral or neurological origin, nutritional, herbal and homeopathic remedies can reduce inflammation, pain and debility. Often a proper course of holistic treatment can result in complete reversal of paralysis, given that no severing of the spinal cord has occurred.

Homeopathic Remedies for Paralysis

- D'Toxifier contains *Arsenicum* with complementary remedies which help the nervous system through improved nutrient utilization and waste elimination; given every five to fifteen minutes apart for one hour will provide initial relief of many symptoms. Also helps lessen the anxiety and irritability often felt by animals with pain and disabilities. Reduces chronic conditions of a toxic lifestyle to prevent spinal cord and nerve deterioration; general restorative to help improve nervous system.

- *Gelsemium* is an outstanding homeopathic remedy indicated for various degrees of muscular weakness and motor paralysis. This is a good remedy for the sudden onset of paralysis. Benefits the depressed, withdrawn pet.

- *Hypericum* is indicated when nerve involvement or damage is suspected.

Herbal Remedies

- Yucca Intensive is as effective as steroids in most applications. If needed, yucca can even be used in conjunction with steroids to reduce the need for heavy doses of this potentially harmful medication, until the herb alone can be used for long-term maintenance—generally within seventy-two hours.

- Stress & A'drenal Plex promotes vitality, restoring integrity to the adrenal glands when paralysis has exhausted the animal. As an adaptogenic formula, these herbs reduce the stress on a body that is constantly exposed to excessive physical or emotional conditions preventing or reversing a severe loss of energy, with anemia, low blood pressure and anxiety.

(see Arthritis, Degenerative Disc Disorders, Inflammation, Pain)

Parasites

(see Pest's name or Symptom-specific subjects)

Parvovirus

PARVOVIRUS is a viral infection which produces a multitude of symptoms with a high percent of cases fatal. The virus is highly contagious—especially to very young puppies or older, debilitated dogs. It can affect the gastrointestinal (digestive) system, the immune system and heart. The virus attacks cells which are rapidly dividing, such as those in the intestines, lymph nodes and bone marrow hence these become targets for infection. Very young puppies can be left with permanent digestive or heart conditions due to cellular damage in these developing gastrointestinal and heart muscles.

The most notable difference in this viral disease is an extremely foul smelling stool (and at times the same metallic odor is also coming from the mouth). These bouts of bloody diarrhea, where septic intestinal tract tissue is shed, can predispose a dog to a future of irritable bowel syndrome and wasting dis-ease, especially if the initial symptoms are treated with veterinary-prescribed steroids (anti-inflammatory) and antibiotics.

Early signs of this infection include loss of appetite, diarrhea and fever. The dis-ease progresses and takes hold of the body very quickly; with exposure to death occurring in as little as seven to nine days. Secondary symptoms are more obvious as lethargy, vomiting and diarrhea with bloody, metallic smelling stools become more extensive. Heart failure, due to loss of blood and fluids (from diarrhea and vomiting) plus septic infection, is often the end result of this progression. There is also a silent form that can affect the heart muscles with no other outwardly symptoms shown. This can result in a sudden-death heart attack situation of no apparent cause—until blood workup is completed.

The veterinary community does not have high expectations for an infected dog. They generally believe twenty-five percent will die, twenty-five percent will survive with no lasting side effects, twenty-five percent will survive with non-life-threatening side effects such as chronic flatulence and another twenty-five percent will survive with life-threatening side-effects such as gastrointestinal deterioration (a condition often diagnosed as irritable bowel syndrome), ending in wasting dis-ease (slow starvation). But many veterinarians admit that approximately fifty percent of dogs who recover from infection will suffer some type of life-long gastrointestinal dysfunction.

I know the horrors personally—my first "push" into holistic pet care was when my own fully-vaccinated nine month-old Rottie puppy became infected and died in 1982. We did everything we could to save her: fluids, steroids, antibiotics, anti-nausea drugs, etc. I had trouble believing the scientific puppy diet (full of chemicals and by-products) that my veterinarian had recommended had damaged her intestinal tract and immune system (read **Step One:** Detoxification and Nutrition; *regarding Ethoxyquin*). But this left her prone to intestinal illness despite her vaccination record with no noticeable symptoms of vaccinosis. I have never vaccinated since or fed chemically preserved foods, and have raised many puppies parvo-free ever since, even those who were exposed to other sick puppies in my care.

Dr. Wendell Belfield, a noted orthomolecular (nutritional therapies) veterinarian, studied the benefits of 1000 mg. of ascorbate acid (vitamin C) a day as a preventative against parvo—it was highly effective. Of the many breeders who follow my LifeStyle™ approach, the only ones who still fight parvo (and other viral infections) are the ones who had a sick puppy shipped into their kennel. None of their holistically-raised puppies ever get sick. Even better news is the fact that my holistic protocol for parvovirus infection is very effective and free of side-effects.

As with distemper, I have read a common prognosis that up to fifty percent of severely ill dogs die despite "good" supportive veterinary care such as fluids, antibiotics and steroids. This is why they push prevention through vaccination, although the parvo vaccine has a high number of complaints, such as fever, vomiting and diarrhea that accompany the shot. In my case, infection happened anyhow. Vaccination is recommended to start as early as six weeks of age—this is such a tender young age for a body that is still adjusting to *being*. The digestive tract is still maturing and strengthening, therefore, more susceptible. No wonder we see cases of vaccinosis in puppies shortly after they begin their "routine" vaccinations.

Of course, the odds of both these outcomes (preventing vaccinosis and reversing infection) are better with the LifeStyle™ approach. Not only can this naturopathic approach reverse severe symptoms related to infection but the outcome of its general preventative program is to build up the immune system response to these (and all) invading organisms—killing them off before they have a chance to "infect." No need to sicken the body first through vaccination.

Parvo Preventative

- Follow The Holistic Animal Care LifeStyle™!

- Newton's Homeopathic Labs® *Parvo Nosode* works well in lieu of yearly vaccination.

- A dilution of 1:30 of bleach can kill the virus on contact. It is recommended that you wash your shoe soles, floors and kennel runs (or other sources of contamination) with this when there is any sign of the virus.

- In case of exposure, herbal Viral D'Tox can be used as a preventative to avoid a full blown infection from occurring. It is recommended as a daily supplement during parvo season (fall and spring) for puppies in high risk situations such as those who walk on neighborhood sidewalks and paths or who play at dog parks and day care. Especially stay away from kennels and other areas canines congregate in stressful situations.

Parvo Reversal

- Newton's Homeopathic Labs® *Parvo Nosode* and Azmira®'s herbal Viral D'Tox also works well when fighting the viral infection.

- D'Toxifier contains *Arsenicum* with complementary remedies which help the immune system through improved nutrient utilization and waste elimination; given every five minutes apart for up to one hour will help stimulate suppression of most parvo symptoms. Reduces chronic conditions of a toxic lifestyle to prevent infection; general restorative to help improve immune response and repair damaged intestinal tissue. D'Toxifier is an excellent general remedy for all parvo-related symptoms, including vaccinosis.

- Homeopathic *Phosphorous* reduces bleeding in the intestines.

- Fast the symptomatic puppy or dog while force-feeding fluids; make a solution of two ounces each of apple juice and purified water. Add one teaspoon of raw honey (for energy and intestinal repair) and one teaspoon of fresh lemon juice (anti-septic). Use a syringe (without the needle) and place towards the back of the pet's mouth, in the corners, to get the fluid on the back of the tongue. Give one ounce of solution per pound of body weight per day. This will compensate for spillage. It is best to give some fluid every hour or two during the height of symptoms (fever, vomiting, bloody diarrhea, exhaustion) to ward off dehydration and keep up the puppy's energy needed for healing. Daily supplements and herbal remedies can be added to fresh fluid solution to be used within the next twenty four hours. Do not give whole capsules to swallow or it will come back up. Instead, empty contents and mix well into the solution.

- As symptoms improve <u>oatmeal water</u> can also be used in this solution instead of plain water, eventually thickening it into a soup once the fever has ended. To make oatmeal water soak two handfuls of oatmeal overnight in a pint of water and strain.

- Once the vomiting has stopped, chicken broth can be substituted for plain water to make the oatmeal water. This will provide easily digestible fats and encourage the digestive tract to function.

- Feed cooked oatmeal as appetite and digestion stabilizes to help break the fever-fasting period. Give four small meals the first few days. A tablespoon or two of yogurt can be added for acidophilus or add Acidophilus to meals. Tuna can water or meat-based baby food can be added for flavor. Oatmeal is soothing to irritated intestinal tissues and will help eliminate dead tissue from the colon.

- Canned Chicken & Beef or Ocean Fish formulas can be added later to the oatmeal as stools firm up and appetite is stronger. These are the easiest to digest and given in three smaller daily meals, they will help bring digestion back on line. After a week of recovery, return to normal daily schedule and meal planning for the pet's age.

Recommended Supplements for Parvo Symptoms

- Azmira®'s Viral D'Tox contains herbal compounds which effectively fight off the parvovirus and help reverse symptoms of infection. Use triple the daily recommended dose in severe cases. Helps prevent the virus from spreading further and infecting additional healthy tissue. This shortens the course of infection and lessens the severity of most symptoms. Protects the liver and digestive tract from long-term viral damage.

- Yucca Intensive provides anti-inflammatory compounds for ulcerated, bleeding intestines. Reduces pain and intestinal discomfort.

- Seek veterinary diagnosis and support if you suspect parvo! It can be a deadly infection as the heart can fail due to electrolyte imbalance from chronic vomiting and diarrhea (preventable when you provide a **Mega Pet Daily,** rich in potassium, magnesium and calcium, in the fluid solution).

- **Acidophilus** is given once the crisis is over. This helps reestablish friendly flora in the digestive tract that was destroyed by the virus. Give as directed for six weeks.

(See Vomiting, Diarrhea, Infection—*for related symptom support*)

Pneumonia

(see Coughs, Infections, Respiratory Ailments)

Pregnancy

PREGNANCY is mentioned here because many pets first develop health or emotional symptoms while pregnant, or shortly thereafter, especially allergies or anxiety. This is understandable, given the amount of toxins produced by supporting the growing litter, changes in hormones and nutrient requirements not being met. Some never have a reoccurrence of toxic reactions, although it is more common to find pregnancy was the genesis of chronic "allergies" for many animals. Please do not breed any pets which have a history of severe health, structural or emotional conditions or you probably will pass on this genetic weakness. Allow a season in-between litters or foals to give the female a chance to strengthen fully prior to carrying another pregnancy. Dis-ease is common in over-bred animals as each litter takes its toll.

Research carefully any herbal supplements you use during pregnancy, since many herbs can be dangerous for both mother and babies, even while nursing.

Herbs to Avoid During Pregnancy

- *Angelica, Goldenseal, Pennyroyal* which can cause uterine contractions.

- *Mugwort, Wormwood, Rue* also stimulates mild contractions.

- *Barberry, Cascara Sagrada* can be too strong a laxative during pregnancy, when used full strength. It is safer when combined with other herbs, as in our **Herbal Wormer.**

- *Buchu, Juniper Berry*, because it is a strong diuretic, is too dehydrating.

- *Ephedra (Ma Huang)* is too strong an anti-histamine to use during pregnancy

- *Pennyroyal and Neem* are too powerful in antiparasitic herbs for pregnancy in their undiluted state. For severely infested pregnant females, where the fleas, mites or ticks must be brought under control—use Azmira®'s Neem Dip with confidence in its regular recommended dilution. Do not use prior to giving birth or right after birth or allow residue to form on the nipples where babies will nurse.

In the event that you suspect your pet is currently pregnant and exhibiting symptoms, apply the alternative fasting program with one and a half times the recommended Mega Pet Daily allowance.

Administer *safe* herbal remedies. You can also safely rely on the effectiveness of homeopathic remedies at this time. Whatever you are doing—whether or not it has been the same for your pets entire life, you must expect *the unexpected* during pregnancy. Be careful, always keep a close eye on the mother-to-be for any reactions or stress so you can alter her feeding, supplementation and remedy use as needed before there is a full-blown crisis.

Beneficial and Safe Herbs to Use During Pregnancy

- Daily Boost is a must for the pregnant animal! Provides a variety of herbs which cleanse and tone the blood (prevents anemia and septicemia), stimulate digestive functions and improve nutrient assimilation (improves milk production), reduce digestive upsets and flatulence, build resistance to dis-ease and allergies, have anti-fungal properties and prevent a drop in blood sugar (vital to both moms and babies).

- Garlic Daily Aid is wonderfully supportive and nourishing to the growing fetus. Helps repel pests and worms while promoting exceptional organ tissue and skin support, iron and antifungal/antibiotic properties for mom.

- NaturFiber helps keep the colon functioning well for pets prone to imbalance or with a history of irritable bowel. Prevents flatulence, constipation and colon stress.

- **Yucca Intensive** is a safe alternative to steroid or pain medication use.

- **Aller'G Free** is a wonderful anti-histamine, a good alternative to *Ephedra.*

- **Aller'G: Skin & Digestive** will control digestive upsets and/or poor skin conditions.

- **Skin & Liv-A-Plex** improves iron assimilation and skin conditions. Prevents hormonal imbalance, cleanses the blood, is a safe antibiotic to use, and aids liver metabolism.

- **Grape Seed Extract** is a powerful antioxidant, reverses growths and improves resistance to allergens or dis-ease.

- **Herbal Calm** is good for situational use. Great for hyperactivity, anxiety, or stressful situations such as traveling which come up during pregnancy.

- **Herbal Wormer** is a safe alternative to chemical wormers.

Beneficial and Safe Homeopathic Remedies to Use During or After Pregnancy

- **D'Toxifier** contains *Arsenicum* with complementary remedies which help the pregnant animal through improved nutrient utilization and waste elimination; given every fifteen minutes for one hour will help lessen many symptoms associated with pregnancy, whelping and nursing the young. D'Toxifier is safe for exhaustion, restlessness, detoxification/septic infections, dry itchy skin, irritability, incontinence, discomfort, and loss of weight (impaired nutrition) despite growing fetuses. Addresses appetite issues and digestive upsets such as diarrhea, constipation and vomiting. Contains *Phytolacca* which prevents and reverses mastitis and weakness or pain in the lumbar regions. Promotes milk flow. Used as a weekly maintenance dose it reduces possibility of a miscarriage. Promotes wellness; general restorative to stimulate healthy fertilization, pregnancy, and lactation.

- *Alumina* is used for abnormal cravings, small hard knotty stool, or difficulty passing stool of any shape or consistency.

- *Apis* benefits the pregnant animal who becomes listless with inflamed eyes, is without thirst yet urinates frequently. Helps reverse whole body edema. Reduces excessive licking, scratching and skin eruptions.

- *Helonias* benefits the animal with a tendency to abort. For prolapse or poor positioning of the uterus. Helps balance blood sugar and stabilize pregnant pets with diabetes. Reduces irritability and depression during pregnancy.

- *Hydrastis* is a necessary remedy for any breeder or caregiver of a pregnant animal to have available; Discharges a retained placenta after birth. Helps to stimulate resistance against infection.

- *Nux Vomica* is good for old symptoms which have recurred with pregnancy and are not responsive to D'Toxifier. Acute digestive upsets, especially nausea after eating, are also markers of Nux. Bad tempered (irritable) with constipation and liver inflammation are common symptoms for pregnant pets living a toxic lifestyle. Use apart from D'Toxifier.

- *Pulsatilla* relieves diarrhea during pregnancy, especially if pet is highly excitable or suffers exhaustion from symptoms that are worse during the day.

- *Phytolacca* prevents or reverses mastitis, cracks or small ulcers about the nipples. An ingredient of D'Toxifier.

- *Phosphorous* helps reduce uterine bleeding.

- *Sepia* is used for threatened abortion preceded by severe allergic or toxic reaction.

- *Urtica Urens* benefits the mother who can not lactate or suddenly has a diminished flow. Promotes milk production and improves nutrient and naturally-occurring antibody availability in the milk. One dose, used as a preventative, of Urtica Urens 30C as soon as the babies are born is an excellent choice.

Pulse; Irregular function

PULSE; IRREGULAR FUNCTION of the pulse can be the reaction to an imbalance in the body's water/electrolyte balance. Stress of any kind coupled with a toxic lifestyle renders the heart susceptible to many disorders including an acute reaction resulting in an irregular pulse.

Normal Heart Rate/Pulse: Taken inside the thigh on femoral artery.
Small dogs—90 to 120 beats per minute
Large dogs—65 to 90 beats per minute

Cats—100 to 140 beats per minute
Horses—25 to 40 beats per minute

Homeopathic Remedies for Irregular Pulse

- *Digitalis* in the homeopathic form or *Arsenicum* (in a pinch), are the wonder remedies for heart irregularities, especially the pulse. Give one dose every five minutes for fifteen minutes, then once an hour till the pet is resting.

- D'Toxifier contains *Arsenicum* with complementary remedies which help the pulse through improved nutrient utilization and waste elimination. Excellent first-aid remedy for an irregular pulse. Reduces chronic conditions of a toxic lifestyle to prevent heart irregularities; general restorative to help improve circulatory system.

- *Iberis* is the most influential remedy that I have ever worked with on the pulse. Quickly regulates and rebalances; given in a weekly dose of 30C it helps maintain proper pulse.

(see Heart Conditions)

Rattle Snake Bites

RATTLE SNAKE BITES can have serious long-term side-effects, if the animal survives. Symptoms include raised, red, inflamed area with one or two puncture wounds or deep depressions. The pet will exhibit increased anxiety.

- Immediately tell your vet you're on the way into the emergency clinic.

- Start a crisis dose (every five minutes for the first hour then every hour after until stable) of homeopathic *Crotalus Horridus* 6X (for the venom) and *Hypericum* 6X (for the pain) on the way in and continue a maintenance dose (twice per day) for two weeks. Have these on hand in your first aid kit if you live near snakes or hike the desert with your dogs!

- For a tumultuous, violent heart beat with labored breathing give a crisis dose of *Belladonna* and/or *Aconite*.

- Feed herbal Yucca Intensive, a natural steroid alternative, to reduce swelling and pain.

- Supplement with **Blood & Lymph D'Tox** and/or **ImmunoStim'R** for six to twelve weeks to help repair internal tissue and skin damage through catabolic and metabolic waste removal.

- Spray the wound frequently with **Rejuva Spray** to reduce swelling and discourage infection.

(see Symptom-specific subjects, i.e. Fever, Infection)

Respiratory Disorders

Respiratory Disorders are common to many pets today due to the toxic environment in which we all live. They are constantly bombarded with chemicals right under their noses; insecticides, lawn treatments, chemical fertilizers, carpet cleaners (or new carpet out-gassing), floor products (if it smells strong it's toxic!) and hundreds of other forms of pollution. Too often a diagnosis of "allergies" or "upper respiratory disease" is given and the body suppressed through steroids and antibiotics, sometimes year after year, only to progress to a more serious condition such as cancer. It doesn't have to be that way. The Holistic Animal Care LifeStyle™ promotes optimum respiration (including on a cellular level) and elimination of the very toxins which disturb and imbalance the respiratory process, while promoting the improved utilization of nutrients to strengthen the organs and tissues of the respiratory system.

(see Symptom-specific subjects, Asthma, Pneumonia)

Ringworm

Ringworm is a fungal infection often mistaken for a skin parasite. It can create many of the same symptoms, such as skin inflammation, itching, and hot spots, associated with allergies or fleas. Ringworm looks like a small, circular area with hair loss and irritation. Scratching can lead to bacterial infection.

- Treat ringworm <u>topically</u> with an undiluted application of herbal **Yeast & Fungal D'Tox** to infected areas and <u>supplement</u> twice daily with recommended dosage. Double this dose for the first forty-eight hours. Supplement for an additional six weeks past the time of the last noticeable patch. The fungus can easy re-infect the pet if this is not followed.

- Double the recommended dose of **Garlic Daily Aid** and feed **Yucca Intensive** if the skin is very inflamed and the pet is scratching a lot.

- Use homeopathic *Sepia* to stimulate the curative response against ringworm. This can also be given preventatively for the whole family when someone in the household is infected.

- Be watchful of the other family members, both human and animal, as ringworm is highly contagious.

(see Symptom-specific subjects)

Roundworms

ROUNDWORMS can be very destructive, especially in young puppies and kittens. This is one of the most common parasitic infestations known. They are thick-bodied, whitish-to-cream-colored worms which inhabit the small intestines, interfering with nutrient absorption and irritating the intestinal tract. Chronic infestation can lead to malnutrition and irritable bowel syndrome. In severe cases there has been rupture of the intestinal wall due to an impaction of adult worms.

Immature roundworms can also cause dis-case in the rest of the body as they travel through the lungs, liver and other organ tissues of the body before settling in the intestines to grow. This accounts for the birth of puppies or kittens with roundworms—the larvae travel via the umbilical cord while the babies are still in the womb. Other babies get infected through larvae which settled in the mammary gland tissues to be passed on through the mother's milk, later maturing in the pup's or kitten's intestines.

Roundworm eggs are shed in feces and can lay dormant for years in the environment prior to being consumed by an animal. The best defense is a strong immune system which immediately sees the larvae as a foreign invader and quickly mounts an anti-parasitic attack. This is why I recommend Garlic Daily Aid in the daily foundation supplements. Garlic has wonderful anti-parasitic action and is particularly effective against roundworms while soothing the digestive tract. If a proper defense has not happened due to a toxic lifestyle and further support is necessary, I have had good success with this protocol.

- **Herbal Wormer** is quite effective in reducing both the intestinal worms and minor larvae infestation. It can be safely used for pregnant bitches and queens as well as week-old babies. For severe infestations or debilitated pets.

- The *addition* of **Giardia & Parasitic Cleanse** for six weeks will strengthen the anti-parasitic actions to completely eliminate blood larvae and prevent a relapse.

- **Yucca Intensive** reduces inflammation in the intestinal tract.

- Homeopathic **D'Toxifier** contains *Arsenicum* with complementary remedies which help stimulate anti-parasitic activity through improved nutrient utilization and waste elimination. Promotes the reversal of many symptoms associated with infestation, including constipation and colon irritation.

(see Digestive Disorders and other Symptom-specific subjects, i.e. Constipation)

Seizures

SEIZURES are the result of a trauma to the brain including inflammation, damaged tissue or blood clots from accidents and allergic reaction to vaccinations, chemicals or medications—especially from chronic use of over-the-counter antihistamines and monthly ingested or topically applied pest control products. It has been reported that within three to six months of chronic use, particularly of antifungal and anti-inflammatory drugs, a pet developed seizures, which stop as abruptly as they started, when medication is ceased and detoxification is complete.

Some pets may actually have an allergic reaction to the chronic assault of histamine or adrenaline (as a glandular response to ongoing allergy conditions). This is why it is so important to control toxic reactions and allergies quickly, and not allow the chronic suffering of symptoms.

Unfortunately, it is now quite genetically common especially among many popular breeds or mixes of: Chihuahuas, Chow Chows, Dalmatians, Poodles, Min Pins, German Shepherds, Labs, Cocker Spaniels, Dobermans and Lhasa Apsos. Cats heavily in-bred, especially Siamese, can also develop seizures. But all animals are prone to developing epileptic seizures from ingested chemicals, viral infections or trauma to the brain. I believe that yearly vaccinations, especially that aggressive puppy schedule—are more at fault in triggering seizure activity—than the veterinary community is willing to acknowledge at this time.

Also, so many other issues influence seizure activity (including sensitivity to yeast and urea toxicity), that I believe "epilepsy" has been given out too freely as a diagnosis—and pets are drugged unnecessarily—leaving them prone to other dis-ease.

Epileptic seizure activity seems to be most active when the animal is resting. There is no set pattern or warning system—some pets suffer frequent fits, others more occasional ones. Heavy anti-convulsion drugs are often prescribed but with debilitating side-effects. Regardless of the cause, seizure activity can be reversed through a natural approach.

Nutritional Supplements To Help Control or Eliminate Seizure Activity

- L-TryptoPet contains the amino acid l-Tryptophan; when given in daily doses of 1500 mg.—regardless of size of animal—this supplement helps rebalance brain chemistry to prevent seizure activity. This is a particularly excellent remedy for those who suffer great depression, irritability and fear around their seizure episodes.

- B-Complex 50 is given to increase the dose available in Mega Pet Daily to a daily total of up to 200 mg. for cats & small dogs to 400 mg. for large dogs. Seizure activity and severity have been known to cease with only the addition of B-Complex 50. These vitamins are vital to the proper function of electrical impulses and sponsoring brain chemistry responsible for seizure activity.

- MSM is a nutritional sulfur supplement which aids in repairing and strengthening the tissues of the brain. MSM benefits the animal whose seizure activity can be traced to traumatic damage to the brain, caused by drugs, chemicals or traumatic injury to the head in a car accident. In addition, it is helpful in protecting and repairing damage from the seizure activity.

- Coenzyme Q-10 is a nutrient which replenishes the strength and vitality to brain cells, particularly those in the aging or severely epileptic pet. This is an excellent supplement to prevent deterioration which may lead to seizures in a prone pet or help slow the spread of damaged cells during seizure activity.

- Vita E 200 provides therapeutic doses of vitamin E to help repair and strengthen cellular tissue or a compromised brain. Especially benefits the animal who has a history of a toxic lifestyle or other chronic health conditions. In addition to Mega Pet Daily, feed an additional 100 I.U.'s for cats and small dogs (giving half a capsule each morning) to 400 I.U.'s per day for large breeds.

Herbal Remedies for Seizure Disorders

Herbal supplementation can quickly reverse the underlying hormonal and stress-related imbalance triggering the fits. Herbs promote tissue repair and cellular regeneration.

- Calm & Relax is a combination of standardized extracts known for reducing and possibly eliminating seizure activity. I have been using this remedy with great success since 1994. These herbs will help normalize and restore the nervous system while providing a sense of calm and reducing seizure activity (regardless of its cause), without the sludgy side-effects of drugs. Rebalances hormones that can stimulate seizures. These are *relaxants* that reduce the severity of seizure activity (instead of drugs resulting in digestive upsets, liver inflammation and stupor). This formulation has successfully weaned many pets off the heavy narcotics used for seizure elimination—allowing them to live seizure-free *and alert* enough to enjoy their lives.

- Yucca Intensive is a natural alternative to steroids. Proven effective in reducing inflammation; the nervous system and brain can have inflammation from dis-ease or trauma resulting in seizure activity.

- Blood & Lymph D'Tox is an excellent combination to aid in blood purification and detoxification in general. Ammonia (from metabolic and catabolic waste) can develop on the brain, hastening the degenerative process, damaging healthy brain cells and encouraging seizures. Nutrients, such as B-vitamins, are malabsorbed due to these toxins, further rendering the brain weaker and more prone. This should be *added* if the Calm & Relax has not made significant improvement after six weeks or used at the beginning of your protocol along with the Calm & Relax to encourage rapid response in a body that has been living a very toxic lifestyle.

- Grape Seed Extract is a powerful antioxidant. Benefits include reducing the recurrence of seizures from a toxic reaction by eliminating free radicals which encourage brain deterioration.

- Immuno Stim'R should be used to maintain a catabolic waste and ammonia-free environment for healthy brain tissue, significantly reducing the likelihood that seizures will return.

Homeopathic Remedies for Seizure Disorders

- D'Toxifier contains *Arsenicum* which can reverse seizure activity in many cases. It is formulated with complementary remedies which help the nervous system through improved nutrient utilization and waste elimination; given every five to fifteen minutes apart for one hour will help stimulate suppression of seizures and resulting side-effects. This product addresses many symptoms associated with seizures including digestive upset, anxiety and withdrawal. Weekly dosing can help prevent epilepsy, use daily with severe episodes; general restorative to regulate brain function.

- *Absinthium* addresses the pet with nervous tremors which precede the attack. These seizures include much twitching and trembling, especially when the fit or fits are coming in small clusters.

- *Arnica / Hypericum,* when used in combination, works wonders in reversing seizures related to trauma—such as car accidents.

- *Belladonna* is helpful for nausea or vomiting that follows a fit. It can minimize the violent nature of an episode. Belladonna is a particularly productive remedy when it comes to the reversal and prevention of seizures. Some animals have remained seizure-free with a single weekly or monthly 30C dose. Helps reduce seizure activity following constipation. Straining to evacuate bowel (as well as the toxins being absorbed) can trigger episodes, so maintaining proper colon health is vital to treating these seizures.

- *Bioplasma,* a combination of the twelve *tissue cell salts,* should be incorporated into daily supplementation for general support—to rehabilitate the nervous system.

- *Silicea* is good for seizures that occur during sleep or as the pet is waking.

- *Thuja* should be used when vaccinations are the suspected injurious agent. *Thuja* is included in D'Toxifier.

Shaking

Shaking can be a secondary symptom to pain, fever, cold, eliminatory or digestive system upset, nervous system dysfunction, fear or emotional shock. Therefore, it is best addressed as part of the protocol for that primary health condition or behavioral situation.

- D'Toxifier contains homeopathic *Arsenicum* with complementary remedies which help the body through improved nutrient utilization and waste elimination; given every fifteen minutes for one hour will help suppress shaking from physical or emotional symptoms. Reduces chronic conditions of a toxic lifestyle to prevent shaking; general restorative to help improve wellness.

- R&R Essence, a few doses given every five to fifteen minutes, will quell the majority of shaking symptoms due to fear, anxiety, shock, etc.

- Calm & Relax is an herbal extract which promotes deep relaxation and lessens shaking in more severe, chronic cases.

Shock (and resulting Grief)

Sudden onset, including states of panic, terror or shock, the result of an accident or difficult experience such as the death of a beloved owner, can trigger loss of concentration, inability to learn or retain appropriate behaviors and withdrawal. Some pets will vocalize their shock and grief with howls. Many pets react aggressively when stressed or taken by surprise, become quick to react or maybe seem desperate.

Homeopathically-potentized Flower Combination for Shock

- R&R Essence

This Azmira® homeopathic flower combination, given before a difficult event, during stressful situations or following a traumatic experience reduces the fear and shock experienced and minimizes the long-term effects, such as grief or loss of appetite, that shock might have on the emotions or body (both emotional and physical stress cause dis-ease).

This helps to return the pet more quickly to a clear mind, offers them a sense of security and gains their attention; important especially if they need emergency medical treatment. Minimizes negative reactions by pets overwhelmed by their experiences. Reduces the likelihood of a depressive immune response—common consequence of trauma or severe stress is the onset of disease—just as emotional stress can often result in the relapse of a physical condition such as cancer or allergies.

NOTE: This remedy should be in every first aid kit, excellent for accidents, onset of illness, general stress, and to minimize the effects of any other difficult situations you and your animals may encounter.

Homeopathic Remedies

- D'Toxifier contains *Arsenicum* with complementary remedies which help the nervous system through improved nutrient utilization and waste elimination; given every five minutes for fifteen minutes then every hour for four hours, will help reduce the negative side-effects of shock and grief. Benefits the anxious and fearful pet. Excellent general remedy for emotional and physical shock.

- *Aconite* benefits the pet who has experienced an emotional shock such as the death of a family member or a physical/emotional shock as during an accident, attack or beating.

- *Gelsemium* is indicated for the animal who has suffered a physical ailment relapse following the shock-producing event. This pet may withdraw and seem paralyzed by the experience. Can become very clingy and needy of attention, vocalizing their displeasure during their grieving stage.

- *Phosphorus* reverses restlessness in the animal recovering from shock, especially the result of loud noises such as during a thunderstorm. This animal becomes depressed from his experiences. Phosphorus is beneficial for the sudden onset of all physical or emotional symptoms.

Nutritional Remedy

- Use B-Complex 50 to soothe the nervous system and protect it from the effects of long-term shock. Use 100 mg. for small pets and 200 mg. for large dogs and horses daily, two to four weeks following the traumatic event.

Behavioral Guidance

- These pets need reassurance that they are in good hands and need calm around them. Minimize sudden or excessive stimuli to allow the nervous system to rebalance and the pet to regain its strength. A bed of their own and a comfort toy, pillow or blanket is very important to pets suffering from shock or grief. At times this may even seem to border on obsessive behavior once they begin clinging to this comfort object, but it will pass as they grow emotionally stronger.

Sinusitis

(See Infections, Upper Respiratory Problems)

Skin and Coat Conditions

SKIN AND COAT CONDITIONS occur frequently with many other health or behavioral conditions. I am very frustrated at the amount of "allergy" diagnoses I hear about when two weeks of homeopathic detoxification and double the recommended dose of Garlic Daily Aid reverse many of the symptoms, but the medical recommendation instead is steroids and antibiotics which create a host of additional side-effects! The skin, the largest eliminatory organ, can manifest many symptoms due to toxicity and hormonal imbalance. What the liver and kidneys cannot eliminate is exuded through the skin. Certainly regular grooming is essential to a beautiful coat but to have a truly healthy shine, you must detoxify and nourish the tissue cells of the skin and coat which is why **Steps One** and **Two** are so successful in reversing eighty percent of all skin conditions.

Animals living a toxic lifestyle bombarded with poor quality pet food, vaccinations, shotgun medications and an emotionally stressful home or training environment often manifest their physical and emotional stress in skin dis-eases. Vaccinations, in addition to other side-effects, do account for a high percentage of skin tags, cysts and small growths due to the tremendous effect they have in unbalancing a healthy body, while suppressing the immune response and digestive/eliminatory systems. The LifeStyle™ approach is the best way to prevent and reverse these skin and coat problems:

DRY COAT, DANDRUFF, CRACKED SKIN and THIN SKIN that bleeds easily should be addressed through liver support and improved nutrient absorption. Thyroid function should be checked and addressed if needed. These are the classic symptom markers of a toxic pet. Poor digestion (with a toxic lifestyle) creates nutrient imbalance and toxic overload for the liver and kidneys. Additional nutrients are blocked by metabolic waste or putrefying food matter while others are excessively mined by the body in trying to maintain balance in other bodily functions that are vital and need the nutrients—such as the heart and brain. The skin suffers, the coat misses out on sulfur, selenium, biotin, vitamin A and E, just to name a few, and so the overall condition of the animal looks poor.

HAIR LOSS, POOR COAT CONDITION and EXCESSIVE SCRATCHING are similar to dry coats and thin skin (please read above) and respond well to the LifeStyle™ approach. In addition to improved digestion and nutritional supplementation; proper grooming is of paramount importance for supporting tissue, stimulating dead coat or skin removal and circulation to bring more nutrients to the skin and coat for tissue repair. A daily brushing, followed by a rub down with a damp terry cloth towel can work wonders. Supplementation promotes the growth of new, healthy fur cells and improves skin tissue elasticity to reduce scratching and hair loss.

PIMPLES, CYSTS, FATTY TUMORS and WARTS are pockets of toxins, bacterial or viral organisms and other irritants which the body has formed protective tissue around to ward off the spread of the injurious agent to the surrounding tissue, instead of breaking down and eliminating the culprit through a healthy and strong immune response. It is common to treat these with antibiotics or surgical intervention only to find it hastens the spread of the offending growths. Surgery should only be resorted to in the case of a growth becoming too big and threatening to burst, or smaller growths seriously irritating the eyes, under the tail or other sensitive parts after a naturopathic protocol has been tried.

ECZEMA and HOT SPOTS are also commonly found on animals living a toxic lifestyle. As excessive bodily waste is exuded through the skin, it becomes an irritant to malnourished skin causing the animal to bite and scratch. In some cases the skin may have been bitten by a flea or penetrated by a foreign object like a cactus needle causing the animal to chew it. This, plus excessive licking, can create a raw wound which is referred to as a hot spot. Often these symptoms are initially treated as an *allergy* and the pet is bombarded with antihistamines, antibiotics and steroids which suppress the immune system and cause the symptoms to get worse over time. Although allergies can occur, I have found them to be less a cause than toxicity or flea and tick bites.

GREASY COAT OR OFFENSIVE ODORS can be addressed through a twenty four-hour fast followed by proper grooming (shedding out of old coat) and shampooing. This will cleanse all impurities the skin has exuded during the fasting period, and before. These impurities create offensive body odor.

Caring for the Skin and Coat Topically

- Use Rejuva Spray to eliminate skin irritation from flea and tick bites, pimples, rashes, pustules and other wounds. Promotes tissue repair while preventing or reducing bacterial infection. Spray on burns and painful, angry wounds every fifteen minutes for the first hour to reduce pain and inflammation.

- Apply Rejuva Gel to reduce scarring for burns, scraps and scabs. Reduces irritation and promotes tissue repair. Can use Rejuva Spray to lessen acute pain then switch to Rejuva Gel to prevent scarring.

- Avoid the use of coal tar-based or chemically medicated shampoos, the toxins of which will be absorbed into the blood stream through the skin.

- Do not bathe too often. When the skin is severely irritated, no more than every two to four weeks. Too frequent whole body bathing can actually worsen the condition by drying out the skin, thereby encouraging greasy skin. (Body oils will try to replenish themselves quickly and heavily to counter such drying.)

- Spot clean with Organic Shampoo and disinfect the skin with Rejuva Spray whenever needed. Add twenty drops of Goldenseal Extract if needed for infection control and ten drops of Yucca Intensive to two ounces of concentrated Organic Shampoo for serious inflammation and/or infection.

- Use Organic Conditioner to replenish elasticity to the skin and soften the coat until nutrients can work from the inside.

- For body odor, apply a final antiseptic rinse—one lemon (cut up, rind and all) boiled in one pint of distilled water for 5 minutes then covered and simmered for twenty minutes, left to sit in the water over night. Do not use unfiltered tap water which is chlorinated and irritating to the skin. Strain in the morning and refrigerate.

Nutritional Supplements

- Super C 2000; feed up to bowel tolerance. Start at 1000 mg. for cats and small dogs, 2500 mg. for medium-sized dogs and 4000 mg. for large breeds and horses. Increase daily by 500 mg. until the stool loosens—then cut back 500 mg. for a few days until the stool firms up. Repeat as needed. Vitamin C repairs coat and skin cells quickly and builds resistance to environmental pollutants which can compromise good health.

- **Mega Pet Daily**; following a twenty four hour fast, feed up to twenty five percent more of daily recommended amount for six weeks—this protocol generally helps address the nutritional healing of the skin and coat even in severe cases. Mega Pet Daily is rich in vitamin A, E, B-complex with biotin, selenium, potassium and copper, all nutrients which easily become depleted from a toxic lifestyle and result in a poor skin and coat condition.

- **Mega Omega-3** fatty acids are vital to healthy skin and coat tissue. Helps reduce the itch from allergies and a toxic lifestyle. Older pets especially need this supplementation as they maintain lower levels in the blood as they age.

- **MSM** is a nutritional sulfur supplement which replenishes the elasticity in skin, reversing the aging process. This is a vital nutrient for the reversal of hot spots and other chronic wounds or rashes.

Herbal Remedies

- **Aller'G: Skin & Pimple** is a general skin and coat restorative, perfect for the classic symptoms of a toxic lifestyle—dry coat and flaky skin with rashes and/or pustules. Generally, a month or two of this formula with the foundation supplements and symptoms reverse themselves. This remedy can be used as a spring tonic each year to promote detoxification and circulation to the skin, helping to prepare for the onset of allergens and environmental assaults such as fleas or lawn fertilizers, which can irritate and burn the skin causing a reaction.

- **Skin & Liv-A-Plex** promotes detoxification to improve fatty acid metabolism while it purifies the blood. This formula is an antibacterial remedy to help eliminate skin infections. For disorders associated with hormonal imbalance or stress. Aids liver metabolism—vital to a healthy skin and coat.

- **Blood & Lymph D'Tox** addresses the severe cases of chronic skin and coat problems including infections and open wounds that refuse to heal. It can be used in conjunction with **Skin & Liv-A-Plex** when needed for serious cases.

Homeopathic Remedies

- D'Toxifier contains *Arsenicum* which is a good general homeopathic choice for most skin irritations, poor coat conditions and hair loss since its primary action is on the liver and unhealthy skin is generally a window to a toxic liver. It is formulated with other remedies which improve skin and coat condition through nutrient utilization and waste elimination. Aids with thyroid balance, also needed for a healthy coat. Reverses a congested liver; for inflammation and detoxification. Helps eliminate dandruff, skin rashes, pimples, hot spots or tags, plus warts, cysts and fatty growths.

- *Apis* addresses rashes and general irritation, resulting in scratching or rubbing.

- *Belladonna* is for dry, inflamed skin that can be visibly swollen and painful to the touch. Sudden, rapidly spreading rash or pustules. This is good for skin conditions caused by a toxic substance reacting with the skin, either ingested or topically applied. Whether the contact occurred months ago, or yesterday, this is a good choice.

- *Calcarea Carb.* is an outstanding wart eliminator. It is good for an animal who has suffered malnutrition resulting in a poor coat and skin condition. Excellent remedy or for any small wound that won't heal readily. For diabetic pets: a weekly dose of 30C promotes proper digestion resulting in a better skin condition.

- *Hepar Sulph.* is indicated for weepy, painful wounds on the skin such as a chronic, infected hot spot.

- *Lycopodium* has a marked regulating influence on sebaceous cysts. This remedy can also be given in a monthly 30C dose for maintenance, to prevent a recurrence.

- *Psorinum* is beneficial when the skin has an acrid odor with discharging pustules or hot spots that are slow to heal; reduces production of sebaceous glands associated with a greasy coat and sebaceous cysts. Is also indicated for dirty and dingy coat that is brittle and lackluster.

- *Rhus Tox* is beneficial for red, swollen, intensely itching skin. Burning eczema with the tendency to heavy dandruff and scale formations. I call this my *Cocker Remedy* because so many

Cockers suffer from these markers and respond so well to Rhus Tox.

- *Sepia* works well on irritations, especially cracked toes and feet that itch badly with no relief from scratching.

- *Silicea* works well for eliminating growths under the skin, including cysts, abscesses or ulcers. Promotes the expulsion of splinters, boils, etc. under the skin.

- *Sulphur* addresses circular-patch irritations, pimples and pustules with dry, scaly and unhealthy skin; often the cause of scratching and hair loss. Itching is worse after bathing. Skin irritation or eruption is the result of a course of steroids, antifungal or antibiotics given to treat another condition.

- *Thuja,* also in D'Toxifier, will eliminate warts, cysts, and fatty growths that are associated with a bout of vaccinosis or have developed within three months of the last vaccinations and/or are growing on the vaccination site. This is a good remedy to add to others if the reversal of skin symptoms is occurring but not quickly.

(see Allergic Reactions, Immune Dysfunction-*infections*)

Skin Parasites

SKIN PARASITES can trigger your pet's skin or coat symptoms and leave pets susceptible to allergy reactions. When you have an acute skin problem, it is prudent to have your pet examined to find out whether a skin parasite is present so that it may be addressed as one of the underlying problems. Avoid the use of medicated or chemical-based topical pest control treatments, which could possibly depress the immune system and increase your pet's sensitivity to allergic reactions.

Regardless of your findings, an immune system imbalance needs to be addressed. Healthy, non-toxic pets do not encourage infestation. Waste products exuded through the skin will invite and feed fleas and ticks. Yeast (even nutritional yeast), commonly used to ward off fleas and ticks, may become toxic to the liver, increasing instances of infestation. Ear wax and debris also develop, providing an area for bacterial and yeast infections, which attract ear mites.

(See Ear Problems, Fleas, Mange, Mites, Ringworm, Skin & Coat Problems, Ticks)

Snake Bite

(see Rattle Snake Bite)

Spinal Problems

(see Arthritis, Intervertebral Disc Disease, Degenerative Disc Disorders)

Spraying (marking territory)

Pets who feel a compulsion to continue doing wrong, visiting the same spot even after punishment, are often driven by a strong primal urge to make their point and stand their ground. Feelings of inadequacy or being overwhelmed by a situation, such as changes in litter or box location, foods, household routines, and family dynamics can trigger this urge. Strong willed pets, who want to make a point, may also seek attention any way they can. These remedies help to stabilize negative emotions during transitions, new pets, or hormonal reactions and can help heal strong feelings of resentment and bitterness that are being acted out more aggressively than seen in the jealousy/resentment dynamic. These strong emotions and reactions can exacerbate medical conditions associated with glands (especially thyroid and adrenal glands), digestion and the eliminatory system.

Whenever addressing any urinary behavior be sure to rule out any urinary dysfunction first and seek veterinary diagnosis if needed.

- Homeopathically-potentized Flower Remedy—Spraying

Homeopathic Remedies

- D'Toxifier contains *Arsenicum* which is for the pet who is also exhibiting great anguish and restlessness. Urinates when left alone. Wanders the house. Vocalizes for no known reason. Formulated with complementary remedies, D'Toxifier also helps the pet through improved nutrient utilization and waste elimination. Reduces chronic conditions of a toxic lifestyle to eliminate house training accidents; general restorative to help improve wellness.

- *Apis* is for the fidgety, hard to please pet. Sudden shrill, piercing vocalizations (very beneficial with high strung Siamese cats who urinate outside their box). Jealousy in which the act of urination seems specifically for a certain person (i.e. urinating on your partner's pillow).

- *Gelsemium* helps the pet who hides to urinate or defecate. Will go in the corner of your closet or behind the furniture rather than in their box or outdoors.

- *Nux Vomica* is indicated for the irritable pet who is overly sensitive about changes in their routine and environment. Benefits the pet who was put off by a strong cleaning solution in their box and began to void outside of it, or the aged pet who begins to go anywhere for no apparent reason other than they are becoming a bit "senile." Use apart from D'Toxifier.

Behavioral Guidance

- These pets need reassurance that things will remain the same and do better with a set routine, such as being fed in the same place at the same time each day.

- You can try several litter boxes around the house and install doggie doors, but usually homeopathic remedies and set training/play/exercise times to focus the pet's attention, improving communication and lavishing some individualized praise on them works wonders.

- Be sure to treat any urine spots with enzymes (available at a pet shop or vet clinic) or white vinegar—no ammonia, which has the same base odors as urine and will continue to attract the pet back to the spot!

Staph Infection

(see Infections)

Stomach Problems

(see Digestive Disorders)

Stool Eating

STOOL EATING is an unhealthy thing, to say the least. Dis-ease and parasitic infestation can occur. There are various reasons why an animal would resort to eating stool, their own or other animals. In general, it is a nutritional imbalance in which they are seeking the predigested protein (in meat-eater's feces) or minerals, a chemical imbalance or obsessive need resulting in this behavior. Dogs love to eat horse manure and this is the only healthy response to eating another's droppings—manure provides digestive enzymes and fiber (which is what creates flatulence afterwards). Stool eating should clear up on **Steps One** and **Two** alone but if it should continue then follow these recommendations:

Herbal Remedies

- **Daily Boost** is an herbal blend which promotes proper digestion to lessen the urge to eat stool while detoxifying the body from the waste previously ingested.

- **Calm & Relax** will help rebalance brain chemistry associated with stool eating. Lessens the anxiety of a pet who is eating their stool out of stress or boredom.

- **Digest Zymez** provides digestive enzymes to promote nutrient assimilation.

- **Aller'G: Skin & Digestive** benefits the animal who is toxic and malnourished from poor absorption of nutrients.

- **Sea Supreme** is a trace mineral supplement which reduces the need to eat stools in an otherwise healthy pet.

- **Yucca Intensive** is an herb which detoxifies the liver and imparts a bitter taste to the stool.

- **Immuno Stim'R** is excellent in herbal detoxification and rebalancing the body while improving nutrient use; beneficial in preventing stool eating from returning.

Homeopathic Remedies

- **Obsessive** reduces a pet's obsessive interest in playing with and eating stool.

- **R&R Essence** is indicated for the pet who eats their stool out of stress.

- **D'Toxifier** contains *Arsenicum* to help to prevent a toxic reaction from stool eating while lessening the urge to eat non-food objects. Formulated with complementary remedies which help the pet through improved nutrient utilization and waste elimination; a few doses prior to turn-out in a pen will help suppress the urge to eat stool.

Using Homeopathic Remedies and Behavioral Guidance to Change This Habit

- Give them a dose or two of your chosen homeopathic remedy, five to ten minutes apart, let them out to play and watch.

- As soon as they approach a stool to eat it: reprimand them.

- If they go back to it: reprimand, bring them inside and dose them again.

- Wait a few minutes: give another dose and try again. Repeat until they leave the stool alone.

(see Appetite, Digestive Disorders)

Strains and Sprains

STRAINS AND SPRAINS occur when a tendon, ligament or muscle is stretched beyond its normal range causing tissue damage and an inflammatory response with pain and stiffness. Rest, ice and remedies are proven quick healers of sprains and strains.

Nutritional Supplements

- Increase Super C 2000 (up to 2000 mg. per twenty pounds of body weight per day, 6000 mg. for horses) helps strengthen ligaments and tendons and reduce inflammation or tissue deterioration.

- MSM is a sulfur-based product, which not only helps reduce inflammation, repair connective tissue and strengthen it to prevent future strains, but is also wonderful for the poor skin and coat conditions which often affect weakened animals. This is a great supplement for the hips, knees and shoulders.

- L-Pheny Pet is a powerful, non-addictive analgesic. Seems to be responsible for increasing the brain's endorphins. Is beneficial to add when Yucca Intensive and Calm & Relax are not enough.

- Coenzyme Q10 may be used to aid in the prevention or reduction of strains in older or debilitated pets. This supplement is an excellent over-all nutrient for older, arthritic animals.

Herbal Remedies

- Yucca Intensive is a very effective anti-inflammatory. The roots contain steroidal saponins, which react in the body as chemical steroids do, without the side effects; they also reduce tissue inflammation and pain. Be sure to use a cold-pressed extract found in Azmira®'s rather than the low potency by-product powder or even weaker, teas or tincture. Standardized extract contains up to eighty-five percent more bio-available saponins and is easier on the digestive tract then any other forms.

- Garlic Daily Aid, *double the daily dose,* is a wonderful supplement for ligaments and tendons affected by inflammation. Provides sulfur for connective tissue repair and strengthening.

- Daily Boost contains six excellent dietary herbs for liver and blood detoxification, reducing free radicals that can irritate joints, and improving nutrient utilization for structural support.

- Blood & Lymph Detox helps detoxify the body of impurities which, when left circulating in the blood, feed the inflammatory response by settling in the joints and surrounding tissues. Weakens ligaments, muscles and tendons leaving them susceptible to strain. This formula works more towards a reversal of the weakness which leads to chronic inflammation and joint deterioration. Helps repair damaged tissues and regulates the body's immune system. Excellent to use when a pet suffers strains due to autoimmune disease.

- Immuno Stim'R also removes the catabolic waste which feeds the inflammatory response and makes the joints stiffer and hotter, leaving them prone to strains. This formula is well suited for maintenance of an arthritic pet, especially one who suffers chronic sprains. Can be used to give the other herbal remedies a boost when needed for severely debilitated pets.

Homeopathic Remedies

- D'Toxifier contains *Arsenicum* with complementary remedies which help connective tissue through improved nutrient utilization and waste elimination; given every fifteen minutes for one hour, then every hour after reverse discomfort and swelling. This will stimulate anti-inflammatory action and tissue repair. Helps prevent connective tissue damage. When given as a weekly maintenance dose D'Toxifier will encourage the strengthening of connective tissue.

- R&R Essence reduces the shock and physical stress associated with an accident or sudden strain to reduce the side-effects and quickly bring the body into a curative response.

- *Ruta* reverses lameness after strains. Benefits flexor tendons especially. Legs give out or the animal can't get up easily.

- *Rhus Tox* is for severe stiffness in the joints/ligaments resulting from chronic strain; painful movement.

(see Arthritis)

Stress

STRESS is a killer of our pets as well as us. Stress creates hormonal imbalance (in the endocrine system) and muscular tension which leads to a weakening of the digestive system (resulting in malnutrition), the eliminatory system (resulting in toxic build-up of blood wastes which create dis-ease), the cardiovascular system (creates heart dis-ease) and the nervous system (creating more stress). It is a vicious cycle and most dis-ease is founded in a stressful environment.

- The use of homeopathic R&R Essence before, during and after stressful times (accidents, training, transitions, car rides, etc.) will help to minimize stress' negative side-effects.

- Homeopathic D'Toxifier contains *Arsenicum* which can reverse stress-producing chemicals in the body. It is formulated with complementary remedies which help the nervous system through improved nutrient utilization and waste elimination. This product addresses many symptoms associated with stress including digestive upset, anxiety and physical pain. Weekly dosing can help prevent stress from becoming a degenerative process; a general restorative to promote wellness.

- For severe, chronic stress, the use of herbal Calm & Relax can help rebalance brain chemistry and prevent future negative health or behavioral effects.

- Double the recommended B-vitamins by adding B-Complex 50 to the foundation levels in Mega Pet Daily during times of severe stress. Use in addition to Mega Pet Daily: 50 mg. per twenty pounds of pet per day. Use 200 mg. per day for horses.

You will see that the majority of my recommendations, regardless of the condition described, include remedies to lessen the "stress" on that particular organ system to help encourage healing and reduce the likelihood of relapse.

(see Symptom-specific subjects)

Strokes

STROKES can come on suddenly from a variety of causes. Symptoms can be minor at first but the overall condition can rapidly deteriorate, and often strokes become frequent occurrences until the pet is totally debilitated. It is not certain whether strokes occur in animals as they do in humans, but the symptoms are very similar. Most noticeable is a marked pulling of the head to one side, droopy eyelids or twitching. The animal may walk around in circles or get stuck in a corner and just sit and stare. Partial paralysis—especially of the mouth, making eating and drinking difficult—requires more home care.

Nutritional Supplements for Strokes

- B-Complex 50 is given to increase the dose available in Mega Pet Daily to a <u>daily total</u> of up to 200 mg. for cats & small dogs to 400 mg. for large dogs for the first three months following the stroke.

- MSM is a nutritional sulfur supplement which aids in repairing and strengthening the tissues of the brain. MSM benefits the animal whose stroke can be traced to traumatic damage to the brain, be it by drugs, chemicals or traumatic injury to the head in a car accident. In addition, it is helpful in protecting and repairing damage from the stroke itself regardless of cause.

- Coenzyme Q-10 is a nutrient which replenishes the strength and vitality to brain cells, particularly those in the aging or severely debilitated pet. This is an excellent supplement to prevent deterioration which may lead to strokes in a prone pet or help slow the spread of damaged cells due to the stroke.

- Vita E 200 provides therapeutic doses of vitamin E to help repair and strengthen cellular tissue and a compromised brain. Especially benefits the animal who has a history of a toxic lifestyle or other chronic health conditions. In addition to Mega Pet Daily feed an additional 100 I.U.'s for cats and small dogs (giving half a capsule each morning) to 400 I.U.'s per day for large breeds.

Herbal Remedies

- Yucca Intensive is as effective as corticosteroids in most cases where anti-inflammatory support is required. If needed, yucca can even be used in conjunction with steroids to reduce the need for heavy doses of this potentially harmful medication, until the pet can be weaned solely onto the herb for long-term maintenance.

- Calm & Relax benefits the pet who has become highly sensitive and vocal with anxiety following a stroke. Helps rebalance brain chemistry and regenerate brain tissue. Promotes sound sleep to recover from the episode while regaining function and coordination.

- Grape Seed Extract is a powerful antioxidant. Benefits include reducing the recurrence of strokes by eliminating free radicals which encourage brain deterioration. This should be every older pets' supplement protocol to help prevent strokes.

Homeopathic Remedies

- R&R Essence will help reduce the physical and emotional trauma which coincides with a stroke, often making the secondary symptoms worse. Use immediately after the stroke and for at least the following two weeks. Can be used in addition to any other remedies.

- D'Toxifier contains *Arsenicum* which is indicated for the pet who wanders the house with great anguish and restlessness following a stroke. Additional complementary remedies help the body through improved nutrient utilization and waste elimination; given every fifteen minutes the first hour, then every hour until the pet is resting, will help reverse symptoms of stroke. Continue daily for two weeks following the stroke. Reduces chronic conditions of a toxic lifestyle to prevent stroke; general restorative to help improve wellness.

- *Aconite* is a good homeopathic remedy for strokes in general.

- *Bufo* is used if paralysis is the result of a stroke.

Surgery

Surgery can be a stressful time for the owner, often due to the owner's fears and loss of control. A few things should be considered to make the situation easier on the pet and to prevent long-term side-effects from occurring.

Pre-Operation

- Do NOT vaccinate for at least six weeks prior to surgery! The stress of the surgery can increase the possibility of vaccinosis.

- Speak to the veterinarian regarding what to expect when the pet returns home. Do they need confinement? Stitches protected? Force-fed fluids? Be prepared.

- Feed Milk Thistle (in general) or Skin & Liv-A-Plex (for older or debilitated pets) for forty-eight hours prior to the surgery. This will help protect the liver from the gas and any medications used during surgery.

- Give homeopathic R&R Essence (for stress) and Phosphorous (will prevent bleeding) every fifteen minutes for an hour prior to surgery. If this is not possible, dose as closely to the time of surgery as you can.

Post-Operation

- Absolutely Do NOT vaccinate for at least six weeks post surgery. This will reduce the possibility of vaccinosis.

- Homeopathic D'Toxifier contains *Arsenicum* which can reverse the gas and other stress-producing chemicals in the body. It is formulated with complementary remedies which help the body and skin repair through improved nutrient utilization and waste elimination. This product addresses many symptoms associated with surgery including digestive upset, anxiety and physical pain. Works as a general restorative to promote a quick recovery and general wellness.

- Increase Super C 2000 by 25% to 50% and double Garlic Daily Aid to prevent infection and promote tissue repair.

- Feed Milk Thistle (in general) or Skin & Liv-A-Plex (for debilitated or older pets) for two to six weeks post-surgery. This will help protect the liver from the gas used during surgery and any medications used after surgery.

- Feed MSM to increase nutritional sulfur available to the body for tissue repair for deep or damaged cuts.

- Apply Rejuva Spray to wound to promote tissue repair and reduce infection and inflammation. Will help "dry" the wound. Decreases scratching and biting at stitches.

- Use Rejuva Gel, beginning one week after surgery, on the stitch site to minimize scarring.

- VitaE200 both as a supplement and topically (once stitches are removed) to minimize scarring.

Teeth (& Gums)

TEETH (& GUMS): Diseases of the mouth often revolve around gum problems (gingivitis), abscesses, and bad teeth. Proper oral care is vital to good health. Poor teeth and painful gums can contribute as much to your pet's poor health and chronic condition as chemicals. Proper chewing becomes difficult; therefore the digestive process begins poorly. Food gets swallowed whole, which is more difficult to break down further for assimilation. Vital nutrients are lost, regardless of how good the diet is.

If chewing is too painful—your animal may be refusing to eat—lack of food can quickly exacerbate an immune weakness. I have seen too many pets starve to death because of bad teeth. Bacteria, which grow well in the warm, moist environment provided by the mouth and feed off the yeast and sugar available in the animal's standard diet, can trigger a severe systemic infection, if not addressed.

Weekly cleaning of your dog or cat's mouth, availability of a high quality dry kibble food (home prepared if preferred), chew toys and bones will provide the tools necessary to keep the teeth free of tartar. Avoid rawhide! It contains formaldehyde and can become lodged in the digestive tract as it swells with fluid. Chemical-based diets or treats for tartar control—may actually keep the teeth white, but at what expense—kidney or liver failure? It is still too soon in their popularity to tell, but I suspect that these chemicals will prove to be just as burdensome as others. Proper maintenance is the best, safest route to take to assure that your pet's teeth won't be the cause of disease or death.

Examining & Brushing Your Pet's Teeth

To prevent tooth decay and oral problems, examine your pet's teeth weekly. Check for any signs of redness, ulceration or discharge between the teeth and around the mouth and tongue. Note any cracked or chipped teeth and if they are secure in the gum. Your veterinarian must immediately treat abscessed, cracked, loose or dangling teeth.

Follow this examination by a dental brushing with a child's toothbrush for smaller pets and soft adult toothbrush for dogs over fifty pounds. If your bigger dog has problems opening their mouth wide enough, then a child toothbrush can easily reach the back molars. You can also wrap a thin wet washcloth around your index finger to rub the teeth clean—which some pets might feel more comfortable with—especially in the beginning, until they become accustomed to the idea of having their teeth brushed. Apply a small amount of natural toothpaste. Adult's or kid's is fine as long as you avoid fluoride. Use one that includes tea tree, grapefruit or goldenseal extract, if gum infection is suspected. I prefer this to pet-specific dental paste, which can be full of chemicals, sugars and artificial flavors.

Start the toothbrush at the back of the mouth, working your way to the front teeth. Try to open the mouth slightly so you can get behind the teeth and to the back bottom molars—a prime decay area. Wipe away any leftover toothpaste with a wet cloth. You do not need to use a lot of toothpaste to begin with, so there should not be much left over to wipe away or swallow.

I keep a glass of clean water to rinse the brush in and then apply the clean brush *with water in the bristles* to scrub away whatever toothpaste remains between the teeth. It is safe for your pet to swallow a little of the natural toothpaste; many actually enjoy the taste, but do not overdo it. You do not need to foam up the mouth to get it clean. Pets, especially cats, don't like the foam and will fight you.

Remove any accumulated tartar that brushing has left behind, with a dental scraper available in many pet catalogues. You can also safely remove heavy tartar by applying a flat edged scraper to the crown of the tartar build-up (at the gum line) and flicking it away from the gum line. It will usually come off in a large chunk. Try not to allow your pet to swallow these chunks if possible. Once the majority of tartar has been cleaned, weekly brushing and proper diet should keep them tartar-free and pearly white.

As a side-note, many have begun to floss their pet's teeth, and I highly recommend this. Always approach your pet gently when introducing anything new, even the brushing. Start by getting them accustomed to having you rub a clean finger over their teeth and gums. Once they have become comfortable with this, you can proceed to brushing and flossing. I love the new pre-strung-flossed dental picks available. It is a small plastic holder for floss so you can easily maneuver it in between the teeth with one hand and hold the pet with the other.

Never force your pet to do anything, but rather slowly introduce them to it. If you force them, they will only fight you and then avoid you—with toothbrush in hand—in the future. Use a homeopathic "rescue" flower remedy like *R&R Essence* and/or homeopathic *Aconite* to calm them if needed, and proceed to clean them as best as you can. If your animal is very difficult to handle you can use *Calm & Relax* for a few days prior to the cleaning and follow the homeopathic suggestions at the time of need. Use R&R Essence (to reduce stress) and/or Fear remedy if needed.

Yearly teeth cleaning under anesthesia—where animals are actually put on a breathing tube, as they would be during major surgery—could weaken your pet's immune system and interfere with their good health in general.

Many pets have had a recurrence of various chronic symptoms shortly after having their teeth cleaned under gas. There is always the risk of dying during any surgical procedure, which should not be taken lightly. Your dog should be put under anesthesia for life-threatening conditions only—not for elective procedures. Unless it is life threatening or teeth need to be removed and pus pockets drained, avoid anesthesia, which can further weaken your pet's immune system. During anesthesia, animals are completely under and on a respirator, not breathing on their own, having lungs pumped. I have heard of too many animals having relapses of old conditions or symptoms and becoming severely weakened following a veterinary dental cleaning, many of them having nothing more than "dirty" teeth to warrant taking such a chance with the pet's health.

Personally, I know of eight clients' dogs and two cats who died under this procedure! Some veterinary, grooming or alternative practitioners will clean your pet's teeth without anesthesia, so seek them out if needed.

Most problems can be prevented, but if needed—oral problems generally respond well to home care:

- **Bad breath** is mainly associated with poor dental hygiene. Certainly, rotting and infected teeth will have an offensive odor, but I have found that most cases of bad breath actually occur in the digestive tract, not from unsightly tartar build-up. If dental hygiene does not get rid of the offensive odor—be sure to detoxify and check what diet you are feeding. Brushing (including the tongue) will eliminate the majority of oral odors, while the addition of a liquid chlorophyll breath product will also help temporarily mask the odor. Clean teeth and gums do not smell.

- **Painful, bleeding gums** that might be too sore to touch—apply clove teething gel (or standard drug store gel) and give a dose of homeopathic *Hypericum* a few minutes before cleaning. Wait at least thirty minutes between the clove gel use and any homeopathic remedy dosing, as clove essence is an antidote. Continue with the Hypericum twice per day, until gums are normal. Homeopathic *Mercurius* benefits pets that are very irritable with swollen gums that might bleed easily.

- **Preventing Tooth Decay**—is easily accomplished through weekly cleaning and basic nutritional support, as well as chewing products. Avoid rawhide, which produces a sticky film adding to build-up in addition to being a digestive tract no-no, as it could cause intestinal blockage and death. Raw soft bones (chicken, beef, lamb, pork, etc.) are a choking hazard and also a digestive tract no-no, but large baked-hard or raw beef shanks or knuckles provide a good surface to chew on. Azmira® has a full line of "human-grade" smoked bones that are perfect for keeping a pet's mouth healthy (knuckles for dogs and turkey necks for the cats).

  This helps remove tartar from the surface of the teeth; as well as stimulate the gums. Several hard natural and plastic chew toys have been recently developed for dental care. These are appropriate, as long as they are of good quality food-grade materials although I do not believe that they can do a proper job alone without the weekly cleanings.

Homeopathic Remedies to prevent TARTAR and Tooth Decay

- D'Toxifier helps counter the effects of a toxic lifestyle which may lead to tartar. Improves the health of gums through nutrient utilization and waste elimination. Helps stimulate suppression of many symptoms of tooth decay (i.e. painful gums, bleeding or infected).

- Several remedies have been touted as a preventative tartar control remedy. I have seen some success with *Calcarea Phos.* both in a lower daily dose (10X to 3C) and/or higher potencies (200C), dosed weekly. But to be safe… keep brushing!

(see Gingivitis-*gum disease*, Infections)

Thyroid Problems

THYROID PROBLEMS can be very common to animals that exhibit chronic symptoms, especially in chronic skin, liver or weight conditions. Often the thyroid problem can be caused by previous cycles of steroid medications—the very drugs most commonly used to suppress most chronic symptoms.

Testing for hormonal levels will benefit you in general, regardless of what you decide to do, but be wary of the veterinarian who recommends a thyroid medication for a "border-line imbalance." Look at the numbers on the test. They always list the range it should be in and if it is only slightly out of range, forget medication, at least at first. Too many pets are put on medication (and suffer their serious side-effects) for border-line conditions that are regarded by naturopathic science to simply be a symptom of imbalance (dis-ease)—easily corrected with **Steps One** and **Two**. Utilize thyroid medication *carefully* and only when appropriate for you *and* your animal, especially if nothing else seems to work.

Raw glandulars with thyroid and supportive organs such as adrenal and pituitary glands, plus proper nutrition, can often reverse thyroid weakness and rebalance function.

Nutritional Supplements

- Coenzyme Q-10 promotes greater organ resiliency in the older or weaker pet.

- MSM helps to strengthen the thyroid gland.

- Seasupreme provides iodine to promote thyroid function.

Homeopathic Remedies

- D'Toxifier contains *Iris, Phytolacca and Arsenicum* with complementary remedies which help the thyroid gland through improved nutrient utilization and blood waste elimination; given as a weekly maintenance dose it helps regulate thyroid function. Reduces chronic conditions of a toxic lifestyle to prevent thyroid imbalance. Works for both "hypo" and "hyper" thyroid conditions.

Herbal Thyroid Remedies

- Yucca Intensive seems to help the thyroid respond quicker to nutritional support.
- Blood & Lymph D'Tox is good for goiter and <u>hypo</u>activity.
- Calm & Relax helps rebalance the endocrine system and is appropriate for <u>hyper</u>activity.
- Stress & A'Drenal Plex benefits the animal with adrenal exhaustion in addition to a hyperactive thyroid.

(see Symptom-specific subjects)

Ticks

TICKS create a lot of health problems for owners and their pets. These blood sucking pests can suck the health right out of a dog or cat if left untreated and can bring on the quick demise of a weak and compromised host. In addition, they transmit the bacterial infection resulting in tick fever. Like fleas, they used to scare me; once an infestation began inside the home and yard it took cans of chemical foggers and toxic dips to eradicate them. I saw many a pet, especially puppies, get very sick from the chemical warfare. But don't worry! Over the years natural remedies have been proven effective in preventing and eliminating tick infestations.

(follow recommendations for Fleas; see Skin Conditions)

Tick Fever

TICK FEVER, or Ehrlichiosis, can be fatal if left untreated. This parasitic bacterium is transmitted through the bite of an infected tick and takes up residence on a weakened host. Clinical symptoms including lethargy, fever, weight loss, bleeding disorder, eye and ear discharge and swollen lymph nodes can be very debilitating. In severe cases liver or kidney failure and seizures are possible. Once you have a diagnosis, address the symptoms as you would any other condition following the **Three Simple Steps** of detoxification, fuel to heal, and remedies to stimulate and support the process.

Herbal Tick Fever Remedies

- Viral D'Tox has a misleading name, as it is very effective against bacteria as well. This herbal combination has reduced Ehrlichiosis titers quickly, often within six weeks. Helps minimize general symptoms and promotes vitality.

- Blood & Lymph D'Tox is a good addition to the Viral D'Tox for chronic cases or severely debilitated dogs who are not responding quickly enough.

- Yucca Intensive reduces pain and inflammation associated with tick fever.

Homeopathic Remedies

- D'Toxifier contains *Arsenicum* with complementary remedies which help the body through improved nutrient utilization and blood waste elimination; given as a weekly maintenance dose, it helps regulate immune function. Reduces chronic conditions of a toxic lifestyle to prevent infestation and general symptoms of ehrlichiosis for symptom reversal. Helps with the recovery period.

- Newton's Homeopathic Labs® Ehrlichiosis Nosode can be used both as a preventative during times of high exposure or to aid in titer reversal.

(see Symptom-specific symptoms, i.e. Immune Dysfunction, Lethargy)

Training Problems

TRAINING PROBLEMS are possible to undo, even prevent, with a few simple steps. To prevent trauma from occurring during training and to teach an animal to trust again, never force an animal to do anything they truly fear until you have desensitized them to it. Use the homeopathically potentized R&R Essence prior to teaching new or difficult lessons to reduce the likelihood that fear will replace reason in your pet and will interfere with their learning or provoke negative behavioral outcomes which can then become chronic behavioral reactions.

To reverse behavioral problems, you must first identify the emotional triggers and behavioral traits, such as fear, aggression and neediness that your animal is exhibiting. Azmira® has a remedy for each of these traits and more. It does not matter if your pet is feral, too old, or you do not have its history. Use the proper remedy in conjunction with behavioral modification, through the desensitizing exercise described in the section: Behavioral Problems, and your animal will quickly gain a new attitude.

Upper Respiratory Problems

UPPER RESPIRATORY PROBLEMS can be the most difficult chronic symptom to reverse, since the lung and nasal tissues can be so easily irritated by allergens and toxins. Damaged from chronic symptoms such as wheezing and discharge, these tissues become even more sensitive. Daily cleaning of the nostrils with a warm, damp cloth to keep discharge and crusted mucous clear of nasal passages will help facilitate healing. Homeopathic and herbal supplementation can successfully address these symptoms.

(See Asthma, Allergy Reactions, Infections.)

Vaccinosis

VACCINOSIS is the condition the body is subjected to when there is a negative reaction to a vaccine. The vaccine, more notably the ingredients which stabilize the vaccine such as mercury and formaldehyde, can trigger an allergic reaction and weaken the immune system enough to lower resistance to other allergens and toxins in general. Many chronic conditions of allergies, arthritis, liver or kidney problems and autoimmune dysfunction started with vaccinosis.

If you suspect that this is the case, use D'Toxifier containing homeopathic *Arsenicum* and *Thuja* in frequent daily doses until symptoms begin to reverse themselves. Then use this remedy combination once a day for one month, switching to a higher potency *Thuja* 200C once a week for an additional three months. Acute symptoms which will be addressed include lethargy, mental confusion with digestive upsets including loss of appetite and fever. You may also see a discharge from the anus, the nose, the eyes or the injection site within twelve hours of the shots. Seizures are a possibility, especially with the rabies or the all-in-one vaccines. Use these homeopathic remedies as a preventive and to lessen the likelihood of a reaction: begin dosing a few days prior to the shots. Newton's Labs® Nosodes made from the actual diseases, such as rabies, distemper, parvo, Feline Leukemia or FIP can also be used to effectively reverse vaccinosis or, when used as a preventative prior to and after giving the vaccine—will definitely help minimize the likelihood of a negative reaction.

Some dogs, like my friend Richard's dog Laney, have a recurrence of cancerous growths after a vaccination. It is a very stressful time when he has to renew her license and must have a rabies shot (the only vaccine she gets) and measures are taken to protect her from the side-effects. This past year Laney, who is now ten years old, had a reaction despite the nosode and suffered a recurrence of a growth on her lip within two weeks of the shot. This growth had been in "remission" for over four years. She was fasted, detoxified and Richard increased her foundation supplements as well as followed recommendations from the cancer protocol. Within six weeks the lip was noticeably better. Sometimes the body just needs a bigger boost than we anticipate. Hopefully someday the law will be changed to reflect what they realize in Europe; that one shot and a booster is all that is needed for a lifetime of protection.

Reducing the Risks of Vaccinosis

- Do not vaccinate if you absolutely do not have to by law. This is especially true for indoor-only cats.

- Seek a veterinarian who will draw a titer on your pet to determine if vaccination is even warranted. Many will accept a high titer count as proof of protection.

- Ask the veterinarian to only prick the skin and not discharge the full vaccine. Some will accept this as a vaccination sufficient for licensing.

- Do not give vaccines during illness or recovery from trauma. Avoid vaccinating six weeks prior to or following surgery. The body is already stressed and more likely to have a negative reaction.

- Avoid giving all-in-one vaccines at all costs! This causes the most serious reactions. Stagger the individual doses over a few weeks.

- Give rabies vaccines to mature, healthy pets only; very young, infirmed or old animals are most prone to reaction.

- If you must vaccinate, avoid giving yearly vaccinations during the seasons your pet is most sensitive (stressed) if they suffer allergies or arthritic conditions.

- Avoid vaccines altogether if the pet suffers from cancer or other serious dis-eases. The vaccine will only weaken the body and allow the condition to flourish. Many chronic symptoms or conditions, some reversed for years, reappear within six weeks to three months of a vaccination.

Vaccine Avoidance

- To avoid vaccinations altogether, begin by researching homeopathic nosodes. Newton's Homeopathic Labs® makes outstanding nosodes for all the infectious dis-eases. I have had great success with this type of homeopathic protection and I do not vaccinate otherwise, except to stay in compliance with my canines' rabies licenses.

- For maximum protection these remedies are to be used in conjunction with **Step's One** and **Two**.

- Viral D'Tox is an outstanding product of herbal compounds with properties which help build resistance to viral *and bacterial* infections such as Feline Leukemia, Parvovirus, and Kennel Cough. I start supplementing with it a week before exposure or at first notice and I have never had an infection take hold.

(see Symptom-specific subjects, i.e. Fever, Digestive Disorders, Seizures)

Valley Fever

VALLEY FEVER is a serious, often-fatal, fungal infestation, found in the arid southwestern states and Mexico. Pets who dig and those with chronic allergy conditions are most prone to developing Valley Fever. The fungal spores grow deep in dry desert dirt and are released by any type of digging. It is inhaled or absorbed through the skin. During clinical studies most healthy dogs tested had a low 1:4 titer with no symptoms; Valley Fever symptoms only manifest themselves in weakened hosts. Treatment with chemical anti-fungal drugs often suppresses symptoms only to have them return with a vengeance once medication is ceased.

The side effects of anti-fungal drugs can be permanently damaging to the liver and kidneys, and they suppress the appetite and the immune system as well. Therefore it is not uncommon for pets being treated for Valley Fever to develop immune suppressed-related symptoms, including reactive arthritis which worsens an already inflamed structural system. Herbal treatment is effective in reversing the fungal count. Often, with veterinary medical care, the count may end up in the low end (1:4), but it will never reach zero since the body retains antibodies. This is not true with The Holistic Animal Care LifeStyle™ Valley Fever protocol. We have proven that within a year of Lifestyle™ changes with this protocol the antibody count can be zero and stay at zero as long as the body is supported! Nevertheless, a holistically supported pet can remain free of symptoms or weakness, regardless of a "positive" titer count.

Full reversal is not possible when medication has been used first—with or without the protocol; either antifungal, antibiotic or steroid drugs (suppress the immune function and allow some infestation to remain to resurface at the first sign of physical or emotional stress). Relapse is especially high when treated with medication only.

Herbal Remedies for Valley Fever

- Yeast & Fungal D'Tox is a very powerful anti-fungal and anti-yeast therapeutic formula, and is beneficial in reducing Valley Fever spore infestation and secondary infections. For reversal, use at least six weeks prior to drawing another titer count (it should be lowered by then to 1:4 or even eliminated as we see in a number of cases that use the full protocol). Continue using for another three months after the count is zero to avoid a relapse. One or two bottles a year (preferably right after the rainy season or during construction when spores are at their most infectious state) can prevent infestation or recurrence.

- Garlic Daily Aid has anti-fungal activity and is very valuable to use for the prevention (at the recommended dose) or reversal (double the dose) of Valley Fever and related symptoms such as lack of appetite and other digestive disorders.

- Yucca Intensive relieves the inflammatory response often associated with Valley Fever, since the spore infestation can settle within the brain, lungs, bones and joints, irritating healthy cells.

- Stress & A'Drenal Plex is excellent for addressing the secondary symptoms of infestation—lethargy, thyroid imbalance and general poor condition with exhaustion.

- Immuno Stim'R helps to reduce symptoms in a severely debilitated pet and prevents recurrence when used as part of your daily maintenance protocol.

- Daily Boost has anti-fungal properties, but most importantly, is a blood purifier and toner which helps build up healthy red blood cells, boosts energy and immune function. This is an excellent daily supplement to help prevent fungal infestation. Reverses the ravages of Valley Fever in severe cases when combined with

Yeast & Fungal D'Tox. Promotes good appetite, often lost from anti-fungal medications or fatigue.

(see Symptom-specific subjects, including Appetite, Arthritis, Inflammation, Pain)

Vestibular Disease

VESTIBULAR DISEASE is a severe disorder of the nervous system portion responsible for the maintenance of balance and coordination of muscle activity. Chemicals, infectious diseases, trauma and chronic ear infections can contribute to symptoms including head tilting or rolling, disorientation, vomiting and actually falling over when attempting to walk.

Genetically, Burmese and Siamese kittens are prone to developing **congenital vestibular syndrome** within the first month after birth. These kittens can not develop enough neuro-muscularly to walk properly. Although the Siamese kittens will often also be deaf, they will recover some coordination by six months of age. The Burmese will not recover and often warrant euthanasia. Supporting the queen nutritionally, including tissue cell salts, during gestation is vital to preventing the possibility of this development.

Vestibular ataxia syndrome is seen in kittens born to a queen who is stricken with feline parvovirus during pregnancy. Kittens seem to have trouble learning to walk, although the condition may or may not get worse over time. Holistic nosodes and remedies for structural inflammation or viral conditions may reverse these weaknesses.

(see Symptom-specific symptoms)

Viral Infections

VIRAL INFECTIONS are marked with fever and often nervous system dysfunction as viral infections can quickly settle in the brain, spinal column and nerves (i.e. Distemper, Parvovirus). Antibiotics are often recommended despite the fact that they DO NOT reverse viral infections. They are given to quell secondary symptoms of infection to prevent bacteria from infecting, yet they do much more damage to the digestive tract interfering with nutrient absorption and weakening the immune response! Viral infection responds well to nutritional supplementation, herbal remedies and homeopathic immune response stimulation.

(see Infections)

Vomiting

Vomiting can be the result of a recently ingested object or bad food, a viral infection, vaccinosis or indicative of a chronic digestive disorder, just to name a few causes. The important thing to remember is not to allow the vomiting to weaken the pet further through dehydration or depletion of their energy. Whenever in doubt as to the cause or the vomiting has become uncontrollable, then seek proper diagnosis and medical care immediately but I have found very rare instances of when naturopathy can not help.

Homeopathic Remedies for Vomiting

*part of Azmira®'s D'Toxifier

- D'Toxifier contains *Arsenicum* with complementary remedies which help the digestive and eliminatory system through improved nutrient utilization and waste elimination; given every five minutes apart for one hour will stimulate symptom suppression. Reduces chronic conditions of a toxic lifestyle to prevent digestive problems; general restorative to help regulate the liver which is often a trigger in many vomiting instances.

- *Arsenicum* is used for digestive imbalances from poor quality diets or general toxicity and will alleviate most vomiting, especially if there is liver or spleen involvement. This remedy is especially effective when the disorder has been triggered by a season of ingesting monthly flea and tick control medications or other drugs. Alternate weekly doses of Arsenicum 200C with daily doses of D'Toxifier for severe cases of toxic reactions.

- *Belladonna* is for the sudden onset of gastrointestinal symptoms. After initial use, should be tapered off slowly and then followed by a more specific remedy. Belladonna is indicated for "fatty" loose stools and lack of appetite resulting from pancreatic imbalances that also cause vomiting.

- *Berberis Vulg.* stimulates liver function, reduces uric acid and reduces the urge to vomit.

- *Carbo Veg* is helpful when the pet is also overweight, has chronic stool problems, seems to have trouble digesting well, and burps soon after eating. This is a good senior pet tonic. Pets vomit following meals.

- *China* supports pets that have chronic liver involvement with digestive imbalances who are very sensitive to touch and open air. They chill easily and seek to hide, especially after meals. Although they may crave cold water, it will cause them to burp up partially digested food.

- *Colocynthis* is indicated for pets who are cramping or whose stomachs are rumbling. There may be other symptoms. They want to lie on a hard surface or they will respond to positively when you rub their belly. Movement, drinking or eating will aggravate symptoms.

- *Nux Vomica* also addresses the majority of digestive imbalances, including vomiting, gas, lack of appetite or stool problems (especially alternating between constipation and diarrhea along with vomiting). Use this when D'Toxifier is not available.

- *Phosphorous* is indicated if the digestive problems include great debilitation, fluid loss or frequent vomiting with or without diarrhea soon after meals. Partially digested food often comes up immediately. Pet has difficulty in expelling stools which leads to a toxic reaction and vomiting.

- *Pulsatilla* aids when symptoms, such as nausea or vomiting are not too severe. Food is often the culprit, especially if it is high in animal fats or rancid ingredients. The offending food might be vomited up partially digested. The tongue may become coated with a thick white or yellowish material.

- **Taraxacum* stimulates liver function and proper bowel evacuation. Promotes general rest and recovery of the digestive system, reducing urge to vomit.

- *Ipecac* can quickly subdue vomiting, especially when it is related to food or ingested chemical allergies.

Fasting With Fluids During Vomiting (associated with viral infection, etc.)

- Fast the symptomatic pet while force-feeding fluids to prevent dehydration; make a solution of two ounces each of apple juice and purified water. Add one tablespoon of raw honey for energy. Use a syringe (without the needle) and place towards the back of the pet's mouth, in the corners, to get the fluid on the back of the tongue. Give one ounce of solution per pound of body weight per day. This will compensate for spillage. It is best to give some fluid every couple of hours during the height of symptoms (fever, vomiting, bloody diarrhea, exhaustion) to ward off dehydration and keep up the pet's energy needed for healing. For severe vomiting you may not be able to give much fluid before triggering more vomiting. Give the minimum amount your pet can handle and as frequently as you can until their vomiting subsides through homeopathic dosing. Daily supplements and herbal remedies can be added to fresh fluid solution to be used within the next twenty four hours.

- As symptoms improve <u>oatmeal water</u> can also be used in this solution instead of plain water, eventually thickening it up to a soup once the fever has ended. To make oatmeal water soak overnight two handfuls of oatmeal in a pint of water and strain.

- Once the vomiting has stopped, chicken broth can be substituted for plain water to make the oatmeal water. This will provide easily digestible fats and encourage the digestive tract to function.

- Feed cooked oatmeal as appetite and digestion stabilizes to help break the fasting period. Give four small meals the first few days. A tablespoon or two of yogurt can be added for acidophilus and use Azmira®'s Acidophilus. Tuna can water or meat-based baby food can be added for flavor. Oatmeal is soothing to irritated intestinal tissues and will help eliminate dis-eased tissue from the colon, reducing the urge to vomit.

- Chicken & Beef or Ocean Fish canned formulas can be later added to the oatmeal as stools firm up and appetite is strong. These are the easiest to digest and given in three smaller daily meals, they will help bring digestion back on line. After a week of recovery, return to normal daily schedule and meal planning for the pet's age.

(see Digestive Disorders)

Warts

(see Skin and Coat Problems)

Weight Problems

WEIGHT PROBLEMS are not uncommon in pets also struggling with chronic health or behavioral symptoms. Improper digestion and assimilation (also at the root of dis-ease) can interfere with the body's ability to utilize calories properly for energy. The brain is responsible for deciding if the body is being fed enough. If nutrients are not available to the blood through proper assimilation, the brain will think that the body is starving and decides to store calories as fat, rather than use them as energy to repair tissue and support the immune system.

This is why reduced calorie diets fail in the long-term. A sound nutritional supplement protocol, with appropriate calories fed daily for the desired weight limit, fuels the brain to burn calories instead of storing them. The weight gradually comes off with no negative effects.

Pets who suffer great anxiety or debilitation along with their conditions suffer improper digestion and can have trouble maintaining proper weight, regardless of what they are fed. The LifeStyle™ approach helps rebalance the endocrine system, promotes proper nutrient assimilation and puts healthy weight on the pet.

Be sure to exercise your pet daily. Playing games such as "chase" or taking a walk, for as little as fifteen minutes a day, can help improve their metabolism and burn fat. When inactivity has been the norm, be sure to start with shorter periods of time exercising until your pet is comfortable and does not strain itself.

Always weigh your pet prior to starting a weight gain or loss program. Smaller pets can be weighed by you stepping on the scale first then with them in your arms and subtracting the difference. If your dog is too large to hold, bring them to your veterinarian's office. Most will weigh you pet at no cost, provided you are not visiting with the veterinarian for advice. Weigh your pet every month for comparison. Slow, but steady, weight changes are best. In addition, measure your pet at the beginning. Some may not lose as much weight initially, but should be firming up. Measure your pet first around the front of the chest, from elbow to elbow. Proceed to measure all the way around the chest and back, holding the tape just behind the legs. Then measure around the waist, just behind the last rib. Repeat this monthly. This way, if the weight has not changed much, you will be able to see if the body is responding. It is not uncommon to see these changes first without much weight loss or gain. This is a good sign that the body is responding, and the scale will soon reflect it. Measuring the body is the best way to see changes in a horse when a scale may not be available to you.

- **D'Toxifier** contains *Arsenicum* with complementary remedies which help the body through an increase in metabolism, improved nutrient utilization and waste elimination. Reduces chronic conditions of a toxic lifestyle to prevent both over and under-weight problems; general restorative.

- **DigestZymez** helps improve nutrient absorption in either cases of over or under-weight pets.

- **Herbal Slim** works to melt pounds away naturally and rebalance the digestive tract for greater assimilation.

- **Stress & A'Drenal Plex** has herbs which work synergistically to restore integrity to the adrenal and/or thyroid glands to promote weight gain and maintenance of proper weight during crisis. This acts as an adaptogen to counter chronic stress, which may be resulting in weight loss.

- **Dairy & Egg Protein Powder** adds calories and amino acids to promote weight gain and improved muscle mass.

(see Digestive Disorders)

Wobblers Syndrome

WOBBLERS SYNDROME is often diagnosed in Dobermans and Great Danes, although Shepherds and Rottweilers are also prone. Horses are also affected. It is a condition of instability and deformities of the neck vertebrae which places pressure on the spinal cord, causing hind end weakness, with or without pain, and eventually, paralysis.

(see Degenerative Disc Disorders, Paralysis)

Worms

WORMS can seriously compromise the body; interfere with proper digestion and assimilation, which leaves the body more susceptible to toxic reactions. Internal parasitic infestation can, more often than skin parasites, become deadly. Avoid chemical dewormers which are so harsh they can permanently damage the sensitive linings of the digestive tract, especially of young animals.

Herbal worming can be successful if you follow the directions carefully. Often, products should be administered along with fasting for optimum effect. Read instructions carefully.

- Herbal Wormer contains herbs which are effective against roundworms, tapeworms, whipworms or pinworms—helps eliminates eggs plus prevents infestation when used weekly.

- Garlic Daily Aid, in double the recommended dose, is an excellent antiparasitic against intestinal worms and will help the body to shed them faster when combined with Herbal Wormer. Used daily, in the recommended dose, it will help to prevent infestation.

- D'Toxifier contains *Arsenicum* with complementary remedies which help the body through improved nutrient utilization and waste elimination; given every fifteen minutes for one hour (especially twelve and again twenty-four hours after supplementing with Herbal Wormer) will help stimulate elimination of worms. *Arsenicum* is for the animal who becomes irritated when infested. Reduces chronic conditions of a toxic lifestyle to prevent infestations; general intestinal restorative.

(see Digestive Disorders)

Wounds

(see Infections, Skin Conditions)

CHAPTER ELEVEN

How To Be Your Vet's Best Friend

The most important ally you need to share the job of taking care of your pet is a trusted veterinarian. Although I am very much a proponent of at-home naturopathic care through a healthy lifestyle, I trust in the wonders of modern diagnostic tools and veterinary medicine when warranted. You should never, ever, think that you could handle each and every health concern by yourself. Please be happy to assume *control* of your pet's health care and weigh all medically-related decisions carefully, based on the expertise and guidance of a competent professional in addition to the knowledge you have gained.

Yearly health exams and occasional blood work can help catch an imbalance early, before it ever becomes a health problem. Often an imbalance in the endocrine system, protein assimilation, or blood sugar irregularities can be spotted in a simple blood test long before the actual symptoms appear and a chronic physical or emotional condition develops. When facing specific symptoms, proper diagnosis to verify a specific imbalance can make the difference between addressing the problem head-on and/or trying a "hit or miss" therapy that can go on for months. Monitoring the body as it responds to the chosen therapy will also help you quickly identify what is, or is not, working.

The more you know and understand, the more successful you will be—the healthier and safer your animals' lives will be.

Today there are more holistically-oriented veterinarians who are well versed in the complementary modalities of nutritional therapy, herbs, homeopathy, acupuncture, massage and chiropractic care. Some have even expanded to incorporate esoteric therapies of sound, light and energy healing. In addition, a high number of allopathic (traditionally trained) veterinarians are now accepting that natural pet care has its place within their traditional, medically-based practice. Based on what you have learned, it is now up to you to decide how well a veterinarian is practicing medicine naturopathically, is well educated in holistic care versus using a holistic shingle outside his office door to bring in business, while still symptom-treating. Or even worse, is he treating with drugs first and remedies second to control the side-effects? Don't just *trust*—your pet depends on you.

Unfortunately, many of us have had very negative experiences with veterinarians, especially those allopathically trained veterinarians who are not familiar with natural care and are uncompromising in their views. Possibly, a vet has spoken to you as if you did not have a clue in your head about your pets' health care needs and dismissed your attempts to seek a chemical-free life for your pets. It's more likely that they simply failed to address your pets' past conditions successfully, and you have lost faith in the medical approach.

I am hoping that by giving you a little insight into what veterinarians might be experiencing at their end, and encouraging you to join forces with them, it will help empower you. Knowledge is power. Let's be perfectly clear—I am not encouraging you to give your vet unchallenged authority over your pets' medical care. By becoming your vet's ally, you can successfully incorporate proper veterinary care into your pet's holistic lifestyle.

Vets are frustrated by a client's lack of knowledge as to what their pet's symptoms actually are.

One of the most common complaints that I have heard from veterinarians is that when they ask an owner for a pet's medical history, they can't get a straight answer. It's probably true that many pet owners do not care or do not realize how important a medical and lifestyle history is. Although a pet often is treated as a possession, they do not get the general maintenance a family car would get. Most people know the brand of engine oil they use, but can not tell you the food they feed their pet. Even those pets that are lucky enough to be considered a member of the family often are not given this consideration.

This has made clinical visits frustrating for many veterinarians. Sometimes, owners will tell a vet that they fed their pet whatever was on sale last week at the grocery store or it was "the blue bag, you know which one." Or when the pet has been on medication from another clinic, the owner cannot identify the medication, let alone the classification of the medication, whether it was an antibiotic, antihistamine or steroids. Who can blame the vets for becoming jaded about some of their clients!

Also, many owners often come into the veterinarian's office with half-baked ideas about treating disease naturally and will argue with the veterinarian, who may be open-minded at first, but when she/he is given conflicting information, will respond with an ultimatum: Do it my way or find another veterinarian. Obviously, there are some veterinarians who are simply close-minded, who will refuse to even consider natural alternatives. Believe me, there are still plenty out there, but the majority of allopathic veterinarians whom I've interviewed made it clear that they are willing to do what works best for each pet. They stressed that they really appreciated a pet owner who was responsible, well informed and knowledgeable about the choices for a naturopathic therapy protocol, based on the clinical diagnosis.

With this in mind, I have prepared a ten-point health checklist that I recommend you read carefully and put to good use. Please observe your pets daily so that you understand what they look and feel like when they are healthy. Answering these questions will enable you to quickly identify and address naturopathically any weakness or imbalance when it occurs; this improves your chances of *complete* symptom reversal. If a more serious, underlying issue is at hand, the information will quickly make itself clear to you and you can seek a diagnosis. Always have this information available the next time you visit your veterinarian, as it will help them assess the situation correctly.

Dr. Newman's Holistic Animal Care LifeStyle™
Ten-Point Health Check List

1. ENVIRONMENTAL CAUSES OF DIS-EASE

- Has your pet been given a new medication or recent vaccination?
- Is your pet wearing a chemically-based flea/tick collar or suffering chemical dips? Receiving monthly prevention of heartworm medication or other ingested pest control products?
- Have you recently sprayed the yard for weeds, or applied chemical pest control solutions in the house or yard?

- Are there any other poisons, radiator fluid, or toxic plants, such as Poinsettias, available to your pet to chew on or ingest in some way?

- Have you recently moved into a new home or installed new floor covering that might be seeping formaldehyde or other toxins that your pet is directly exposed to?

- Has the quality of your pet's drinking water or diet changed?

- Is your pet exposed to second-hand smoke?

- Is your pet an "out-door-only" pet? *This exposes them to additional stress and pollutants which diminish the immune response.*

2. <u>NUTRITIONAL CULPRITS</u>

- Has your pet's diet changed recently?

- What type of food do you feed? How often do you feed?

- Is it well balanced? Any yeast, sugar, salt or by-products? *Bring in the label if needed and read Chapter 4:* **Step One**.

- Have your pet's eating habits recently changed?

- Do they seem satisfied or always hungry?

- Has the pet's food gone rancid due to age or heat? Does it smell bad? *These are the number one reasons for appetite changes.*

- Have you introduced any new supplements, treats, chewable toys, rawhide or food ingredients that may be creating the problem?

All of these issues can trigger a toxic reaction, weaken the immune system or cause actual organ failure. Symptoms of "infection" (fever, digestive upsets and withdrawal) may actually be caused by a toxic reaction from a poor diet, not an organism. This can cause you to waste time treating the body with an antibiotic when a twenty-four hour detoxification is all that is needed. Look at the whole picture before jumping to any conclusions or using medications (in non-life threatening situations).

Because ninety percent of health problems today are caused by pets' environment and diet, it is vital that you become aware of what it is exactly that your pet has been exposed to or is ingesting. Just because your pet seemed to do well on its previous diet for four years (with a beautiful coat that you washed and brushed to look good) does not mean the diet did not cause this "sudden" digestive upset or toxic reaction. It is simply a fact that the body is now older (weaker) and unable to keep fighting the chemicals and by-products. The same can be said for years of toxic pest control products.

Once you can answer these questions honestly and have explored the additional *specific symptom causes and progressions or markers* by asking the next questions—you will become more familiar with your pet's ongoing health and be able to keep your pet in optimum condition.

Identifying where the imbalance is manifesting itself most, despite the obvious symptom, will also help you quickly address the root of the problem by focusing on the predominant weakness first. This is also valuable information for your veterinarian; when exactly did the symptom first manifest itself? Has it been ongoing or intermittent and for how long? In addition, by making the necessary changes in your pet's lifestyle and health care before a serious problem or chronic condition arises, you will be able to keep them healthy, and save money to boot. Prevention IS the best cure!

3. <u>DIGESTIVE SYSTEM</u>

- Does your pet have daily bowel movements? Is flatulence a problem and when; after eating, sleeping or exercise?

- Has the stool smell, volume, color or consistency changed recently?

- Have there been intermittent episodes of digestive upsets for no apparent reasons?

- Is there a poor coat condition or weight loss indicating chronic malabsorption?

Major signs of dis-ease can include vomiting, diarrhea or constipation for more than 24 hours. Pancreatic imbalance (fatty, discolored stool) and internal parasitic infestations (rice or string-like bodies within the stool) can be quickly diagnosed by your veterinarian, thereby making these symptoms much easier to reverse, and preventing them from developing into more serious conditions such as diabetes or irritable bowel syndrome.

4. <u>URINARY FUNCTION</u>

- Has your pet's normal daily intake of water changed? Increased or decreased?

- Do you allow free access to a potty area? Based on their urges?!

- Do you impose set potty times around your own schedule? Has this schedule changed?

- Is your pet refusing to use the same litter or potty area as before? Was it cleaned with a strong smelling chemical? Is the litter too aromatic or toxic such as with cedar or newsprint?

- Is the urine now painful, scant, or bloody? Is there a metallic or sweet odor to it?

- Has the flow of urine increased? Is the urine almost colorless or darker? Is it thicker, even gelatinous; with gravel or pus? Which color is the pus—whitish, yellow-greenish or reddish?

- Has your pet recently become incontinent? Did it follow a specific event such as a viral infection, vaccination or spaying? Or are they just older having suffered years of toxic living?

- Have they recently become more withdrawn, naughty, fearful or jealous?

5. <u>SKIN AND COAT MARKERS</u>

- Have there been changes in sheen or general condition?
- Dry flakes, dull coat or greasy with hot spots, pimples or rashes?
- Excessive shedding, hair loss, scratching or licking, fur pulling, etc.?
- Is the coat rougher, patchy or breaking off?
- Infected, raw, irritated or foul smelling pustules or hot spots on the skin?
- Any general "pet odor" or an unclean smell?

Coat and skin condition can give you good general information about your pet's health. Functions of the digestive, endocrine or immune systems, especially the adrenals, thyroid, intestines, kidneys and liver are shown in the skin and coat cells. Toxic waste will often be eliminated through the skin if these systems are not kept in peak condition, interfering with nutrient absorption vital for a truly healthy coat.

6. <u>EARS</u>

- Is their hearing diminished? Do they seem over-sensitive to sounds?

- Are external pests, such as mites (small dark specs like pepper) present for months prior to the immune system taking a serious dive? Have the ears begun to smell?

- Are symptoms related to allergy seasons or weather changes? Any swimming?

- Has there been a history of infections? A recent round of antibiotics or antifungal medications?

A toxic reaction, vaccinosis, allergies and yeast or bacterial infections will often first manifest themselves in the ears. Immersion in water (in pools or lakes) can also create swimmer's ear in dogs. When ears are inflamed or have a waxy discharge, it is often the first sign of immune imbalance, generally toxicity or an external parasitic infestation. The use of antibiotics or antifungals, for a previous infection elsewhere in the body, can leave a pet prone to developing an ear infection within three months after the use of the drugs. Some vaccinations, particularly distemper and rabies, also have this side-effect.

7. <u>EYES & NOSE</u>

- Is there chronic dryness? A lack of tearing with excessive rubbing?

- Have infected eyes quickly become matted and painful?

- Is discharge from eyes or nose chronic? Or seasonally related?

- Does the nose looks smooth and moist or have dry ridges formed recently?

- Is the color of the nose a solid black or has it begun to fade to a pinkish tone?

Red, swollen eyes are a window upon the immune system, especially symptomatic of improper liver function and detoxification. Irritated eyes can create blocked tear ducts, manifesting nasal discharge and respiratory difficulties. Genetic conditions, such as turned-in lashes, can be addressed early on before they can cause permanent damage and even blindness. By the time the nose begins to dry and form ridges across the top, the body has been exposed to months of a toxic lifestyle and malnutrition—or a digestive imbalance which interferes with the proper assimilation of vital nutrients. A lack of pigment also indicates a nutritional or immune system imbalance.

8. NERVOUS SYSTEM, BODY, JOINTS & MUSCLES

- Has your pet recently shown signs of confusion, lethargy or uncontrollable shaking? Difficulty drinking or eating? Any rapid weight changes?
- Has there recently been a severe behavioral change?
- Is there any fever or body odor present?
- Has their gait or movement changed, especially getting up or down?
- Noticeable pain or limping? Restless sleep or exhaustion?
- Any chewing or licking on the extremities with no signs of pests or allergies, possibly indicating nerve impingement?

9. RESPIRATORY AND CARDIAC

- Has your pet's breathing changed? Can they play as long before becoming winded? Have they developed a cough or wheezing?
- Has their resting pulse rate or breathing pattern changed?

10. EMOTIONAL AND BEHAVIORAL

- Has your pet recently become withdrawn, fearful, nervous or aggressive?
- Have they become more destructive in chewing on themselves, furniture, walls or are they suddenly soiling in the house?
- What changes in the family dynamics or location have occurred?

There can often be a physical problem behind these behavioral issues, just as stress can lead to health problems. Have you or your family recently gone through divorce, moving, death (even of another pet), or other stressful events? Your pets will surely suffer the increased stress in their environment. Often, they suffer more than humans do in such a change—all they understand is that there's a problem. *They can not reason that it might soon be resolved.* Nor do they know why the change may have occurred. They just worry about the change in their environment and the fact that you, as the center of their universe, are now different in a negative way.

Remember, for your own protocol development—the nuances of dis-ease, as addressed in these questions and answered in Chapter 10: Symptoms A to Z, will help you identify the correct remedies to apply first which will quickly promote proper symptom reversal, if possible, and will improve your chances of a long-term benefit. The longer the body is left to fight on its own, the weaker it can become. It takes tools (detoxification, nutrition and remedies) to build up the body's resources to suitably fight dis-ease. A process of "wait and see" affects all other organ systems and they too will become out of balance—dis-eased.

By being able to identify any health or behavioral issues that have changed in your pet, giving proper naturopathic care first when appropriate and when not successful, realizing that there is a more serious imbalance, will serve you well. This information and process of elimination will also help your veterinarian to assess the underlying problem more quickly than if they have to guess. Often due to guilt, an owner will minimize just how long a symptom has been present or how severe the condition has actually become. This will only confuse the veterinarian during the intake exam and possibly lead them to make a wrong diagnosis and prescribe an inappropriate course of treatment.

It is best to address all changes in your pet's health as quickly as possible, but in the event that you have waited or simply did not notice such changes until it became a serious problem, report these facts honestly so that your veterinarian can take this into account. It makes a difference!

Blood in the urine is a symptom to notice but it isn't considered *as serious* when it happens for a day or two due to detoxification—*with improvement in the animal's overall condition.* This can be either a process that you have initiated or the natural cleansing process (part of a curative response) promoted by your pet's immune system in reaction to an injurious agent. As I have described in **Step One**, the cleansing process (as seen during urinalysis) can produce traces of blood. This is due to the release of old tissue, crystals and even bacteria that has been stored in the urinary system and have irritated the urinary tract. The responding white blood cells additionally found in the urine may initiate concern but don't worry if all the other markers indicate it is a process of detoxification (a curative response) and not a healing crisis such as an episode of FUS. This is a good thing! Getting rid of these waste by-products is exactly why you should detoxify your animals on a regular basis and support their self-induced cycles of detoxification.

Blood in the urine for a few days with changes in fluid intake and painful urination—*as the cat weakens in general*—is more serious. If you don't know what trigger is associated with the bleeding, it's smarter for the veterinarian to know that the bleeding has been ongoing, rather than assume, based on erroneous information, that it is less serious.

In addition, certain foods, supplements, remedies or herbs that you have been recently using for another condition such as allergies or arthritis (especially within the last six to eight weeks) may have created a natural curative response. Remember, detoxification **IS** the first step the body will take to rebalance and strengthen itself. Taken at face value, these symptoms may lead the veterinarian to suspect a more serious chronic problem. But once you inform the vet about these changes and their known effects, she/he may feel more confident to *support* the curative process, rather than *suppress* the symptoms with medication or a change in remedies.

Also, when you are better informed, your veterinarian will probably have more confidence in your judgment. Many veterinarians, even holistically-oriented ones, will rely on drugs to suppress symptoms easily (one or two pills a day), rather than suggest a holistic protocol (fasting, dietary changes, frequent supplementation or remedy dosing) because they suspect that the owner will simply not be willing to comply and follow through.

Certainly, it can be difficult to decide when to seek veterinarian care or when to try to support your pet's own curative abilities by yourself. Whenever in doubt, do seek professional support. Just be sure that the vet is someone that you know is competent, who can be trusted, and who is *willing* to support you in treating your pet naturally.

It is ultimately up to you to decide what is best for your animal. You can still follow a LifeStyle™ protocol regardless of whether your vet recommended medication, as long as you are not in a life-threatening situation—and I mean acute (as in <u>today's</u>) life-threatening symptoms and not the potential of death later on as in the case of cancer. But it is important to verify with them a proper diagnosis if you are not getting the results to which you are entitled.

What is a *Trusted* Veterinarian?

It is not as vital that you seek out a holistic or alternative care veterinarian, as it is that you find someone who is <u>willing</u> to listen to you, is <u>thorough</u> in their examination and diagnosis, <u>will explain</u> what it is that they recommend and, most importantly, <u>will treat you and your pet with respect</u>. If you do not like the way a veterinarian approaches your pet or speaks to you, then find another, regardless of how well they were recommended to you.

A Trusted Veterinarian Will Always:

- Allow, even request, that you are present during the exam. *Many clinics today ask that you wait in the lobby since an anxious owner can make a pet more unruly, which takes attention away from the diagnostic process. Educate your pet to be handled and be prepared to stand quietly next to the table out of the way when needed to, so your veterinarian can work uninterrupted.*

- Make your pet feel safe and comfortable by not towering above them.

- Be calm and respectful toward the animal and you.

- Move the animal carefully and not abruptly.

- Speak to you and your pet in soothing, respectful tones.

- Be willing to discuss your views and desire to treat your pet naturally and cost-effectively.

- Answer all your questions honestly without being condescending.

- Take a complete history, prior to giving you their opinion.

- Give you a realistic prognosis and explain the stages of disease and treatment.

- Discuss the alternatives available, medical or holistic, with the costs of each.

- Explain the use of certain medications, including shots <u>prior</u> to prescribing them.

- Ask for your consent before giving your animal a shot or drug during the exam.

- Avoid unnecessary testing, invasive procedures, and surgeries.

- Be someone both you *and* your pet feel comfortable with and can trust.

The best way to have your vet work with you as a trusted ally is to be clear about what you want and what kind of veterinarian you want to take care of you and your pet. I mention both of you here. Isn't the fact that the veterinarian treats your pet well the main issue? Absolutely not!

You will also be in crisis when your pet is in crisis. You will be fearful of the unknown (dis-ease, death, medical costs), concerned about the pain and what suffering your companion (for many it is their child) may be experiencing. Often, you will be just as overwhelmed by the situation as your animal is. Therefore, it is crucial to your pet's well being that the veterinarian is capable of taking care of *your* needs and fears. If she or he doesn't do so, confusion and fear will most certainly interfere with your judgment and ability to follow through with the prescribed care.

Anyone who has come home to discover a sick animal and rushed him to the veterinary clinic will tell you what it felt like. Even though they may be clear-headed professionals, when faced with this emergency they let experts make all the decisions for them. And those decisions are very important. Man or woman, it makes no difference, we are all vulnerable at one time or another including me and it's very important to have allies. Please do try to make your vet an ally. A trusted veterinarian who will support you and your pet can make the difference between life and death.

First, you must find this wonderful human being—a qualified veterinarian who will cater to you and your pet. My recommendation is that you begin by asking your friends who they like and trust (assuming that your friends are like-minded). You might also ask your breeder, groomer or trainer as well. Then make a phone call. Is the veterinarian willing to call you back when she/he has the time and spend a few minutes on the phone to speak to you regarding your needs? Or can you only speak to a secretary or vet tech about the clinic's services and philosophy before scheduling your first visit? If they won't make an effort now, it's probable that they won't care later. Think about it. I'd call others. Certainly, some vets may simply be too busy to talk because they are so good they are heavily booked. If you are pleased with the way you are treated over the phone, make an appointment for a health check up (well-check) in order to feel them out and allow your pet to get to know them without the additional pressure of being injured or ill. This is crucial; that you and your pet have the opportunity to trust the veterinarian before crisis hits! It will help the veterinarian as well, since they will have a picture of your pet in good health, and therefore be better able to determine what is out of balance when dis-ease or injury hits.

Don't forget to interview the staff also, and take mental notes about how well they work with each other and the veterinarian. Are they respectful of each other or argumentative? How clean is the clinic? Does it smell or have ground-in dirt? Is there urine or stool left on the floor? Do the trays and sinks look well kept? Always ask to see the kennels where they keep pets overnight and for recovery after surgery. Does the clinic have separate areas for cats and dogs so they don't hassle each other, soft lighting or covers to minimize stress, and (I can not stress this enough) a clean environment? Ask if they are willing to give your pet's usual diet if she has to remain overnight. At one time or another this will be important to you—you may need to board them overnight or leave them for a procedure—so you better know up front what is going on back there.

One last consideration: Ask if there is another veterinarian whom you could turn to in an emergency if your regular vet was not available. Knowing you have a backup plan will come in handy if you are faced with an emergency.

Being your vet's "best friend" through open, honest communication and team work will help assure that you are totally prepared to address any preventative or rehabilitative issues regarding your pet's health quickly, efficiently and successfully. You may only see them once a year for a check-up (which should include blood work every other year for older or prone animals), but in the case of a more serious condition or emergency, you need to know whom you can count on because your best friend is counting on you!

CHAPTER TWELVE

PRODUCT DESCRIPTIONS

<u>AZMIRA® HOMEOPATHIC DETOXIFICATION</u>

D'Toxifier

<u>Therapeutic Actions</u>: The **Step One** remedies in this homeopathic formula are classic stimulants of glandular, organ, blood and lymphatic node cleansing. They bring about an improved state of well-being through enhanced metabolic and catabolic waste elimination. The influence of these remedies gradually alters the constitution of the body by promoting the utilization of nutrients being supplemented in **Step Two** and herbal remedies in **Step Three**. This formula protects vital organs especially the heart, brain, spleen, pancreas, thyroid, liver and kidneys. It balances and cools excess heat in the blood.

D'Toxifier may be used to promote a period of detoxification when used alone or in conjunction with a fast or given as a weekly maintenance dose. It will further stimulate the process of self-induced detoxification to promote symptom reversal rather than suppression. For example, in the case of fever in response to bacteria: this allows the fever to work quickly without much discomfort (symptoms) to the body.

This is accomplished through the removal of metabolic and catabolic wastes that build up in the circulatory fluids. These cause organ congestion, joint inflammation, a reduction in nutrient assimilation, digestive upsets and poor immune response with degenerative tissue conditions and mutating cells. This is at the root of all dis-ease from allergies and premature aging to cancer.

Indications: Life! This remedy can help build the pet's resistance to the daily barrage of toxins and allergens in the environment and those ingested with many commercial diets. It is especially beneficial when drugs are necessary; it decreases the likelihood of side-effects. D'Toxifier also contains Thuja which aids in the prevention and reversal of vaccine-induced symptoms, past and present. Use with all LifeStyle™ protocols to encourage improved organ function, nutrient utilization and blood waste removal.

AZMIRA® DIETS

CANINE NUTRITION

Classic Dog   Dry Kibble

Recommendations: All Life Stages and Breeds; can be fed alone or with Azmira® canned food. Foundation diet of LifeStyle™ approach to optimal pet health. For best results follow package directions.

Ingredients: Beef Meal, Whole Ground Barley, Oatmeal, Whole Ground Grain Sorghum (millet-type grain), Flax Seed, Alfalfa Meal, Natural Flavors, Canola Oil, Lecithin, Menhaden Fish Meal, Apples, Carrots, Garlic, Kelp, Mixed Tocopherols (natural antioxidant), Yucca Schidegera Extract, Ester-C®, Vitamin & Proteinated Mineral Supplements

Guaranteed Analysis: Crude Protein 22% (min), Crude Fat 8% (min), Crude Fiber 4% (max), Moisture 10% (max), Calcium 1.5% (min), Phosphorus 1% (min), Linoleic Acid 2% (min)

Other Nutritional Information: 3300 Kcal/kg approximately 445 Kcal/cup; pH 5.9 - 6.3; Sodium .16%; Phosphorus 1.33%; Magnesium .15%; Potassium .61%; Manganese 38 ppm; Omega 3:6 ratio = 1:4

LifeStyle Dog   Dry Kibble

Recommendations: All Life Stages and Breeds; can be fed alone or with Azmira® canned food. Foundation of LifeStyle™ approach to optimal pet health. For best results follow package directions.

Ingredients: Lamb Meal, Whole Ground Barley, Oatmeal, Whole Ground Grain Sorghum (millet-type grain), Flax Seed, Alfalfa Meal, Natural Flavors, Canola Oil, Lecithin, Menhaden Fish Meal, Apples, Carrots, Garlic, Kelp, Mixed Tocopherols (natural antioxidant), Yucca Schidegera Extract, Ester-C®, Vitamin & Proteinated Mineral Supplements

Guaranteed Analysis: Crude Protein 22% (min), Crude Fat 8% (min), Crude Fiber 4% (max), Moisture 10% (max), Calcium 1.5% (min), Phosphorus 1% (min), Linoleic Acid 2% (min)

Other Nutritional Information: 3100 Kcal/kg approximately 406 Kcal/ cup; pH 6.0 - 6.3; Sodium .21%; Phosphorus 1.34%; Magnesium .14%; Potassium .70%; Manganese 38 ppm; Omega 3:6 ratio = 1:4

Beef & Chicken Formula (Dog)   Canned, wet food

Ingredients: Beef, Beef Broth, Chicken Liver, Chicken, Mackerel, Tuna, Oat Bran, Whole Brown Rice, Kelp, Lecithin, Garlic, Vitamin & Chelated Mineral Supplements

Guaranteed Analysis: Crude Protein 10% (min), Crude Fat 5% (min), Crude Fiber 1% (max), Moisture 78% (max)

Other Nutritional Information: 1217 Kcal/kg approximately 456 Kcal/ can; pH range 5.9 - 6.26; Sodium .09%; Phosphorus .28%; Magnesium .03%; Potassium .19%; Manganese 6 ppm

Ocean Fish Formula (Dog)   Canned, wet food

Ingredients: Ocean Fish, Ocean Fish Broth, Chicken Liver, Turkey, Tuna, Oat Bran, Whole Brown Rice, Kelp, Lecithin, Garlic, Vitamin & Chelated Mineral Supplements

Guaranteed Analysis: Crude Protein 10% (min), Crude Fat 5% (min), Crude Fiber 1% (max), Moisture 78% (max)

Other Nutritional Information: 1082 Kcal/kg approximately 406 Kcal/ can; pH range 5.9 - 6.26; Sodium .09%; Phosphorus .28%; Magnesium .03%; Potassium .22%; Manganese 6 ppm

Lamb & Barley Formula (Dog)   Canned, wet food

Ingredients: Lamb, Lamb Broth, Tuna, Chicken Liver, Pearl Barley, Whole Brown Rice, Peas, Carrots, Kelp, Lecithin, Garlic, Vitamin & Proteinated Mineral Supplements

Guaranteed Analysis: Crude Protein 10% (min), Crude Fat 5% (min), Crude Fiber 1% (max), Moisture 78% (max)

Other Nutritional Information: 1324 Kcal/kg approximately 497 Kcal/ can; pH range 5.9 - 6.26; Sodium .09%; Phosphorus .28%; Magnesium .03%; Potassium .20%; Manganese 6 ppm

FELINE NUTRITION (can feed Ferrets as well, with 20% more meat and fat added)

Classic Cat   Dry Kibble

Ingredients: Chicken / Turkey meal, Whole Ground Yellow Corn, Full Fat Soybeans, Whole Ground Wheat, Whole Ground Brown Rice, Chicken Fat (preserved with natural mixed tocopherols, Citric Acid and Rosemary extract), Oatmeal, Whole Dried Egg, Menhaden Fish Meal,

Natural Flavors, Flax Seed, Ester-C®, Taurine, Vitamin & Proteinated Mineral Supplements

Guaranteed Analysis: Crude Protein 30% (min), Crude Fat 12% (min), Crude Fiber 4% (max), Moisture 10% (max), Ash 6.5% (max), Magnesium .12% (max), Calcium .8% (min), Phosphorus .65% (min), Linoleic Acid 2% (min)

Other Nutritional Information: 3350 Kcal/kg approximately 530 Kcal/ cup; pH range 5.5 - 6.3; Sodium .26%; Phosphorus 1.56%; Magnesium .14%; Potassium .66%; Manganese 23 ppm; Omega 3:6 ratio = 1:4

Beef & Chicken Formula (Cat)   Canned, wet food
Ingredients: Beef, Beef Broth, Chicken Liver, Chicken, Mackerel, Tuna, Oat Bran, Whole Brown Rice, Kelp, Lecithin, Garlic, Vitamin & Chelated Mineral Supplements

Guaranteed Analysis: Crude Protein 10% (min), Crude Fat 5% (min), Crude Fiber 1% (max), Moisture 78% (max), Ash 2% (max), Magnesium 0.03% (max), Taurine 0.05% (min)

Other Nutritional Information: 1217 Kcal/kg approximately 456 Kcal/ can (13 oz.); approximately 191 Kcal/can (5.5 oz); pH range 5.9 - 6.26; Sodium .09%; Phosphorus .27%; Magnesium .03%; Potassium .19%; Manganese 6 ppm.

Ocean Fish Formula (Cat)   Canned, wet Food
Ingredients: Ocean Fish, Ocean Fish Broth, Chicken Liver, Turkey, Tuna, Oat Bran, Whole Brown Rice, Kelp, Lecithin, Garlic, Vitamin & Chelated Mineral Supplements

Guaranteed Analysis: Crude Protein 10% (min), Crude Fat 5% (min), Crude Fiber 1% (max), Moisture 78% (max), Ash 2% (max), Magnesium 0.03% (max), Taurine 0.05% (min)

Other Nutritional Information: 1082 Kcal/kg approximately 406 Kcal/ can (13.2 oz); 1082 Kcal/kg approximately 169 Kcal/can (5.5 oz); pH range 5.9 - 6.26; Sodium .09%; Phosphorus .29%; Magnesium .03%; Potassium .22%; Manganese 6 ppm.

Lamb & Barley Formula (Cat)   Canned, wet food
Ingredients: Lamb, Lamb Broth, Tuna, Chicken Liver, Pearl Barley, Whole Brown Rice, Peas, Carrots, Kelp, Lecithin, Garlic, Vitamin & Proteinated Mineral Supplements

Guaranteed Analysis: Crude Protein 10% (min), Crude Fat 5% (min), Crude Fiber 1% (max), Moisture 78% (max), Ash 2% (max), Magnesium 0.03% (max), Taurine 0.05% (min)

Other Nutritional Information: 1324 Kcal/kg approximately 497 Kcal/can; 1324 Kcal/kg approximately 207 Kcal/can (5.5 oz); pH range 5.9 - 6.26; Sodium .09%; Phosphorus .28%; Magnesium .03%; Potassium .20%; Manganese 6 ppm.

AZMIRA TREATS

Beef Heart Jerky

Dogs love to crunch these great hard jerky pieces for rewards or snack time!

Beef Straps

Wide, long neck tendon makes a wonderful chewing alternative to rawhide. Great for puppies who are teething. Can satisfy cats who have the urge to chew hard and scratch on their toys.

Beef Tendon Curls

Beef Straps cut into small pieces make quick treats or perfect snacks for toy dogs and cats.

Ground Beef Patties

Beef patties just like you would grill, but baked hard for yummy crunchy treats. Great show bait.

Kidney Bits

Our most popular meat treat for cat lovers! Excellent for finicky canines or felines, this is a terrific treat or can be used to enhance a meal. Provides a great bait or training treat.

Liver Slivers

Tender slices of detoxified beef liver, slow cooked and smoked to perfection!

Turkey Necks

Small dogs, cats and ferrets keep their teeth clean with hours of chewing pleasure on our well cooked and smoked turkey necks.

Ostrich & Emu Treats

Low fat, high taste meat treat is perfect for dogs or cats with dietary issues. Easy on the kidneys and digestive tract.

Beef Bones

Slow baked, hard bones in a variety of sizes for a variety of dogs. Great for hours of satisfied chewing, gnawing and teeth cleaning!

Zoomin' Catnip

Wild crafted, pesticide-free catnip provides fun and emotional "feline fine" well being. Excellent toy refill or scratching post training aid.

Azmira® Nutritional Supplements

Acidophilus   viable powder

Therapeutic Actions: Replaces friendly bacteria in intestines to counter side effects of drugs, a poor diet and digestive stress. Aids in the absorption of nutrients and detoxification.

Indications: Use when intestines are compromised by illness, stress, or medications, such as wormers, antifungal drugs, corticosteroids or antibiotics.

For Your Information: Best given on an empty stomach, one hour before meals, mixed into water or in a gelatin capsule. Follow with drinking water to help dissolve the capsule. Can be fed directly in meals if needed. Wait until after antibiotic drug use to begin supplementation, continue for two to four weeks.

Aller'G Free

Herbal Capsules
Therapeutic Actions:

- Reverses inflammation of the digestive tract, lung, skin, throat and swollen lymph glands. Relieves ear and eye irritations and itching.

- For purification of the blood, liver, lungs, kidneys and bladder, pineal and pituitary glands.

- Reduces and protects against chronic irritation of tissue to encourage repair.

Indications: Incredible first line antihistamine for relief of symptoms associated with inhalant or contact allergies including irritated eyes, ears, or skin, wheezing, licking of paws, head shaking or rubbing, scratching, hot spots, pimples, fur pulling, and rashes. Works as a symptom suppressor until resistance is built through **Steps Two** and **Three**.

Airborne or other Sensitivities: Use daily up to every four hours if needed, during times of high exposure to allergens. Can double recommended daily dose on label. Use six weeks on and one week off to maintain effectiveness. Proven safe and effective in managing most allergy sensitivities when combined with Mega Pet Daily, Yucca Intensive, and Super C 2000. Additional B-50 Complex vitamins should also be considered with highly strung pets, or those with very poor coats.

For Your Information: ImmunoStim'R contains additional herbs to cleanse the lymph glands, support vital glands and organs of the immune system and build resistance for improved allergy support.

Aller'G: Grass & Pollen

Standardized Extract

Therapeutic Actions: Hypersensitivity to Airborne Allergens. This extract constricts, condenses, and contracts the swollen mucous membranes associated with hay fevers and airborne allergies. The astringent and anti-inflammatory actions bring tone and firmness to soggy membranes reducing the likelihood of infection or long-term side-effects to chronic irritation. Also, antibacterial activity enables this formula to check bacterial infections associated with the sinus and nasal cavity that cause irritated eyes and ears.

Indications: This compound should be used for the symptomatic relief of hay fever, allergies, and excessive mucous congestion of the sinus, nasal, ear, and throat. Eliminates a runny nose or itchy eyes, throat and ears. Also, specifically indicated for sinus infections associated with excessive discharges and infection of the eyes or ears.

For Your Information: Do not use this extract with pregnant pets. Use Aller'G Free instead.

Aller'G: Skin & Digestive

Standardized Extract

Therapeutic Actions: An Immediate-Type Hypersensitivity, Allergy, and Anti-inflammatory Formula. The herbal extracts in this compound contain active constituents that act as anti-inflammatory, antihistamine, safe bronchial dilators, respiratory antispasmodics, and membrane integrity enhancers. Most importantly, these herbs protect the liver from circulating allergens and antigens (liver dysfunction is symptomatic in skin conditions) to prevent further damage. This compound is formulated to provide adrenal support when epinephrine is needed by the body to compensate for the inflammatory responses generated from the presence of allergens. Excessive adrenaline excretion can lead to exhaustion and adrenal malfunction. Hyper-sensitivity with uncontrollable scratching are symptoms which quickly exhaust the pet who would respond well to this formula. Helps stabilize skin and digestive tract cells to prevent a degenerative process from occurring.

Indications: This compound is specifically indicated for all disorders of immediate-type hypersensitivity including allergies, urticaria (an eruptive skin disease; hives), reactive dermatitis, reactive arthritis, reactive irritable bowel syndrome, anaphylaxis, food sensitivities, sinusitis, asthma, cough and other acute and chronic inflammations, including of the bowel and liver.

Aller'G: Skin & Pimple D'Tox

Standardized Extract

Therapeutic Actions: The herbs in this compound are classic blood and lymphatic supporters that alter the catabolic tissue conditions and bring about an improved state of well-being through improved metabolism and elimination. These herbs target the organs of metabolism, improving their functions and restoring their vitality by carrying more blood and nutrient supply to, and promoting greater excretion from, the cellular level. The influence of these herbs gradually alters the composition and constitution of the blood and lymph nodes.

This is accomplished through the removal of metabolic wastes that build up in the circulatory fluids and through the gentle nourishing and remineralizing effect that these herbs have upon the blood. Also, wasted tissues and cells are sloughed off and directed to eliminative channels for removal from the body. At the same time, new healthy tissue growth is encouraged with this herbal blend. The liver is detoxified and strengthened.

Indications: This compound cools excess heat in the blood and liver and may be used specifically in the treatment of cancer, tumors, cysts, toxemia, lymphedema, swollen lymph nodes, gouty and psoriatic arthritis, eczema, psoriasis, acne, and all skin disturbances. This formula is well suited to the multi-symptom suffering pet.

For Your Information: This compound is recommended as a yearly spring tonic to promote general detoxification and improved metabolism: use for six to eight weeks. Works well with other allergy formulas when additional need arises and ImmunoStim' R has not helped.

B-Complex 50

Capsules

Indications: Exceptional support for the nervous system, digestion, utilizes energy from food, builds hair and tissue, protects the organs, stimulates growth, builds the blood, prevents fatty deposits in arteries, protects against lead and pesticides, supports the eyes and glandular activity, aids in pain control, reduces seizure activity, and can even repel biting insects. Use in addition to foundation supplements, when *extra* B's are needed, as during times of increased stress, traveling, allergy season, and rehabilitation or with older pets.

Biotin

Tablets

Indications & Therapeutic Actions: Promoting growth; mandatory for metabolism of fatty acids and amino acids for tissue repair including coat, nail, and hoof improvement. Aids in natural antibiotic production. Replaces biotin often depleted during antibiotic drug therapy and illness.

For Your Information: Best used short-term in addition to Mega Pet Daily.

Blood & Lymph D'Tox

Standardized Extract

Therapeutic Actions: The herbs within this compound act as blood and lymphatic alteratives and bring about distinct and definite changes in metabolism, eliminating catabolic tissue and other cellular waste. This compound also augments the body's natural defense mechanisms by activating natural immune responses.

Indications: These herbs are indicated for conditions associated with a build-up of catabolic wastes in the tissues. Specifically indicated for all cancers, tumor growths, incipient cancers, blood dyscrasias, lymphatic engorgement, cysts, fluid cysts, ovarian cysts, cervical dysplasia, and skin ulcerations. Also indicated for *those* conditions that are associated with a breakdown of the auto immune system.

For Your Information: *Complementary* Azmira® Compounds: Grape Seed Extract and ImmunoStim'R

Calcium with Boron-3

Capsules

Indications: Necessary for formation and repair of bone and to maintain healthy glands. Essential for proper functioning of the heart muscles and muscular movements of the intestines (peristalsis), aiding digestion. Provides energy and participates in protein structuring of RNA and DNA. Helps blood clot, relieves spasms, promotes liver health and prevents colon cancer, thus making this a good supplement for colitis (irritable bowel syndrome).

Calendula

Standardized Extract

<u>Therapeutic Actions</u>: A natural anti-inflammatory and skin soother. Helps to regulate and lessen fever. Soothes irritated eyes and ears when used diluted as an eye or ear wash. Helps replenish elasticity in membranes.

<u>Indications</u>: Topically and internally useful for many skin disorders, such as rashes and sunburn, as well as neuritis and gum pain. For relief of irritated membranes, including those of the digestive and eliminatory systems.

Calm & Relax

Standardized Extract

<u>Therapeutic Action</u>: Supports the nervous system and controls most seizures. Is a mild sedative and excellent for general pain relief. Reduces anxiety to promote rest while it soothes nerves. Relieves hormone imbalance, also often associated with seizures, glandular dysfunction and incontinence. Helps digestive problems resulting from anxiety. Is an antispasmodic, helps indigestion and is a nerve tonic; rebalances neurological function, slows deterioration.

<u>Indications</u>: Nerve, Trauma, and Sleep formula - our strongest herbal calmer helps support the nervous system and restore balance for more serious or chronic conditions. Excellent in controlling many types of seizures and as a general restorative for pets that have undergone a long and stressful or painful period. Works as a daily tonic for highly stressed pets that may result in digestive problems and loose stools. Reduces the need to "hump" that some pets have regardless of neutering. This compound is specifically indicated for the treatment of nerve and muscle spasms, nerve trauma, nerve injury, and nervous agitation. As a restorative, it repairs the vital force after injury, trauma, or shock. It is specifically useful in the treatment of anxiety, insomnia, hyper-excitability, tension, nerve exhaustion, and nerve disturbances. This compound can also be used as an anti-viral agent both topically and internally for the treatment of herpes, especially those associated with feline viral infections.

Coenzyme Q10

Gel caps

<u>Therapeutic Action</u>: A potent antioxidant and nutrient booster, supports cellular metabolism.

<u>Indications</u>: Excellent supplement for the brain and can be used for Dementia-type disease. A great source of energy, useful for Fatigue Syndromes. Used with canine and equine athletes to increase endurance.

May be used for muscular dysfunction and chronic irritation. Excellent for all types of gum disease and helps to maintain healthy teeth. Shows great promise in the treatment of heart diseases, such as angina pectoris, congestive heart failure, mitral valve prolapse, and hypertension. Overall, CoQ10 is an excellent immune system booster. It is found in every cell in the body, so it makes sense that it is essential in the path to overall good health!

Daily Boost

Herbal powder
Therapeutic Action:

- Reduces flatulence, colic & digestive tract stress.

- Blood, liver and gallbladder tonic, improves condition and function.

- Stimulates proper stomach & intestinal function.

- Adaptogenic herb builds resistance to disease and allergies.

- Detoxification & anti-fungal properties.

- Supports the immune system, colon health and blood sugar regulation, helps prevent colitis (Irritable Bowel Syndrome).

Indications: For additional digestive and detoxifying effects to support optimal digestive and immune system functions. Benefits severely debilitated pets or those simply seeking to reach optimal health. Integral part of ongoing nutritional and detoxification process to assure maximum absorption of daily nutrients. Best used with Azmira® Animal Nutrition diets and LifeStyle™ foundation supplements.

Dairy & Egg Protein Powder

Nutritional protein powder
TO MAKE A HIGHLY NUTRITIOUS LIQUID FORMULA FOR PUPPIES, KITTENS OR SICK AND WEAKENED PETS
Use goat's milk (best choice for added animal protein and calories), purified water, apple juice or carrot juice for base: per 15 lbs or under of body weight use approx. 1 heaping tablespoon of powder per 4 ounces liquid. Feed this four times per day. Very small, young or debilitated pets may consume less per meal, with more frequent feedings needed. Can increase amount fed per day as needed for appetite or caloric intake adjustment. Shake or blend until smooth. Serve room temp. or warmer but do not boil. Can add as needed, blended by hand or electric mixer; canned Azmira® pet foods, cottage cheese (these are needed to introduce more solid animal protein), yogurt (for digestive aid), oatmeal (for stool

support and colon cleansing), banana or apple sauce (energy foods). Can add formula to Azmira® dry pet foods to encourage weaning.

Therapeutic Actions: Easy to assimilate source of calories full of vital amino acids and a supportive nutritional panel to stimulate growth, a good immune response and rejuvenation.

Indications: Excellent source of protein and nutritional supplement for addition to home cooked diets, weaning meals and the liquid feeding of sick or baby pets. For wasting-type diseases: needed for added calories or often is the only source of nutrients a pet can tolerate easily.

Digest Zymez

Capsules

Therapeutic Actions: Increases nutritional assimilation, which in turn helps fuel the body, clear up the skin, stimulate the immune system and support an overall improvement of health.

Indications: To aid digestion, reduce stool eating, intestinal gas, cramping and assimilation problems, prevents fatty deposits, helps kill infections, soothing for ulcerations. Important supportive supplement for pancreatic and bowel problems, or when stress is interfering with digestion. For common, non-responsive diarrhea or loose stool.

For Your Information: For meat eating animals only!

Eyebright

Herbal capsules

Therapeutic Actions: Rich in vitamins A, C, and silicon; high in calcium, magnesium, zinc, niacin, vitamins D and E; contains some B vitamins, small amounts of sodium, iodine, copper, and zinc. Antiseptic, anti-bacterial properties help prevent eye infection and open tear ducts. Can be used externally as a wash and/or internally for eye infections, etc.

Indications: Strengthens eyes, dissolves stys, eases eye strain, and is beneficial for the optic nerve. Prevents excessive secretion of fluids and relieves discomfort from eyestrain and minor irritation. Good for allergies, dry eye, itchy and/or watery eyes, and runny nose. Also used to combat hay fever symptoms and builds some resistance.

For Your Information: Safe to use with Aller'G Free or antibiotics. Do not use this extract with pregnant pets.

Flav'r Shak'r

Powder shaker

Indications: Aids appetite by triggering sense of smell and stimulates basic detoxification to encourage eating and proper digestion. Great general supplement for finicky pets! Simply sprinkle a small amount on food and watch them eat with gusto. Great general supplement for meat eating reptiles and birds.

For Your Information: Can be used with Mega Pet Daily as this supplement is so low in therapeutic potency. For meat eaters only!

Garlic Daily Aid

Gel caps

Therapeutic Actions: A blood purifier, antifungal, antibiotic and anti-parasitic, beneficial to circulation, digestion, liver, kidneys, thyroid and nerves; purges toxins, stimulates the lymphatic system and builds the immune system. Excellent daily tonic, highly recommended for LifeStyle™ foundation protocol.

Indications: Repels fleas and ticks. Can help prevent or reverse diarrhea. Generally detoxifies the body of yeast, fungal, bacterial, and viral infections. Can help arrest the spread of parvovirus, kennel cough and most other infections in general. Can kill internal parasites and other injurious organisms. Excellent supplement for chronic ear infections, arthritis, allergies, skin, liver, thyroid, kidneys and neurological problems. An adaptogenic supplement to help maintain good health and promote weight stabilization.

Giardia & Parasitic D'Tox

Standardized Extract

Therapeutic Actions: This compound contains bitter principles that activate secretions of the digestive and alimentary (entire food passage) canals. The antiparasitic activity is strong acting upon a wide range of amoebas and blood-borne worms including heartworm. Can be used preventatively during active exposure to mosquitoes.

Indications: This compound is indicated whenever there may be a suspicion of amoebic or microbial growth (germs conduct parasitic action on the body) and other general parasitic activity; can also be used to address fungal (ringworm) and yeast growth, both internally as well as topically. Can be used safely to clean out the colon, even with IBS, when intestinal parasites are suspected as a trigger. Can be used as Spring/Fall detox program to protect from seasonal infestations.

For Your Information: To use topically in addressing fungal and yeast growth; Dilute 3 to 4 drops in a tablespoon of water or Rejuva Spray. Apply directly to infected area. Do not use this extract with pregnant pets. For heavy infestations of intestinal worms such as roundworms, tapeworms or pinworms it is best to use **Herbal Wormer** first, or in combination with Giardia & Parasitic D'Tox .

GLA 125 – Borage Seed Oil

Gel caps

<u>Therapeutic Actions</u>: Reduces inflammation during arthritic response, normalizes brain function controlling pain centers and blood pressure, helps skin conditions by replenishing elasticity and may reduce the growth rate of some tumor-causing cancers, especially in breast tissue.

<u>Indications</u>: Provides the same benefits as the Omega-3's found in fish oil, but without fish allergens or placing as much digestive stress on the body.

GlucoMChondro

Tablets

<u>Therapeutic Actions</u>: Highly effective component in the repair of torn ligaments, sprained muscles and traumatized nerves. Combines two top tissue repair nutrients and a joint lubricator (Glucosamine, MSM and Chondroitin) in one convenient tablet.

<u>Indications</u>: Beneficial for arthritis and tendonitis as well as general respiratory weakness, allergies and skin repair. Can be used in symptom reversal or preventive protocols.

Glucosamine

Capsules

<u>Therapeutic Actions</u>: An effective analgesic (pain reliever), stimulates the production of connective tissue, which can repair joints by stimulating the growth of new cartilage, tendons and ligaments.

<u>Indications</u>: Addresses arthritic joints, osteoporosis and tendonitis. Beneficial in degenerative disc conditions. Use in conjunction with Shark'Rah to successfully support bone and joint conditions by promoting lubrication of the joint (producing synovial fluid) to further stimulate the joint's curative response.

Goldenseal Root

Standardized Extract

<u>Therapeutic Actions</u>: Well documented as an excellent herb for fighting viral, bacterial and yeast infections while stimulating the immune system in general. Cleanses the blood, liver, lymph glands, and kidneys. Safe to use in conjunction with antibiotic drugs. Boosts immune response and continues rejuvenation support after use.

<u>Indications</u>: Supplement for infections. Mix with water for wound cleansing and healing of abscesses, gangrene, pus disease, and gingivitis. Wonderful eyewash to fight infection and open blocked tear ducts.

<u>For Your Information</u>: Do not use this extract internally with pregnant pets.

Grape Seed Extract

Capsules

<u>Therapeutic Actions</u>: Nature's most powerful antioxidant! 500 times stronger than vitamin E. Even stronger than pine bark extract (Pycnogenol®). Contains 92% O.P.C. - the highest concentration in the industry.

<u>Indications</u>: Toxic waste build-up resulting in tissue growth such as fatty tumors and skin tags. Reduces the growth of cancerous tumors and slows the spread of cancer in general. For chronic, severe arthritic or allergic responses with poor detoxification. For blood or organ toxicity, especially in the brain (seizures), liver (skin problems, hepatitis, etc.), pancreas (diabetes, pancreatitis) and kidneys/bladder (FUS, nephritis, etc.).

Herbal Calm

Herbal Capsules

<u>Therapeutic Actions</u>: Immediate, yet temporary calming effect appropriate to travel or specific situations that may be stress producing. Does not produce lethargy or cloudiness of mind.

<u>Indications</u>: Symptoms associated with anxiety and stress including excessive salivation, pacing, aggression, grooming or traveling problems and hyperactivity or difficult transitions (training, moving, family changes, introducing new pets, etc.). Use during allergy season to reduce anxiety due to excessive scratching and biting, soothes general nervous conditions. Can help to curb destructive behavior and increase attention span during training. Well suited for daily use to eliminate many other negative, unwanted behaviors (when used with behavior modification). Excellent supplement to use during competitions.

<u>For Your Information</u>: Best to introduce herbs two to four times, twenty hours prior and again dose one hour prior to anticipated event to build up assimilation and optimize therapeutic response. Lasts two to four hours; pets may remain calm even longer and even sleep if allowed. For chronic disorders use Calm & Relax.

Herbal Slim

Herbal Capsules

<u>Therapeutic Actions</u>: Safe Ephedra-free herbal blend for natural weight loss and appetite reduction. Lowering calorie content may actually create a slowed metabolism and increased fat storage. This herbal formula

stimulates the body to burn fat, increases digestion and assimilation, reduces appetite, and generally supports health through proper colon care. The more nutrients that make their way into the bloodstream; the more satisfied the body will be and the more willing to drop weight, without compromising the organs.

Indications: 10% or more overweight, unresponsive to dietary changes or detoxification.

For Your Information: Feed a high quality natural diet at least twice daily to help assimilation. Beware of "lite" diets, which are mostly nutrient-poor fiber (often peanut hulls that can cause colon problems, especially IBS) and feeding too little food to sustain your pet's daily nutritional and caloric needs (causing the body to store more calories to live off).

Herbal Wormer

Herbal Capsules

Therapeutic Actions: Safe herbal laxative has antibiotic effect on harmful bacteria stimulates secretions of the entire digestive system and its saponins are recognized as a deep cleansing agent with an alkaloid berberine that can kill worms. Excellent cancer herb, beneficial for stomach function, relieves cramping and expels gas, mucous and toxins. Anti-parasitic, especially for tapeworms, pinworms and roundworms. Helps reverse constipation, promotes peristalsis to improve colon functions.

Indications: Temporary relief of symptoms associated with worms, amoebas and parasites, including infestation, constipation, diarrhea, mucous, gas and cramping. Can be used regularly to maintain colon health and digestion. Safe and effective alternative to chemical wormers used for infestations or as a seasonal preventative measure. Can be used with very young or debilitated pets. We have successfully used this with week-old puppies and kittens who were so infested that they could not pass anything until they had been wormed.

For Your Information: Works well with horses, ferrets, and rabbits, as well as dogs and cats. Worming should be applied preventatively twice a year, in the fall and spring. Often, pets are infested with parasites yet are not symptomatic. It is best to cleanse the colon regardless, at least once a year. Do not use this extract with pregnant pets.

Immune Factor Colostrum

Capsules

Therapeutic Actions: This compound is used extensively for the successful treatment of degenerative disorders in humans after careful animal studies were concluded. It encourages the processing of nutritional fuel (as found in Mega Pet Daily or our herbal formulations) to help to feed cellular tissue and promote the replacement of wasted tissue with healthy new tissue. Stimulates and maintains a strong immune response for improved curative reactions and symptom reversal.

Indications: Temporary relief of symptoms associated with immune system disorders; addresses depressed immune systems, cancer, cysts, tumors, degenerative diseases, and chronic yeast, fungal, viral and bacterial infections (by improving responses to antibiotic-type herbs such as Echinacea or Garlic). Helpful for allergies, organ problems, arthritis, wasting disease and fighting stubborn infections. Use this compound when there is chronic degenerative illness as a prophylactic (preventative) treatment to slow the process or for maintenance of a healthy constitution.

Immuno Stim'R

Standardized Extract

Therapeutic Actions: Catabolic Waste Elimination, a tribute to Renee Caisse's formula (ESSIAC®) used extensively for the treatment of degenerative disorders, especially auto-immune diseases where the immune system is turning against the body and breaking tissue down. This compound "stimulates" the "balancing" of the immune system; however the body needs to be supported regardless of an overactive or underactive immune system. It alters the process of waste and nutrition, helping to break down catabolic tissue and promote the replacement of wasted tissue with healthy new tissue. If catabolic waste is not detoxified, the immune system will continue to turn against itself or cannot draw enough "fuel" from the body for a strong curative response, such as infection fighting.

Indications: Temporary relief of symptoms associated with immune system disorders; addresses depressed or overactive immune systems, cancer, cysts, tumors, degenerative diseases, and chronic viral and bacterial infections. Helpful for allergies, organ problems, arthritis, wasting disease and fighting stubborn infections.

For Your Information: May be used as a prophylactic (preventative) when dealing with chronic degenerative illness for the maintenance of a healthy constitution.

Joint E'zer

Therapeutic Actions: This supplement contains glucosamine and chondroitin sulfate that promote strengthening of ligaments, tendons or cartilage and lubrication in the joints for pain relief and improved function.

<u>Indications</u>: This supplement is specifically indicated in the treatment of arthritis and joint dis-ease.

<u>For Your Information</u>: Best used with Yucca Intensive for chronic inflammation and pain. Inflammation breaks down the connective tissues surrounding the joint and minimizes the benefits of Joint E'Zer.

Kidni Biotic

Standardized Extract

<u>Therapeutic Actions</u>: This compound contains natural antibiotic and antibacterial compounds that directly target the urinary system, promotes urinary tract detoxification.

<u>Indications</u>: Very powerful and fast acting herbal alternative to antibiotics for urinary tract infections. This compound is specifically indicated in the treatment of bladder infections, kidney infections, urinary tract infections, and cystitis (inflammation of bladder), and nephritis (inflammation of kidneys). This compound may also be used for chronic urinary irritation or chronic bladder irritation.

<u>For Your Information</u>: Do NOT use with cranberry juice, or other acidic juices which will neutralize the actions of the herbs—try apple or carrot juice instead, as they also promote detoxification.

Kidni Flow

Standardized Extract

<u>Therapeutic Actions</u>: This compound contains diuretic, antiseptic, and emollient principles that act to break down stones and crystals, gently stimulate renal excretions, disinfect the urinary tract, and soothe irritated urinary membranes. This compound also functions as a restorative tonic to the entire urinary system.

<u>Indications</u>: Temporary relief of symptoms associated with kidney, bladder, or urinary tract problems, including difficulty or burning during urination and stone formation. This compound is indicated in the treatment of dropsy from renal suppression, cystic catarrh, renal congestion, enuresis, renal obstructions (gravel, bladder stones, calculi), scalding micturition, irritable bladder, cystitis, nephritis, and inability to urinate freely. Beneficial during cleansing periods because it stimulates the removal of catabolic waste from the tissues and encourages elimination via the kidneys. Safe and effective renal support in even the worst cases, regardless of history.

<u>For Your Information</u>: This formula will promote urine flow and the pet will need access to potty areas frequently! Detoxification can also result in temporary urinary symptoms, including actual clinical readings of urine showing increased white or red blood cells, bacteria, crystals and

other debris. This is great! The body is eliminating the very toxins and debris that influences kidney or bladder symptoms.

Temporary irritation can result in some traces of fresh blood. It will pass within a few days to a couple of weeks. It is recommended that, <u>unless life threatening</u>, medications be avoided during this time or detoxification and potential rejuvenation will cease. Do not use this extract with pregnant pets.

Kidni Kare

Standardized Extract

<u>Therapeutic Actions</u>: The herbs in this compound act to strengthen the musculature and tone the membranes of the urinary system. The soothing and restorative properties of these herbs relieve irritation and weakness of the urinary tract. Helps balance some hormones responsible for certain conditions.

<u>Indications</u>: This compound is specifically indicated for urinary incontinence in all life stages. May be used as a restorative tonic to strengthen the musculature of the general pelvic organs.

<u>For Your Information</u>: Can be used with **Calm & Relax** for severe cases of hormonal dysfunction due to spaying, neutering, etc. Do not use this extract with pregnant pets.

L-PhenyPet

Capsules

<u>Therapeutic Actions</u>: A powerful, non-addictive analgesic found in clinical research to be as effective in relieving pain as morphine or opiates. Seems to increase the activity of brain endorphins believed to be involved in the analgesic response.

<u>Indications</u>: Often helps pets have superior responses to other types of pain treatment. May also help alleviate depression from long term pain or illness, and reduce seizure activity.

<u>For Your Information</u>: Can be safely used with Calm & Relax.

L-Tryptopet

Amino Acid Powder

<u>Therapeutic Actions:</u> Essential for regulating brain activity responsible for hyperactivity, aggression, seizures and mood disorders.

<u>Indications</u>: For hyperactivity, aggression, and mood disorders. Helps with pain relief, promotes sound sleep and alleviates depression and nervous conditions. Can significantly reduce seizure activity when combined with Calm & Relax and the LifeStyle™ approach.

Mega Omega-3

Gel Caps

<u>Therapeutic Actions</u>: Provides concentrated fish oil fatty acids for prostaglandin production and cellular tissue repair.

<u>Indications</u>: Helps to reduce inflammation, especially when associated with allergies and arthritis. Aids dry skin and poor coat conditions, while reducing skin damage from scratching and biting. Lowers muscular pain, blood cholesterol, and diabetic complications.

Mega Pet Daily

Capsules

<u>Note</u>: **Multiple nutritional foundation supplement for The Holistic Animal Care LifeStyle™.** Therapeutically-optimum potency. Vitamins, minerals (chelated with amino acids) in a base of alfalfa, watercress, parsley, rice and lecithin. Higher, yet, easier to assimilate potencies of vitamin A, B-complex, C and E than general pet vitamins, with the additional minerals and fatty acids such as iron, selenium, chromium, zinc, choline, fish oils, and EPA's. These nutrients help "fuel" the pet's curative responses for optimum daily health and healing vitality when needed. Most levels found in other pet supplements are too low to maintain optimum health and create a therapeutic response. This is the best supplement you can buy for the price, due to concentration and spectrum of nutrients available.

<u>Therapeutic Actions</u>: All the vital nutrients for stimulating and maintaining optimum immunity and health. Provides preventative properties for pets with weakened or genetically dysfunctional systems, as well as fuel for curative responses. Easy for weakened pets to digest and assimilate. Proper ratio of magnesium to calcium, important in reducing kidney and bladder stones, by being balanced for improved utilization. Fuels the immune response to reverse weakness while protecting the body from further degenerative processes. Supports improved organ and gland function for heart, lung, liver, endocrine system (thyroid, adrenals, etc.) and neurological system; for good digestion, elimination and skin condition. Provides structural strength and rehabilitative "push". Slows degenerative process.

<u>Indications</u>: Daily supplementation prevents dis-ease. Beneficial for all preventative protocols, especially for stressed, illness-prone or older pets. Excellent for chronic cases where an "edge" may be needed to stimulate healing.

<u>For Your Information</u>: Appropriate <u>for all species</u>. Levels are simply adjusted by limiting or increasing daily dose. Sufficient therapeutic levels of the best balance, yet room for the individual adjustment of certain

nutrients. Vitamins B, C and E can be additionally supplemented to boost Mega Pet levels - as needed for specific curative responses and for a limited use at these higher levels. Capsules can be opened and put into food or liquid. Use scissors to snip the end open for easier access if needed. Foundation of sound nutritional plans, higher levels of nutrients provides "all-in-one" supplement, eliminating overdosing or missing vital co-nutrients. Most cost-effective multiple supplement on the market today based on actual levels provided.

Milk Thistle

Herbal Capsules (contain standardized extract for increased potency)

Therapeutic Actions: Liver Support (also first ingredient in Skin & Liv-A-Plex) Protects liver against environmental toxins and allergens, bitter tonic, demulcent, antidepressant, detoxifier, antioxidant, lowers fat deposits in liver. Protects liver from circulating toxins from chemicals, surgical procedures (anesthesia) and drugs.

Indications: Liver or kidney damage, jaundice, parvo recovery, chronic skin disorders, Hepatitis A&B, chronic liver cirrhosis, adrenal disorders, inflammatory bowel disorders, weakened immune system, vaccinations, surgery, cancer, allergies or arthritis with severe inflammation (often liver-related).

For Your Information: Use therapeutically forty-eight hours prior to vaccinations, chemical pest treatments, chemical wormers, or surgery with gas & then for two to six weeks after treatments to reduce-potential toxic side effects.

MSM

Capsules

Therapeutic Actions: Supports tissue strengthening, cellular permeability and rejuvenation, especially elasticity. Increases oxygenation through improved lung function. Stabilizes biological uses for synthesis of connective tissues (especially when paired with Glucosamine, Mega Pet Daily and Super C 2000), improves bioactivity of enzymes and immunoglobulins. Non-toxic and non-allergenic nutritional sulfur supplement (not to be confused with sulfa drugs).

Indications: Organ or tissue damage or inflammation, asthma, arthritis, allergies, chronic skin disorders, Hepatitis, inflammatory bowel disorders, weakened connective tissue and organs.

For Your Information: Best to double-dose during first 2 weeks to build blood and tissue levels.

NaturFiber

Fiber Powder

An easy-to-feed, smooth-tasting bulk producing vegetable, grain, and fruit fiber supplement for all pets. Can be added to moistened food.

Therapeutic Actions: Optimum Fiber Supplement, **#1 Hairball or IBS Remedy**. Straight psyllium powder is considered (through clinical experience) too harsh on the digestive tract when used alone. I have combined other nutritional ingredients with psyllium to assure the finest colon care and nutritional bulk available. Promotes hydration and lubrication in the colon, improves nutrient absorption. Helps promote proper formation and elimination of stool.

Indications: Irritable Bowel Syndrome (regulates mucous lining reducing reactions), constipation (brings more moisture to the colon) or diarrhea (provides bulking action, restores flora), hairballs, and diabetes (fiber combines with sugars to carry them through the digestive tract). Safe to use long term and for pregnancy!

For Your Information: Great for the prevention of horse colic, protocol: Mega Pet Daily, Super C 2000, Garlic Daily Aid, Yucca Intensive, Naturfiber, 1/2 cup of Bran and 1/8th cup of oil (corn, safflower, etc.), mixed into a twice daily snack of soaked pellets or oats/barley mash.

Oxy Pro

Tablets

Therapeutic Actions: Provides multiple antioxidant boost to the body's detoxification and rejuvenation processes. Supports improved immune response and tissue repair.

Indications: Excellent for those times when "a little more" protection is needed, to pump up levels of another multiple (such as Mega Pet Daily), or to give antioxidants a try when reversing chronic conditions, such as arthritis or allergies.

Panc'rse & GlucoBalance

Standardized Extract

Therapeutic Actions: Pancreatic, Digestive Restorative and Blood Sugar (insulin) Stabilizer. This compound acts upon the re-synthesis of glycogen, facilitates in the repair of the Islets of Langerhans of the pancreas, and promotes better production and utilization of insulin. This balancing compound acts to normalize and restore integrity of the organs and glands associated with carbohydrate and sugar metabolism. Every six weeks, or sooner if symptoms dramatically change, have a veterinarian check if insulin shots are still needed.

Dose actually needed may dramatically decrease over time with the LifeStyle approach and nutritional support. Safe to use long-term.

Indications: Temporary relief of symptoms associated with pancreatic dysfunction and blood sugar problems.

For Your Information: Stool problems with long-term discoloration (especially greenish-grey) and excessive mucous should be under clinical examination for proper diagnosis and possible medical treatment.

Pau D'Arco

Herbal Capsules

Therapeutic Actions: Kills viruses, fungus, effective against all types of cancers, Lupus, and leukemia. Stimulates the immune system, heals wounds and combats infections. Anti-fungal, antiseptic.

Indications: Use both topically and internally for ringworm, hot spots, eczema, psoriasis and staph infections. Excellent for general support, in addition to the symptom-specific remedies, with cystitis (inflammation of bladder), colitis, gastritis (inflammation of stomach), diabetes, liver and kidney care. Relieves arthritis and pain. Is easier on very sick, weakened, or older pets.

SeaSupreme

Nutritional Powder

Therapeutic Actions: General low-potency multi-supplement. Supports digestion, reduces stool eating, stimulates coat and color, and aids in proper growth. Sixteen types of sea vegetation, including yellow, blue, green Algae, Spirulina, Deluse and Irish moss are combined with nutritional yeast to provide sixty trace minerals, nineteen essential minerals, twelve vitamins and ten essential amino acids. One hundred percent food-source supplement helps boost thyroid and thymus gland production, which controls the immune, hormone, and enzyme systems. Supports basic nutrient profile.

Indications: Excellent preventative supplement for degenerative structural problems, arthritis, general skin problems, infertility, low stamina, and poor condition. Helps to promote sound legs and hooves in horses. Great for all animals, including birds, horses, ferrets and reptiles.

For Your Information: Less expensive *and less potent* alternative to Mega Pet Daily for maintenance of healthy animals. Excellent for use with farm animals.

Shark'Rah

Chondroitin Powder

<u>Therapeutic Actions</u>: Found to be supportive in lubricating joints (reduces pain) and in the reversal or prevention of arthritis. Sharks are also highly touted for their remarkable anti-cancer genes, which is beneficial to those supplementing with shark tissue.

<u>Indications</u>: For arthritis and joint injuries, helps prevent and eliminate tumors.

Skin & Liv-A-Plex

Standardized Extract
<u>Therapeutic Actions</u>:

- Stimulates liver metabolism and detoxification, protects liver from toxins, drugs and anesthesia.

- Improves fatty metabolism and blocked liver ducts.

- Purifies blood.

- Combats bacterial growth, viral, fungal and yeast infection. Stimulates immune system and improves curative response.

- Reverses hormone imbalance. Aids skin and tissue repair, improves coat.

<u>Indications</u>: Tissue and Liver Restorative. Temporary relief of symptoms associated with liver problems, including hepatitis, skin conditions, inflammation, gas, constipation, and hemorrhoids. This compound is specifically indicated for a broad spectrum of dermatological conditions, including oily acne or coat, cystic acne, hormonal acne (especially in cats), pimples, eczema, psoriasis, seborrhea, psoriatic arthritis, and many other skin disturbances.

FYI: The chemistry and nutrients of the herbs in this compound promote restoration and well-being of the skin as an eliminatory and protective organ. This compound may also be used as a wonderful spring tonic to promote an alteration of catabolic wastes that have built up over the winter. Excellent decongestant and protector of the liver.

Stress & A'Drenal Plex

Standardized Extract

<u>Therapeutic Actions</u>: This compound acts to restore integrity to the adrenal glands and promote a greater sense of energy and stamina. The adaptogenic properties of these herbs help to build up the body's response to stress, such

as allergic reactions or gland dysfunction. These herbs are also nutritive and tonic to the adrenal glands as well as to nerve cells and tissues.

Indications: This compound is indicated as an adjunct therapy in the treatment of Addison's Disease (an adrenal deficient disorder) and Cushing's disease (an adrenal dysfunction). Also specifically indicated for those exhibiting low adrenal function that manifests into low vitality, anemia, low blood pressure, anxiety, physical strain and pressure, and low or depleted energy.

For Your Information: As an adaptogen, this compound is very useful for those who are constantly exposed to stressful environments or situations, overwork, excess strain to mind and body, and those pets involved in weight management and body building programs.

Super C 2000

Therapeutic Actions: Vitamin C has been found to kill bacteria, viral infections, yeast and fungus, making it a vital protector of the body. Boosts immune system by increasing and speeding up the activity of white blood cells. Ascorbic acid has been found to be a good preventative to viral infections such as parvo. Primary role is in the formation of collagen, which binds connective tissue together (muscles, ligaments, tendons, cartilage, and blood vessels) and holds minerals in the bone - especially in large breed pets prone to arthritis.

Indications: Needed for antibiotic or antioxidant protection and tissue repair. This general detoxifier is beneficial against cancer and degenerative diseases, especially arthritis. Protects all vital organs. Acidifies the urine and eliminates bacteria known to cause bladder and kidney problems. Helps build resistance to allergies and toxins. Other ailments responding well to vitamin C intake include respiratory weakness (particularly asthma), atherosclerosis and heart dis-ease, eye or ear infections, heavy metal poisoning, cystitis, hypoglycemia, drug or vaccine reaction, hepatitis, obesity, tooth decay, periodontal disease, radiation.

Depletors of vitamin C: Life! Infection, histamine responses, poison, air pollution, stress, antibiotics, cortisone, antifungal drugs, painkillers, diuretics, second hand smoke, and aspirin (triples the excretion rate of vitamin C!)

For Your Information: The body of even debilitated, young or very small pets, takes much more vitamin C when sick. Safe to use in high doses and during pregnancy, benefits all recovery. Highest dose needed by the body can be reached by supplementing to bowel intolerance. Keep increasing dose by 500 mg. until loose stool is obtained then back off by

500 mg. until stool forms again – this is the body's bowel tolerance factor indicating the body's need for vitamin C is at that point.

Superoxide Dismutase (S.O.D.)

Powder

<u>Therapeutic Actions</u>: Free radical scavenger - general antioxidant.

<u>Indications</u>: Often beneficial in helping in the reduction of chronic inflammation in the joints, especially when used in conjunction with MSM. Reduces arthritic, allergic and asthmatic reactions. Great flavor enhancer for finicky or debilitated pets. For meat eaters only!

Viral D'Tox

Standardized Extract

<u>Therapeutic Actions</u>: This compound contains strong anti-viral (and anti-bacterial or anti-fungal) activity with immune enhancing properties. Many of the herbs in this compound target cellular immunity and liver functions and act to protect the healthy cells from infection, as well as promote a better flow of the vital force (chi) through the liver system. Supports prevention, even when animal is exposed to highly contagious organisms!

<u>Indications</u>: Specifically indicated in the treatment of chronic viral infections including hepatitis and other live viruses that infect pets: Vaccinosis, Feline Leukemia, FIP, Distemper, and other acute (Parvo, Kennel Cough) or chronic viral infections. Also indicated as an adjunct in the treatment of serious bacterial, Candida yeast overgrowth and fungal infections - as well as herpes infections such as rodent mouth in cats afflicted with Feline Leukemia.

<u>For Your Information:</u> Also protects from and eliminates bacterial infection! Very beneficial in reducing secondary symptoms of auto-immune disorders in pets.

Vita E 200

Gel Caps

<u>Therapeutic Actions:</u> Enhances oxygenation of the blood. Antioxidant, promotes tissue repair and elasticity. Strengthens the heart, revitalizes, increases fertility, tones muscles and skin. Protects against radiation and protects B vitamins from rapid oxidation.

<u>Indications</u>: Cardiovascular dysfunction, poor skin and coat condition, poor wound healing or curative response. Prevention of allergic reactions, including reactive arthritic conditions. Supports the body during chronic or acute illness and rehabilitation.

Vita C BioRose

Capsules

<u>Therapeutic Actions</u>: Vitamin C has been found to kill bacteria, viral infections, yeast and fungus, making it a vital protector of the body. Boosts immune system by increasing and speeding up the activity of white blood cells. Primary role in the formation of collagen, which binds connective tissue together (muscles, ligaments, tendons, cartilage, and blood vessels) and holds minerals in the bone

<u>Indications</u>: Natural antibiotic and Immune system support. This general detoxifier is beneficial against cancer and degenerative diseases, especially arthritis. Acidifies the urine and eliminates bacteria known to cause bladder and kidney problems. Helps build resistance to allergies. Other ailments responding well to vitamin C intake include respiratory and heart dis-ease, atherosclerosis, asthma, eye or ear infections, heavy metal poisoning, cystitis, hypoglycemia, drug and vaccine reactions, hepatitis, obesity, tooth decay, periodontal disease, radiation.

<u>Depletors of vitamin C</u>: infection, histamine responses, poison, air pollution, stress, antibiotics, cortisone, antifungal drugs, painkillers, diuretics, 2nd hand smoke, and aspirin (triples the excretion rate of vitamin C!)

<u>For Your Information</u>: Do not give on empty stomach, always with food. See Super C 2000 for information on reaching bowel tolerance (actual level of vitamin C the body needs).

Yeast and Fungal D'Tox

Standardized Extract

<u>Therapeutic Actions</u>: These extracts contain natural anti-fungal, anti-bacterial, and anti-yeast properties. Studies proved superior anti-fungal or anti-yeast action than popular veterinary drugs, with fewer side effects.

<u>Indications</u>: This compound is specifically indicated in the treatment of yeast-based or fungal ear infections, Candida yeast overgrowth (vaginal infections and penis discharge), fungal infections (toenail fungus), and ringworm. Supportive in the prevention and elimination of Valley Fever spores infection (fungal mycosis). This compound may also be used as an adjunct in the treatment of severe allergies resulting in chronic ear or eye infections.

<u>For Your Information</u>: Seek regular blood work every few months, or when symptomatic, to test for fungal titers (Valley Fever) and assure everything is within range. A 1:4 count is possible within eight to twelve weeks. Long-term supplementation may totally rid the body of infestation. This has not been seen with medication use. Results above 1:68 *with very weakened pets* may require short-term medications to reduce infestation

while supplement reduces other symptoms and rebuilds the body's resistance to further infestation. Under 1:68, address solely with this supplement. Do not use this extract with pregnant pets.

Yucca Intensive

Standardized Extract

A Natural Steroid Alternative containing over 85% active saponins, as compared to most powdered products with only 3-7% of bio-available saponins (powders are actually *the waste product* of the extraction process Azmira® uses). The purity and concentration reduces the likelihood of any digestive tract irritation or malabsorption problems associated with other yucca products, making it safer for long-term use. It is actually the fibrous powder which takes too long to digest in the digestive tract and triggers digestive problems for pets! Azmira®'s standardized extract is immediately absorbed and does not last long enough in the stomach or intestines to create any irritation.

Therapeutic Actions: Yucca contains steroidal saponins, which are nature's most powerful anti-inflammatory agents.

Indications: Reduces pain as well as steroids, bute or aspirin without any gastric side effects. Temporary relief of symptoms associated with joint (arthritis, hip dysplasia), disc, soft tissue, skin, organ, and colon inflammation, including pain (colic); reduces the "itch" of allergies. Tissue swelling reduces the blood flow through injured areas, so that toxins build up, irritating the liver and kidneys. Yucca cleanses these organs, promotes blood flow and tissue repair, while preventing further degeneration of injured tissue. May lower swelling of brain areas responsible for seizure activity. Can be used topically for wound and hot spot treatment.

For Your Information: When used topically, its bitter taste can be used as deterrent to chewing.

AZMIRA®'S FLOWER ESSENCES

Homeopathic Fluid Remedies

Abandonment

Indications: Difficulty being left alone with homesickness, or may be depressed. These pets need their emotions stabilized. Can be used even years after the abandonment happened, when the feeling of fear or loneliness remains.

Aggression

Indications: Concerned & possessive with general negative feelings, aggressive pets are often quick to act out, are troubled, or easy to panic. Their behavior may be overbearing, often too difficult to handle.

For Your Information: This formula should be used with behavior modification to prevent bites, etc. It acts as an emotional filter, not a magic cure-all! Use with Calm & Relax for more difficult cases.

Fear

Indications: Vague fears and anxieties in a pet that often can also lack self-confidence. Or fear *of* known things like thunder, fireworks, strangers or strange objects. These pets panic easily and most behavior is without thinking; they are just reacting.

Jealousy

Indications: For general or specific resentments. Stabilizes the emotions and reduces negative thoughts that trigger emotional outbursts and/or destructive behaviors. Great when introducing new pets, kids, partners, etc.

Neediness

Indications: Over-anxious to please the owner, this pet seeks constant reassurance. Overly concerned about things, they become pushy; often need constant attention or stress develops.

Obsessive

Indications: Seems desperate to continue a specific behavior, such as fixating on a ball or vocalizing incessantly; this pet is often quick to act out. May be controlling and pushy.

R & R Essence—First-Aid Remedy

Therapeutic Actions: reduces trauma, shock, grief; panic, fear, terror; reduce fainting or spaciness; stress, tension, and irritability; desperate and impulsive.

Indications: For calming support when in crisis. Sudden emotional or physical trauma, upcoming stressful events that you wish to minimize reactions to and avoid reinforcing negative impression.

For Your Information: This is Azmira®'s *protection from trauma* formula—this remedy is a "must" for all pet owners to have on hand with their first aid kit. Can be diluted (four drops to two ounces of water) and sprayed into the air to calm caged pets or a few drops placed in water dish when stressful situations arise. Dose directly, every five to fifteen minutes for a half-hour, after the trauma, then dose hourly until relief is apparent and stable. Continue dosing two to four times a day for a few days to maintain benefit.

Spraying

<u>Indications</u>: Pets have impulse to continue doing wrong, even after punishment and may be overwhelmed by the situation or litter box. Often strong willed, out to make a point, they seek attention. Stabilizes negative emotions during transitions, new pets, etc. Reverses strong feelings of resentment and bitterness that result in bad acts.

AZMIRA® TOPICAL PRODUCTS

Organic Conditioner

<u>Contents</u>: Organic Kiwi, Papaya, Oatmeal, Palm Extract, Wheat Protein, Yarrow, Mango, Aloe Vera, Calendula, Vitamin E

<u>Recommendations</u>: Multi-species, All Life Stages cream rinse. Helps to reduce coat static, allergy or bite-related irritations. Use for moisturizing skin after bathing. For best results, brush coat completely before bathing to remove loose hair.

<u>For Your Information</u>: May be used weekly, as a rinse, for acute skin irritations or poor coat condition. Dilute 8:1 in a spray bottle to use in-between baths, after brushing, to maintain sheen on a poor condition or unruly coat. Helps to repel dirt.

Organic Neem Dip

<u>Contents</u>: Organic Neem Extract, Orange, Rosewood, Chrysanthemum, Yarrow, Goldenseal Extract, Yucca Extract

<u>Recommendations</u>: Safe, effective alternative to chemical pest control. Use in combination with Dr. Newman's LifeStyle™ approach for optimal resistance to pests. DO NOT use on pets under 10 weeks of age or those severely debilitated without veterinary supervision! Skin test on one leg of cat before use as cats may be allergic.

<u>For Your Information</u>: Safe when used as directed. Do not use undiluted, especially with pregnant pets. Avoid contact with eyes.

Organic Neem Spray

<u>Contents</u>: Distilled Water, Witch Hazel, Organic Neem Extract, Orange, Rosewood, Chrysanthemum, Yarrow, Goldenseal Extract, Yucca Extract

Recommendations: Spot protection when going into known pest hide-outs like parks or the woods. Use in combination with Dr. Newman's LifeStyle™ approach for optimal resistance to pests. DO NOT use on pets under 10 weeks of age or those severely debilitated without veterinary supervision! Skin test on one leg of cat before use as they may be allergic.

For Your Information: Safe when used as directed. Avoid contact with eyes.

Organic Shampoo

Contents: Organic Coconut, Aloe Vera, Oatmeal, Goldenseal Extract, Yucca Extract

Recommendations: Multi-species, All Life Stages shampoo. Helps reduce allergy and bite-related skin irritations. For best results, brush coat completely before bathing to remove loose hair.

For Your Information: For optimum benefit to overall health, do not bathe more than every six weeks; every two weeks if the skin is in crisis. This prevents stripping essential oils from skin. If lifestyle requires frequent bathing, use our Organic Conditioner for after-bath moisturizer.

Para*Clear

100% Food Grade Diatomaceous Earth

Recommendations: May be applied as barrier to doors, windows or other openings used by pests. Must re-apply when wet. May be applied directly to the coat; however it may dry the skin. Avoid prolonged contact and bathe with Azmira Shampoo & Conditioner when needed.

Indications: Eliminates a variety of environmental pests including fleas, ticks, flies, mites, ants and cockroaches. Apply to wet areas to knock down mosquito hatchings.

For Your Information: This is food grade, not "pool" grade! This is safe for pet use. Avoid prolonged inhalation of dust while applying. Avoid contact with eyes.

Rejuva Gel

Contents: Calcarea Carbo 12x, Rhus. Tox. 12x, Apis 12x, Belladonna 12x, Astacus 15x, Chloralum 15x, and Mezereum 12x in a greaseless Aloe Vera base.

Therapeutic Actions: Soothing homeopathic gel for topical care of skin repair, itchy skin, inflammations, irritations and rashes. Safe if licked off.

Indications: Burns, allergies, eczema, dermatitis, insect bites, reactions to plants, soaps, shampoos, cleaners, chemicals, and dips. Excellent for reducing the inflammation of anal glands.

For Your Information: Refrigerate to add cooling properties. Great for clipper burns or rashes. Can be used under bandages. For cuts or deep wounds use Rejuva Spray initially to protect from infection and begin healing tissue, then switch to Rejuva Gel to prevent scarring.

Rejuva Spray

Contents: Witch Hazel, Organic Extracts of Calendula, Yucca, Goldenseal Root and Grapefruit Seed Extract.

Therapeutic Actions: Reduces inflammation, promotes healing, and has antibacterial, anti-fungal and antiseptic properties to address any ear, skin or wound infection. Excellent ear wash.

Indications: Topical spray for all cuts, wounds, skin eruptions, hot spots, ringworm, prickly heat (rashes), pimples, and scrapes.

For Your Information: Bitter taste reduces chewing on self. Refrigerate for cooling properties. Safe to bandage, but leave infections open to air for some time each day to encourage healing.

PRODUCT AND SERVICES RESOURCES

Dr. Lisa Newman is available for consultation.

Please contact her office at 1-800-497-5665, www.info@azmira.com or 2401 S. 34ᵗʰ Place, Tucson, AZ. 85713, USA.

Azmira Holistic Animal Care® Diets, Treats, Supplements & Topicals

Free Product Guide call 1-800-497-5665 or visit www.azmira.com

Azmira®'s Free Product Support and Protocol Education

1-520-886-1727 or 1-520-293-6639 Monday to Saturday 10AM to 6PM MST

Dr. Newman's Holistic Animal Care LifeStyle™ Correspondence Courses

Call 1-800-497-5665 or visit www.azmira.com
Level One: Holistic Animal Care introduces the fundamentals of alternative healing, behavior modification and proven symptom-reversing modalities for animals of all types. This is geared towards providing the graduate with a strong understanding of, and confidence in, natural pet care for personal use. This provides an in-depth background to better utilize the systematic approach of the LifeStyle™ protocols and recommendations.

Level Two: Holistic Animal Care Consultant course builds on Level One's introduction to Dr. Newman's protocols. Expanding the certificant's depth of knowledge, this course is well suited to anyone seeking a profession in consulting and/or the retail of natural pet products or as a vet tech. In addition to developing protocols for individual cases, this level deals with the legalities of consulting (and how to behave professionally in this field to avoid negative repercussions) plus outstanding customer service advice on how to successfully educate and support your customers.

Level Three: Holistic Animal Care Veterinarian course continues developing the graduate's abilities to benefit clinical applications including surgery recovery, confinement stress control, and eliminating vaccinosis and drug related side-effects. Improving condition specific or organ failure therapies, cancer reversal and preventative protocols are also included. Special emphasis is given to proven remedy alternatives for commonly used drugs. This course is open to licensed veterinarians only.

Newton's Homeopathic Labs°

Free Product Guide: call 1-800-448-7256 or visit www.newtonlabs.net

The American Holistic Veterinarian Medical Association

For a list of holistic veterinarians in your area:
Call 1-410-569-0795 or visit www.ahvma.org

REFERENCES

Animal Protection Institute, *What's Really in Pet Food,* **www. api4animals.org, (2004)**

Association of American Feed Control Officials, *Official Publication,* Oxford, Indiana: Association of American Feed Control Officials (A.A.F.C.O.), 2004.

Belfield, W., DVM, Zucker, M., *How to Have a Healthier Dog,* New York, New York: Doubleday & Co., Inc., 1981.

Boericke, W., MD, *Homeopathic Materia Medica & Repertory,* Delhi, India: B. Jain Publishers Pvt. LTD.: 1996

Coulter, Harris 1., Ph.D. *Homeopathic Medicine,* St. Louis: Formur, 1972.

Cummings, Stephen; Ullman, Dana, *Everybody's Guide to Homeopathic Medicines,* Los Angeles, California: Tarcher, Inc. 1984.

de Bairacli Levy, Juilette, *The Complete Herbal Book for the Dog,* New York, New York: Arco Publishing, 1983.

MacLeod, George, *The Homeopathic Treatment of Dogs,* London, England: The Homeopathic Development Foundation Ltd. 1983.

Martin, Ann, *Protect Your Pet: More Shocking Facts,* Troutdale, Oregon: NewSage Press, 2001.

Merck Sharp & Dohme, *The Merck Veterinary Manual,* Rahway, New Jersey: Merck & Co., 1986.

Newman, L., ND, PhD, *Natural Cat,* Freedom, California: The Crossing Press, 1999.

Newman, L., ND, PhD, *Natural Dog,* Freedom, California: The Crossing Press, 1999.

Newman, L., ND, PhD, *Training without Trauma,* Freedom, California: The Crossing Press, 1999.

O'Driscoll, C., *What Vets Don't Tell About Vaccines,* Langnor, United Kingdom: Abbeywood Publishing, 1998.

O'Heare, James J., Ph.D., *Raw Meat Diets for Cats and Dogs?,* prepublication, 2005.

Pinney, C. C., DVM, *The Illustrated Veterinary Guide for Dogs, Cats, Birds, & Exotic Pets,* New York, New York: Tab Books, div. of McGraw-Hill, 1992.

Pitcairn, R. H., DVM, Pitcairn, S. H., *Dr. Pitcairn's Complete Guide to Natural Health for Dogs & Cats,* Emmaus, Pennsylvania: Rodale Books, 1982.

Thomson PDR, *PDR for Herbal Medicines,* Montvale, New Jersey: Thomson PDR, 2004.

Wright, Jonathan V., M.D., *Dr. Wright's Guide to Healing with Nutrition.* New Canaan, Connecticut: Keats Publishing, Inc. 1984.

General Index

Y

PRODUCT INDEX

OTHER TITLES BY DR. LISA NEWMAN

Allergies, Freedom, California: The Crossing Press, 1999.

Arthritis, Freedom, California: The Crossing Press, 1999.

Natural Cat, Freedom, California: The Crossing Press, 1999.

Natural Dog, Freedom, California: The Crossing Press, 1999.

Nutrition, Freedom, California: The Crossing Press, 1999.

Parasites, Freedom, California: The Crossing Press, 1999.

Skin & Coat, Freedom, California: The Crossing Press, 1999.

Training without Trauma, Freedom, California: The Crossing Press, 1999.

About the Author

Dr. Lisa Newman is a renowned pioneer in natural pet care, an experienced speaker and clinician. A Naturopathic Doctor with a Ph.D. in Nutrition, she has researched and applied her findings for better pet health since 1982. The author of eight books and countless articles addressing all types of pet problems, Dr. Newman's depth of knowledge and breadth of experience show through in this, her ninth book.

The Holistic Animal Care LifeStyle™ is Dr. Newman's unique, systematic approach to optimal pet care; the culmination of her many years and thousands of proven results with animals of all types, ages and conditions. The Holistic Animal Care School of Japan uses Dr. Newman's work as the foundation for its core curriculum.